Monographs in Clinical Cytology

Vol. 22

Series Editor

Philippe Vielh Dudelange, Luxembourg

Henryk A. Domanski Lund

Charles S. Walther Lund

FNA Cytology of Soft Tissue and Bone Tumors

109 figures, 108 in color, and 8 tables, 2017

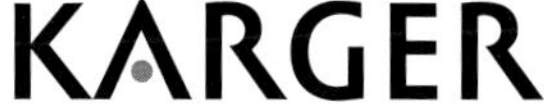

Basel · Freiburg · Paris · London · New York · Chennai · New Delhi ·
Bangkok · Beijing · Shanghai · Tokyo · Kuala Lumpur · Singapore · Sydney

Monographs in Clinical Cytology
Founded 1965 by Georg L. Wied, Chicago, IL

Dr. Henryk A. Domanski
Department of Pathology
Skåne University Hospital
SE–221 85 Lund (Sweden)

Dr. Charles S. Walther
Department of Pathology
Skåne University Hospital
SE–221 85 Lund (Sweden)

Library of Congress Cataloging-in-Publication Data

Names: Domanski, Henryk A., author. | Walther, Charles S., author.
Title: FNA cytology of soft tissue and bone tumors / Henryk A. Domanski,
    Charles S. Walther.
Other titles: Monographs in clinical cytology ; v. 22. 0077-0809
Description: Basel ; New York : Karger, 2017. | Series: Monographs in
    clinical cytology ; vol. 22 | Includes bibliographical references and
    index.
Identifiers: LCCN 2017025751| ISBN 9783318060768 (hard cover : alk. paper) |
    ISBN 9783318060775 (eISBN)
Subjects: | MESH: Soft Tissue Neoplasms--pathology | Bone
    Neoplasms--pathology | Biopsy, Fine-Needle
Classification: LCC RC280.B6 | NLM QZ 340 | DDC 616.99/47107--dc23 LC record available at https://lccn.loc.gov/2017025751

Bibliographic Indices. This publication is listed in bibliographic services, including Current Contents®.

© Copyright 2017 by S. Karger AG, P.O. Box, CH-4009 Basel (Switzerland)
www.karger.com
Printed on acid-free and non-aging paper (ISO 9706)
ISSN 0077–0809
ISBN 978–3–8055–06076–8
e-ISBN 978–3–8055–06077–5

Contents

Preface

An increasing use of minimally invasive diagnostic procedures together with continuously growing ancillary techniques applied to cytological specimens brought widespread acceptance of using fine-needle aspiration cytology (FNAC) in the diagnosis of soft tissue and bone lesions. While cytological examinations have been used in many centers to follow up on previously treated sarcomas or to confirm soft tissue and bone metastases, in the last decade the primary diagnosis of soft tissue and bone tumors has emerged as an important new target for FNAC. As the first-line approach, cytologic examination most often provides diagnostic information allowing the initiation of treatment or guidance of the continued diagnostic investigation.

The purpose of this volume is to describe, illustrate, and summarize the cytological criteria of the most common entities of musculoskeletal tumors and those rare tumors where cytological features have been largely described in case reports and in smaller series. Correlations between cytology and the diagnostic use of ancillary techniques applicable to FNAC, such as immunocytochemical and molecular tests, are detailed on an entity-by-entity basis in order to facilitate the diagnostic workup in the cytological samples. The selection of entities illustrated are based on experience with patients referred to the Sarcoma Centre of the Skåne University Hospital and the illustrations are taken from the considerable cytological material of musculoskeletal lesions, gathered over more than 45 years, which is available in the archives of our institution.

This book provides a comprehensive and well-illustrated review of the FNAC of soft tissue and bone tumors that can be used in the everyday practice of pathologists and cytopathologists in the musculoskeletal field. The content will also be of interest to residents and fellows in cytology, as well as orthopedic surgeons, clinical oncologists, and anyone involved in the diagnosis and therapy of patients with soft tissue and bone lesions.

Acknowledgements

I would like to thank Dr. Måns Åkerman, the pioneer of musculoskeletal cytopathology and former Head of the Department of Pathology at the Lund University Hospital – thanks for teaching and inspiring me to pursue soft tissue and bone pathology/cytopathology.

Henryk A. Domanski, Lund

I would like to thank Dr. Fredrik Mertens for his guidance and help with tumor genetics.

Charles S. Walther, Lund

We would like to thank Dr. Philippe Vielh and Mr. Thomas Nold for recognizing the need for this monograph, and the editorial staff of Karger, particularly Ms. Rebecca Ganz and Mr. Ruedi Jappert, for their excellent administrative assistance during our work on this volume.

Henryk A. Domanski and
Charles S. Walther, Lund

Domanski HA, Walther CS: FNA Cytology of Soft Tissue and Bone Tumors. Monogr Clin Cytol.
Basel, Karger, 2017, vol 22, pp 1–12 (DOI: 10.1159/000475088)

Principles in the Examination and Management of Soft Tissue Lesions

Clinical Features and Team Work

Soft tissue neoplasms comprise a heterogeneous group of lesions with mesenchymal differentiation. Sarcomas are rare, constituting less than 1% of all malignant neoplasms. Benign soft tissue tumors are estimated to be approximately 100 times more frequent than sarcomas. Soft tissue tumors may occur in different planes and locations. However, 99% of benign soft tissue tumors are superficial while two-thirds of the extremity and trunk-wall sarcomas are deep seated. Age-specific incidence rates clearly demonstrate that soft tissue sarcomas are more common with increasing age. There is a slight male predominance, but the gender- as well as age-related incidence is also related to the histologic type and subtype of sarcomas.

In the course of the diagnostic workup of soft tissue masses, a biopsy is necessary in most cases to confirm malignancy and in the case of sarcoma to assess the grade of malignancy and the histologic type. The difficulties in diagnosing patients with musculoskeletal tumors stem mainly from their rarity and to the lack of experience with the microscopic appearance of soft tissue lesions on the part of most pathologists not working in orthopedic-oncology centers [1, 2].

The best approach to a successful diagnostic evaluation of musculoskeletal lesions is to combine clinical data and radiographic findings with the morphologic interpretation of cells and tissue, complemented by ancillary techniques. In specialized orthopedic-oncology centers, orthopedic-surgical, oncologic, radiologic, pathologic/cytologic, and molecular biologic expertise can be combined in a multidisciplinary team to allow the adequate evaluation and therapy, as well as follow-up, of patients with musculoskeletal neoplasms. This multidisciplinary management of musculoskeletal neoplasms favorably influences outcomes for patients suffering from sarcoma [3–7].

Biopsy Techniques

Tumor tissue sampling is necessary for the diagnosis of soft tissue tumors in which malignancy cannot be ruled out by clinical or radiographic means. Open incisional and excisional (local excision for small and superficial lesions) biopsy and core-needle biopsy (CNB) are generally accepted as sampling techniques in the diagnosis of musculoskeletal neoplasms [8]. Open biopsy usually provides sufficient tissue for histopathologic examination as well as for ancillary studies. However, there are risks of intraoperative and postoperative complications and occasional delays in therapy initiation while the surgical wound heals. In addition, incisional biopsy can break natural barriers to tumor growth, which can adversely affect subsequent surgical procedures and increase the risk of the spread of the tumor into surrounding tissues. CNB has become a popular diagnostic procedure since it can be performed in an outpatient setting

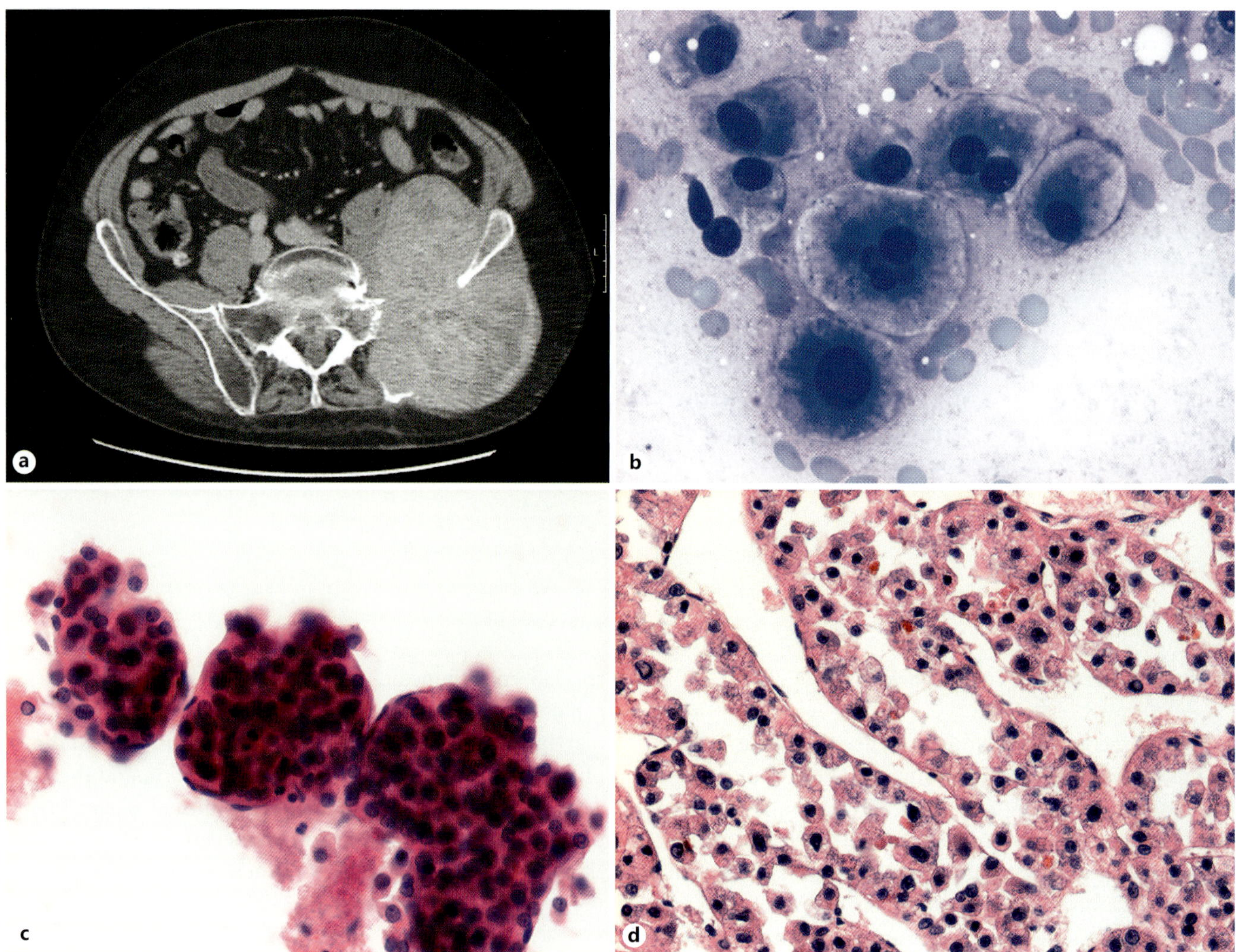

Fig. 1. a MRI with a large pelvic mass extending to the gluteal soft tissue. Clinically suspicious of sarcoma. **b** FNAC of the gluteal mass showing large tumor cells with rounded nuclei and abundant finely granulated cytoplasm, resembling hepatocytes. Binucleated and multinucleated tumor cells. MGG stain. **c** Thick clusters of tumor cells with endothelial wrapping, features of hepatocellular carcinoma. HE stain. **d** Cell block confirms the diagnosis metastasis of hepatocellular carcinoma. HE stain.

and carries a very low risk of morbidity. The evaluation of CNB specimens may be challenging due to limited sampling and the heterogeneity of most soft tissue neoplasms.

An increasing use of minimally invasive diagnostic procedures has resulted in better acceptance of fine-needle aspiration cytology (FNAC) as a first-line approach or as a complementary tool to CNB in the diagnosis of musculoskeletal lesions [9–11]. An FNAC diagnosis is generally accepted in the evaluation of suspected recurrences or metastases of soft tissue neoplasms, as well as in the diagnosis of metastatic carcinoma, melanoma, or lymphoma presenting clinically as primary soft tissue neoplasms (Fig. 1). The ac-

curacy of FNAC in distinguishing benign from malignant soft tissue tumors and sarcoma from other malignancies has been shown to be comparable to that of surgical biopsies, while its accuracy in the grading of soft tissue sarcoma and in establishing a specific histologic diagnosis has been shown to be inferior to both CNB and surgical biopsies. The accumulated experience from centers with expertise in the cytologic examination of musculoskeletal lesions has established additional major indications for FNAC, such as the diagnosis of primary benign/locally aggressive soft tissue tumors and soft tissue sarcomas [7, 9, 11, 12]. The role of FNAC in the initial diagnosis of primary soft tissue is still

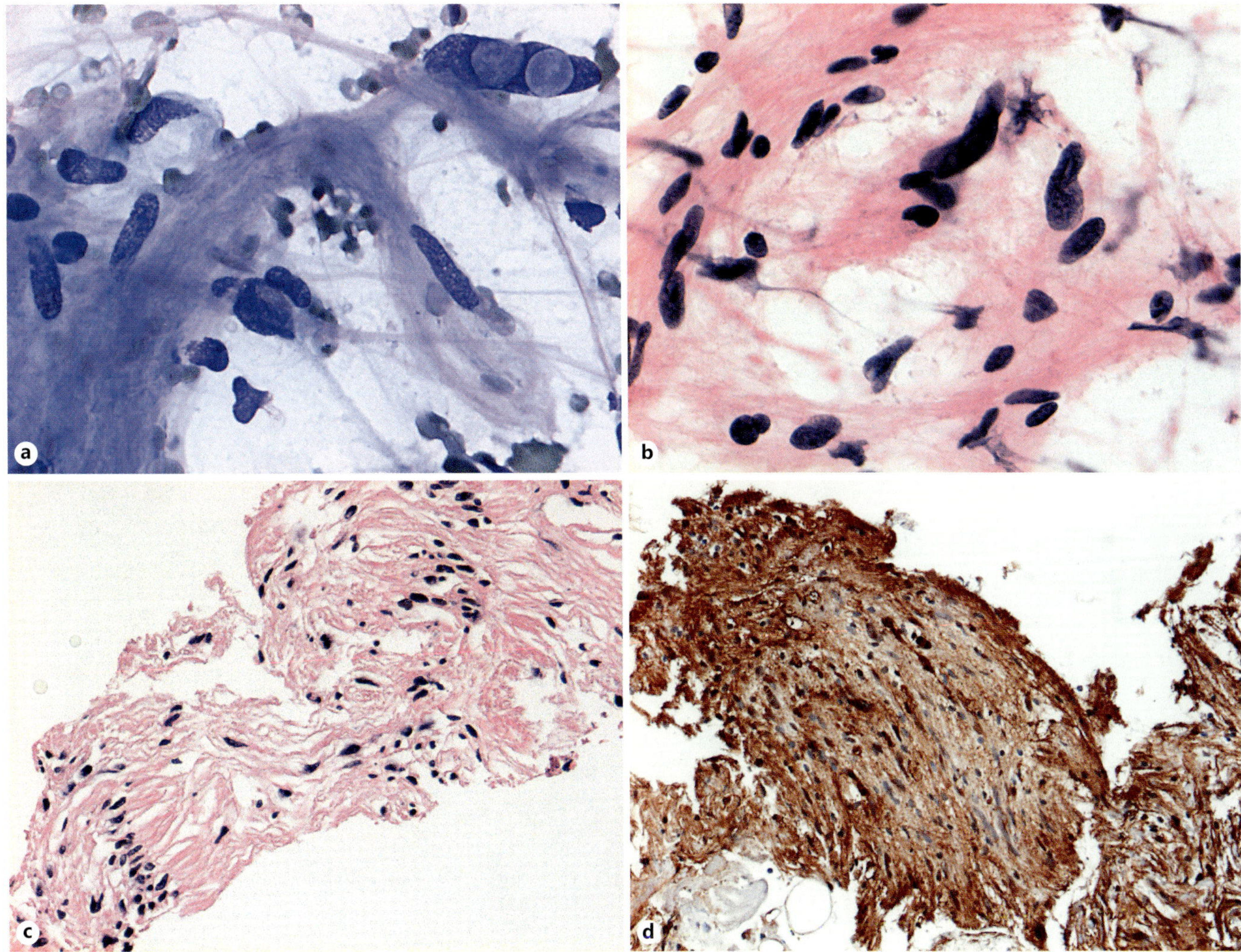

Fig. 2. a ROSE: FNAC of the soft tissue mass in the thigh showing a loosely cohesive cluster of atypical spindle cells. Note the tumor cells with intranuclear inclusions and the fibrillary background of the smears, which are features suggestive of ancient schwannoma. DiffQuick stain. After rapid examination of the first smear, additional passes of FNA were performed in order to obtain more material for ancillary studies. **b** Alcohol-fixed smears showing a loosely cohesive cluster of spindle cells with anisokaryosis and hyperchromasia worrisome for malignancy. HE stain. **c** Cell block showing palisading spindle cells creating a Verocay body and architectural patterns consistent with schwannoma. HE stain. **d** Strong and diffuse positivity for S100 on a cell block section confirms the diagnosis of ancient schwannoma.

debated, however, and the current literature has not completely clarified the optimal biopsy technique for the diagnosis of soft tissue tumors [8, 11, 13–15].

Advances and Limitations of Fine-Needle Aspiration Cytology in the Diagnosis of Soft Tissue Neoplasm

Compared to open biopsy, FNAC has some advantages and also some limitations [2]. Among its advantages, FNAC is an outpatient procedure which is well tolerated by patients and has negligible risks for serious complications. With thin needles, it is easy to sample material from different parts of large tumors, thereby revealing possible tumor heterogeneity. While tumor tissue architecture is better evaluated in surgical biopsies, it can also be evaluated in cell blocks prepared from specimens obtained by FNA (Fig. 2). Through rapid staining applied to aspiration smears, the FNA technique allows for the immediate evaluation of specimen adequacy while the patient waits, known as "rapid on-site evaluation" (ROSE) [16–18]. If necessary, additional aspirations and CNB can be performed in order to obtain material suf-

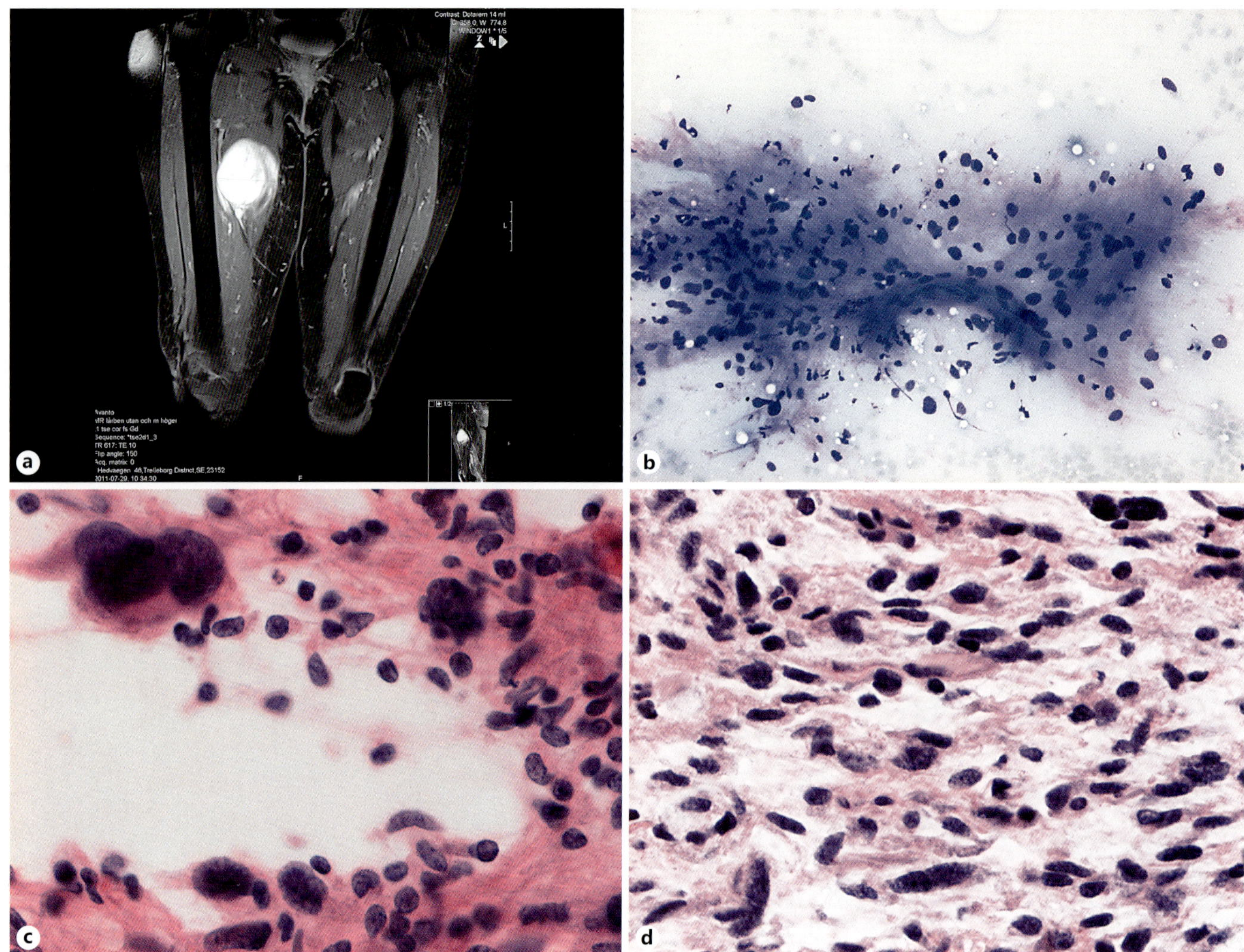

Fig. 3. a MRI showing a deep soft tissue mass in the right thigh suspicious for soft tissue sarcoma. **b** FNAC of the mass shows a loosely cohesive cluster of atypical epithelioid and spindle cells and a capillary vessel fragment embedded in a fibromyxoid matrix, which are cytologic features suggestive of myxofibrosarcoma. MGG stain. Alcohol-fixed smears (**c**) and the cell block section (**d**) show moderate to severe nuclear atypia of tumor cells suggestive of a high grade of malignancy. HE stain.

ficient for microscopic examination and for ancillary studies (Fig. 2).

Generally, the cytomorphology of single cells, in technically satisfactory smears, is superior to that seen in core-needle and open biopsy specimens. The FNA procedure requires fewer resources than other biopsy techniques and is the most cost effective. In addition, the technique of FNA is both easy to perform and easy to learn.

The main disadvantage of FNAC, however, is that samples are very small and it can be difficult to obtain sufficient material for both morphologic examination and all necessary ancillary studies. In addition, there is a lack of pathologists/cytopathologists experienced in the cytologic evaluation of soft tissue lesions.

Fine-Needle Aspiration Cytology according to the WHO Classification

Nomenclature and the classification of soft tissue neoplasms used in daily clinical practice are based on the WHO classification of soft tissue and bone neoplasms.

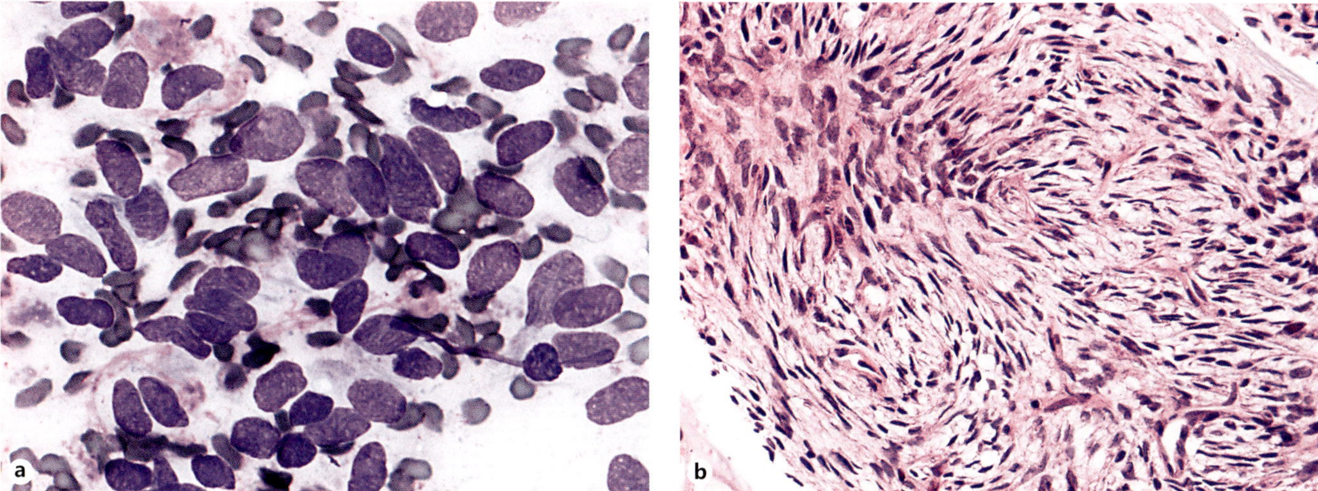

Fig. 4. a The sarcoma grade of malignancy may be determined by the histologic diagnosis. Dermatofibrosarcoma protuberans: low grade (1/3) by definitions. MGG stain. **b** Cell block facilitating examination of the tumor tissue architecture confirms the diagnosis of dermatofibrosarcoma protuberans. HE stain.

During the workup of patients with soft tissue tumors, every effort should be made to establish a histologic diagnosis according to the WHO classification and, in the case of sarcoma, the histologic grade of the neoplasm. A histologic diagnosis of soft tissue yield can occasionally be difficult to establish using routine cytologic smears alone. The aspiration of material sufficient for cell blocks and for ancillary techniques is an important part of the cytologic examination and can require ROSE of the yield. In addition, cytologic examination is an easy and quick method to establish or exclude malignancy, exclude carcinoma, melanoma or lymphoma, and can guide the subsequent diagnostic workup. (Fig. 1–3).

Grading of Sarcomas by Fine-Needle Aspiration Cytology

The most widely used histologic sarcoma grading system is the French FNCLCC system based on tumor differentiation, mitotic rate, and necrosis. Recently, vascular invasion and the pattern of peripheral tumor growth (pushing/infiltrative) have also been shown to be important prognostic parameters. Assessment of these parameters is not always feasible in FNA samples [9, 12, 19–22]. Nevertheless, in technically satisfactory specimens, it is usually possible to categorize a sarcoma into morphologically low-grade or high-grade

malignancy (Fig. 3). In a subset of sarcomas, a specific histologic diagnosis may determine the malignancy grade in an FNA specimen (Fig. 4).

Cytologic Patterns in Aspirates

Apart from classifications focused on clinical management and based on delineating subcategories of therapeutic and prognostic importance, soft tissue lesions can be classified according to their presumed histogenesis or their differentiation towards a predominant cell type based on cytoarchitectural features in smears and the background of the smears. The majority of soft tissue tumors can be placed into 1 of the following 5 categories by the predominant cytologic pattern: pleomorphic, spindle cell, myxoid, small round/ovoid cell, and epithelioid cell [1]. Each of those categories presents certain differential diagnoses (Tables 1–6).

The typical features of the pleomorphic pattern are a marked variation in cellular and nuclear size and shape, and in the case of sarcoma an obvious nuclear pleomorphism with the presence of atypical multinucleated tumor cells and prominent nucleoli. There are benign soft tissue tumors in this category, such as nodular fasciitis and pleomorphic lipoma. Examples of sarcomas in this group are undifferentiated pleomorphic sarcoma, pleomorphic leiomyosarcoma, pleomorphic liposarcoma, and the more infrequent pleo-

Table 1. Cytologic evaluation based on a monomorphic spindle cell pattern

Tumor	Microscopic features	Immunophenotype	Comments
Spindle cell lipoma	Mixture of mature fat tissue and clustered or dispersed bland spindle cells; fragments of collagen-hyaline fibers; occasional myxoid background matrix	Positive for CD34 and BCL-2 Negative for SMA and S100	Variable proportions of each component
Elastofibroma dorsi	Moderate to scanty smears; fat tissue intermingled with collagen fragments/collagen fibers and uniform spindle cells; elastic fibers with characteristic serrated "moth-eaten" edges		Elastic fibers better appreciated in wet-fixed smears using high-power microscopy
Fibrous hamartoma of infancy	A mixture of normal fatty tissue and bland spindle cells, dispersed or in sheets and clusters	Positive for SMA, focal CD34, S100 in the fatty component	
Desmoid-type fibromatosis	Clustered or dispersed fibroblast with elongated fusiform nuclei, insignificant nucleoli, and slight anisokaryosis. Fibroblasts arranged in long, slender fascicles; stripped nuclei and crush artifact	Positive for SMA, MSA, focal desmin, β-catenin Negative for CD34	Collagenous stroma firm for the needle and difficult to aspirate
Dermatofibro-sarcoma protuberans	Tight clusters/fascicles of spindle cells in a collagen matrix; dispersed spindle cells and bland stripped nuclei; poorly defined cytoplasm, bipolar cytoplasmic extensions in better-preserved cells	Positive for CD34 Negative for S100, SMA, and desmin	Cutaneous/subcutaneous tumor
Extrapleural solitary fibrous tumor	A mixture of dispersed cells and tight, fascicle-like clusters of bland spindle cells with inconspicuous nucleoli; stripped nuclei; ropy collagen fibers	Positive for CD34 and nuclear STAT6	Occasionally focal positivity for SMA and EMA
Leiomyoma of deep soft tissue	A mixture of clustered and dispersed, bland-looking spindle cells with elongated, blunt-ended, cigar-shaped, occasionally truncated nuclei and insignificant nucleoli	Positive for SMA, MSA, desmin, rarely focal keratins, ER	Leiomyomas of deep soft tissue are rare targets for FNAC
Spindle cell GIST	No specific features; may mimic smooth muscle tumors	Positive for C-Kit (CD117), DOG-1, and CD34	
Schwannoma	Cohesive tissue fragments. Few dispersed cells; occasional nuclear palisading and Verocay bodies; fibrillary background; slender, wavy (comma-shaped or "fishhook") nuclei with pointed ends	Positive for S100, occasional focal positivity for GFAP	Often sharp, radiating pain at needling
Neurofibroma	Clusters and dispersed bland, fibroblast-like spindle cells and "nerve" cells with indistinct cytoplasm and elongated, slender nuclei with pointed ends	Positive for S100 and CD34; scattered axons positive for neurofilament	Same cells variably positive for claudin-1, GLUT1, and EMA
Monophasic synovial sarcoma	Tight clusters of spindle cells mixed with dispersed cells and stripped nuclei; capillary strands bordered by tumor cells; bland fusiform or ovoid nuclei end inconspicuous nucleoli; mitoses; mast cells	Positive for EMA, keratin, often focally; more than 50% CD99/Bcl-2 positive	

SMA, smooth muscle actin; MSA, muscle-specific actin; EMA, epithelial membrane antigen; ER, estrogen receptor; GIST, gastrointestinal stromal tumor.

morphic malignant peripheral nerve sheath tumor and pleomorphic rhabdomyosarcoma.

The spindle cell pattern is defined by smears showing predominantly monomorphic or atypical spindled cells with fusiform or ovoid nuclei and elongated uni- or bipolar cytoplasm extensions. The cells may be arranged in sheets or fascicles, but dissociated cells or naked spindle-shaped nuclei are often present. Common benign spindle cell tumors are schwannoma and desmoid fibromatosis, while rare examples are deep-seated leiomyoma, spindle cell lipoma, and solitary fibrous tumor. Typical spindle cell sarcomas include a subset of leiomyosarcoma, monophasic synovial sarcoma, malignant peripheral nerve sheath tumor, dermatofibrosarcoma protuberans, and the infrequent fibrosarcoma (infantile and adult).

The common feature in aspirates showing the myxoid pattern is an abundant, viscous yield. Aspirates of myxoid tumors often look like droplets of glue. At low power there

Table 2. Cytologic evaluation based on a moderately and highly pleomorphic spindle cell pattern

Tumor	Microscopic features	Immunophenotype	Comments
Inflammatory myofibroblastic tumor	Tight sheets and dispersed plump or slightly atypical myofibroblasts and occasional ganglion-like cells; inflammatory infiltrate including plasma cells, lymphocytes, and histiocytes	Positive for SMA, variable desmin, and in up to 60% of cases ALK1	
Infantile fibrosarcoma	Tight clusters and fascicles of slightly to moderate pleomorphic spindle cells with bland nuclei but numerous mitoses	Variable focal positivity for CD34 and SMA	
Adult fibrosarcoma	Sheets, fascicles of atypical spindle cells	Positive for vimentin	Diagnosis of exclusion
Pseudomyogenic hemangioendothelioma	Loosely cohesive clusters, sheets and dispersed spindle cells with abundant cytoplasm and long cytoplasmic extensions; variable anisocytosis and anisokaryosis and distinct nucleoli; occasional sparse myxoid background matrix; ganglion-like cells	Positive for cytokeratin AE1/AE3, FLI-1, ERG, CD31; in 50% of cases, retained nuclear INI1	Cytological features resemble those of nodular fasciitis/proliferative fasciitis
Leiomyosarcoma	Fascicles of more or less atypical spindle cells; cigar-shaped/blunt-ended nuclei; segmented nuclei; in tandem position of nuclei; occasional intranuclear inclusions	Positive for SMA, MSA, desmin, h-caldesmon Positive/negative for keratins and EMA	Occasional osteoclast-like giant cells
Spindle cell rhabdomyosarcoma	Smears display predominantly dispersed cells with a spindle cell morphology and variable, usually slight to moderate nuclear pleomorphism	Positive for desmin, myogenin, MyoD1, and commonly SMA and MSA	
Malignant peripheral nerve sheath tumor	Mixture of cell clusters, fascicles, and dispersed atypical spindle cells with elongated, wavy nuclei with pointed ends; hyperchromatic nuclei with large nucleoli and variable presence of pleomorphic and multinucleated tumor cells; fibrillary background	Positive for S100 focally and in less than 50% of cases, and GFAP in less than 30% of cases	

SMA, smooth muscle actin; MSA, muscle-specific actin; GFAP, glial fibrillary acidic protein.

is an abundant myxoid background matrix, blue or blue-violet, occasionally fibrillar in May-Grünwald-Giemsa (MGG) or DiffQuick stains, and faintly pink in hematoxylin and eosin (HE) or Papanicolaou stains. Examples of benign myxoid tumors are intramuscular myxoma, myxoid nodular fasciitis, ossifying fibromyxoid tumor, perineurioma, and mixed tumor of soft tissue. The most common myxoid sarcomas examined by FNAC are myxofibrosarcoma and myxoid liposarcoma, and the less common low-grade fibromyxoid sarcoma and extraskeletal myxoid chondrosarcoma.

Smears showing the small round cell pattern are highly cellular and composed of small- to medium-sized cells with rounded or ovoid nuclei and a variable amount of cytoplasm. The predominant cell type is round, but the cellular shape may be variable, from rounded and ovoid to fusiform or triangular. The nuclei are often bland and the nucleoli small. Sarcomas with a round cell pattern examined frequently by FNAC are extraskeletal Ewing sarcoma, alveolar rhabdomyosarcoma, and neuroblastoma, while pure round cell liposarcoma, poorly differentiated synovial sarcoma, and desmoplastic small round cell tumor are less common.

In the group in which the soft tissue tumors with epithelioid feature, the predominant cell type is rounded or polygonal cells with well-demarcated cytoplasmic borders, a rather abundant cytoplasm, and rounded to ovoid, occasionally irregular nuclei. Nucleoli are often prominent. These cells are arranged in sheets and tight clusters, often with an admixture of dissociated cells and stripped nuclei. The soft tissue tumors in this group are generally rare and infrequent targets for FNA examination. Typical examples of benign tumors with epithelioid morphology are granular cell tumor, adult rhabdomyoma, and paraganglioma, and among the sarcomas, epithelioid sarcoma, clear cell sarcoma, alveolar soft part sarcoma, malignant rhabdoid tumor, and epithelioid GIST. It can be occasionally difficult to distinguish epi-

Table 3. Cytologic evaluation based on a pleomorphic pattern

Tumor	Microscopic features	Immunophenotype	Comments
Nodular fasciitis	Marked pleomorphism in many proliferating fibroblasts/myofibroblasts; ganglion-cell like cells; bland chromatin structure; occasional myxoid background matrix and mitoses	Positive for SMA, occasionally focal desmin, and CD68	Painful or tender, usually rapidly growing; most often spontaneous regress
Undifferentiated pleomorphic sarcoma	Variable cellular morphology, commonly spindle, polygonal, and epithelioid cells with marked cellular and nuclear pleomorphism; multinucleated (bizarre) tumor giant cells; mitoses; necrosis		
Pleomorphic (high-grade) leiomyosarcoma	Pleomorphic cells of variable morphology with an admixture of atypical spindle cells; nuclei with elongated, blunted ends, cigar shaped, and occasionally segmented "in tandem"; necrosis; rare mitoses	Positive for SMA, MSA, desmin, and h-caldesmon Positive/negative for keratins and EMA focally	Positive stains for muscle markers such as SMA, desmin, and/or h-caldesmon required for diagnosis
Pleomorphic liposarcoma	Clustered and dispersed cells, pleomorphic tumor cells including multinucleated giant tumor cells; variable presence of highly atypical, uni- or multinucleated lipoblasts; cells with hyaline cytoplasmic droplets occasionally present; necrosis; mitoses	Lipoblasts are positive for S100, occasionally focal EMA, and keratin positivity Negative for MDM2 and CDK4	Unequivocal atypical lipoblasts in smears required for diagnosis
Pleomorphic (high-grade) MPNST	Hypercellular smears; clusters, fascicles, and dispersed pleomorphic cells of variable morphology with an admixture of atypical spindle cells with wavy, thin nuclei with pointed ends, comma-like nuclei	Focal positivity for S100 in less than 50% of cases and positive for GFAP in less than 30% of cases	
Pleomorphic rhabdomyosar-coma	Marked cellular and nuclear pleomorphism; atypical rhabdomyoblast-like cells, triangular, rounded with eccentric nuclei and eosinophilic cytoplasm	Positive for desmin, nuclear myogenin, and MyoD1	

SMA, smooth muscle actin; MSA, muscle-specific actin; EMA, epithelial membrane antigen; MPNST, malignant peripheral nerve sheath tumor.

thelioid soft tissue tumors from metastatic carcinoma and malignant melanoma, and the use of ancillary techniques in such cases is a necessary part of the cytologic workup.

In addition to these 5 patterns in smears, there are soft tissue tumors showing a mixture of different patterns. For example, smears from biphasic synovial sarcoma show both epithelioid and spindle cell patterns, and from pleomorphic leiomyosarcoma show a mixture of pleomorphic and spindle cell patterns. In most benign adipose tumors, large fat cells predominate and vascular tumors may appear as examples of a pleomorphic pattern, spindle cell pattern, or epithelioid cell pattern. Tables 1–6 list an approach to cytologic diagnoses based on pattern recognition.

Diagnostic Accuracy, Pitfalls, and Complications

If an FNA biopsy is performed by an experienced operator and with adequate samples, the diagnostic accuracy is high. In published reports from the past 20 years, a correct classification of soft tissue tumors as benign or malignant has an accuracy of around 90%. In some reports, the diagnostic accuracy of FNA can reach up to 97% [1, 11, 12, 21, 23–25]. Despite the high degree of accuracy in the diagnosis of malignancy, FNAC has been less successful than open and core biopsies in establishing the histologic type and in the grading of soft tissue sarcomas, and specificity rates for sarcoma have been reported as being between 47 and 98% [1, 11, 26]. In addition, there are some specific limitations connected to the soft tissue tumor area. Heterogeneous composite, hemorrhage, or necrosis of large soft tissue tumors may result in insufficient or suboptimal material being aspirated. In the examination of small and deep-seated, inter- or intramuscular tumors, the lesion can be missed and reactive cells can be aspirated from the tissue adjacent to the lesion. Reactive changes in adipose tissue may mimic liposarcoma, and reactive fibroblasts/myofibroblasts may be confused with a spindle cell or pleomorphic sarcoma. The person performing the examination should be trained in the FNA technique and experienced enough to be able to evaluate whether the sam-

Table 4. Cytologic evaluation based on a myxoid pattern

Tumor	Microscopic features	Immunophenotype	Comments
Intramuscular myxoma	Small, loose cell clusters and dispersed single slender cells with small, round to oval, bland nuclei and long, thin, uni- or bipolar cytoplasmic processes; scattered macrophages and occasional atrophic muscle fibers	Variable positivity for CD34, desmin, and SMA	
Low-grade fibromyxoid sarcoma	Fascicles/clusters and dispersed fibroblast-like spindle cells and naked nuclei with occasional mild anisokaryosis; abundant myxoid matrix; fragments of collagen-rich tissue and curvilinear vessels	Cytoplasmic MUC4 positivity, variable positivity for EMA, CD34, SMA, and claudin-1	It is difficult to render a specific diagnosis of LGFMS based on FNAC alone
Perineurioma	Clusters or dispersed uniform spindle cells with bland, slender, round to oval nuclei and poorly preserved cytoplasm; occasional thin bipolar cytoplasmic processes; myxoid background common	Positive for EMA, claudin-1, and GLUT1, approximately 60% express CD34	
Ossifying fibromyxoid tumor	Mixture of cell clusters and predominantly dissociated cells and rare acinar-like structures in a variable myxoid matrix; often eccentrically situated, rounded (epithelioid) or ovoid nuclei with occasional slight anisonucleosis; naked dispersed nuclei	Positive for S100 in the majority of cases, desmin in less than 50% of cases; occasional focal GFAP, SMA, and keratins	
Myoepithelioma/ mixed tumor of soft tissue	Salivary pleomorphic adenoma-like cytology with epithelial and myoepithelial cells and chondromyxoid or hyalinized matrix in most smears	Positive for keratins, S100, calponin, EMA, and GFAP in about 50% of cases	Difficult to distinguish from chondroid syringoma in subcutaneous locations
Extraskeletal myxoid chondrosarcoma	Dispersed cells, branching cords, strands and cell-balls; abundant myxoid background matrix; uniform bland spindled, fusiform or round cells with ovoid or rounded nuclei; nuclear grooves (coffee-bean nuclei)	Polyphenotypic differentiation; 20% of cases express S100, 30% express CD117	In rare cases tumor cells display neuroendocrine differentiation
Myxofibrosarcoma	Dispersed cells and cell clusters in abundant myxoid background matrix; slightly to moderately atypical spindle cells in low-grade neoplasm, marked cellular and nuclear pleomorphism in high-grade neoplasm; fragments of curved vessels; pseudolipoblasts	Positive for focal SMA, MSA, and CD34 Negative for MDM2, CDK4, desmin, S100, and keratins	Difficult to distinguish low-grade MFS from LGFMS in FNA smears
Myxoinflammatory fibroblastic sarcoma	Spindled to epithelioid cells with variably prominent nucleoli, nuclear pseudoinclusions, and bipolar cytoplasmic extensions; large epithelioid and lipoblast-like cells, bizarre "virocyte" cells; myxoid background material and inflammatory infiltrate	Variable CD34 positivity, positive for EMA, CD117, CD68, nuclear INI1, rare focal keratins	
Myxoid liposarcoma	Clusters of small, round to ovoid, spindled, and stellate nonlipogenic primitive mesenchymal cells with bland nuclei and scant cytoplasm embedded in the myxoid matrix Usually prominent branching, capillary network within the tumor clusters; uni- or multivacuolated lipoblasts	Variable S100 positivity Negative for MDM2, CDK4, CD34, keratins, desmin, and SMA	Size and architectural pattern of capillary vessels in smears are important diagnostic criteria
Lipoblastoma	Fatty tissue fragments usually within a myxoid background matrix; occasional uni- or multivacuolated lipoblast-like cells and hibernoma-like cells; thin capillaries		Lipoblastomas lack the branching capillary network seen in myxoid liposarcoma

SMA, smooth muscle actin; MSA, muscle-specific actin; EMA, epithelial membrane antigen; LGFMS, low-grade fibromyxoid sarcoma; FNAC, fine-needle aspiration cytology; GFAP, glial fibrillary acidic protein; MFS, myxofibrosarcoma.

pling obtained might be consistent with the lesion in question. In addition, a lack of experience in the cytologic diagnosis of soft tissue masses may result in the misinterpretation of even optimal FNA smears [2].

Complications of FNA examination of soft tissue lesions are minor and include small hematomas and localized tenderness. The risk of tumor cell spread in the needle tract must be addressed, even though the

Table 5. Cytologic evaluation based on a small round cell pattern

Tumor	Microscopic features	Immunophenotype	Comments
Glomus tumor	Clustered and dispersed, medium-sized epithelioid cells with rounded to ovoid bland nuclei, inconspicuous nucleoli, and often poorly preserved cytoplasmic borders; variable amounts of a myxoid/fibrillary background matrix in cell clusters	Positive for SMA and caldesmon Negative for desmin, S100 protein, keratin, and endothelial markers	
Alveolar rhabdomyosarcoma	Cell clusters mixed with dispersed cells and stripped nuclei; small- or medium-sized, round to polygonal and ovoid or pear-shaped cells with scanty cytoplasm, coarse nuclear chromatin and often large nucleoli; bi-nucleated and multinucleated tumor cells; mitoses	Positive for desmin, nuclear myogenin, and MyoD1	Requires ancillary tests to distinguish it from other small blue round cell tumors
Poorly differentiated synovial sarcoma of small cell type	Mixture of tight clusters, sheets, and dispersed small round cells resembling those of Ewing sarcoma and stripped nuclei; mitoses	Focally positive for EMA and keratins, positive for CD99 and Bcl-2	Requires ancillary tests to distinguish it from Ewing sarcoma
Extraskeletal Ewing sarcoma	Hypercellular smears; mixture of clustered and dispersed cells with a high N:C ratio and stripped nuclei; common "tigroid" background Double cell population: large, "light" cells with cytoplasmic vacuoles and small, dark cells Rosette-like structures	Positive for CD99, FLI-1 (nuclear), in about 30% of cases focal expression of keratin, S100, and CD117	Requires ancillary tests to distinguish it from other small blue round cell tumors
Neuroblastoma	Predominantly dispersed cells with irregular, hyperchromatic nuclei Small molded clusters of neuroblasts Rosette-like structures with a central neuropil; cells with uni- or bipolar slender cytoplasmic processes; variable presence ganglion-cells; neuropil; necrosis, karyorrhexis, calcifications	Positive for chromogranin, synaptophysin, and NSE; ALK-1 and GFAP variably positive	Requires ancillary tests to distinguish it from other small blue round cell tumors
Desmoplastic small round cell tumor	Uniform or slightly pleomorphic undifferentiated cells with round to oval, slightly angulated, irregular nuclei and scant cytoplasm; nuclear molding and small acinar-like structures; desmoplastic stroma fragments	Polyphenotypic Variable positivity for keratins, desmin, EMA, WT1, neuroendocrine markers, and CD99	Requires ancillary tests to distinguish it from other small blue round cell tumors

SMA, smooth muscle actin; EMA, epithelial membrane antigen; NSE, neuron-specific enolase; GFAP, glial fibrillary acidic protein.

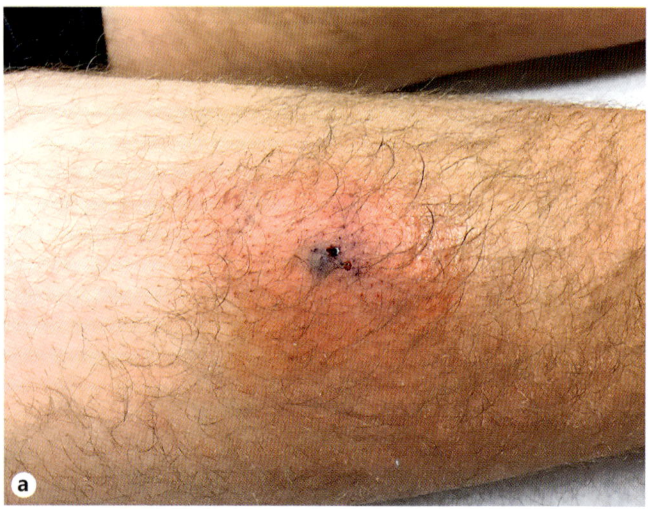
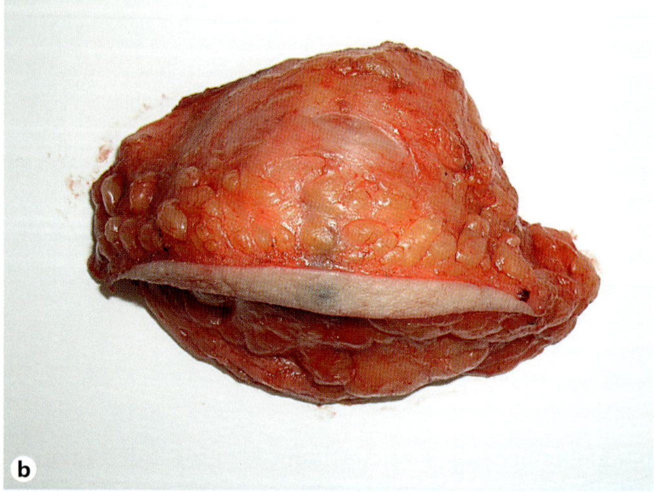

Fig. 5. a Tattoo point after aspiration from a soft tissue sarcoma. **b** An operative specimen showing persistent tattoo, indicating the needle insertion canal.

FNA Cytology of Soft Tissue and Bone Tumors

Table 6. Cytologic evaluation based on an epithelioid pattern

Tumor	Microscopic features	Immunophenotype	Comments
Tenosynovial giant cell tumor	Hypercellular smears, limited yield in tumors with hyalinized stroma; dissociated and clustered mononuclear histiocytoid cells with round to oval nuclei; mild to moderate cellular and nuclear pleomorphism; osteoclast-like giant cells; xanthomatous histiocytes and siderophages	Positivity for CD68 (histiocytes), CD68, and CD45 (osteoclast-like giant cells); occasionally scattered cells positive for desmin	
Adult rhabdomyoma	Clusters or dispersed large rounded, polygonal or elongated cells with abundant granular cytoplasm; small, peripherally located nuclei with prominent nucleoli; occasional cells attached to capillary vessels; occasionally visible cross-striation	Positive for desmin, myogenin, and MyoD1 Negative for S100 and keratins	PAS positive
Epithelioid hemangioendothelioma	Clusters or dispersed epithelioid, polygonal, occasional spindle-shaped cells with variable pleomorphism; binucleated and rare multinucleated cells; dense cytoplasm with occasional intracytoplasmic lumina; nuclei with nuclear grooves, pseudoinclusions and occasional nucleoli; fragments of hyaline and myxohyaline matrix	Positive for CD31, CD34, ERG, FLI-1, and keratin in a third of cases	
Granular cell tumor	Dispersed cells and loosely cohesive clusters of polygonal cells with rounded, small nuclei with insignificant nucleoli and abundant granular cytoplasm; often naked dissociated nuclei in a granular background; occasional cells with moderate anisokaryosis, coarse chromatin and macronucleoli	Strong, diffuse positivity for S100; variable positivity for CD68, CD63, and NSE	PAS-positive diastase resistant
Angiomatoid fibrous histiocytoma	Bloody smears with variable cellularity Clusters and dispersed ovoid to spindled histiocytoid cells with poorly defined cell borders; occasional whorled arrangement of tumor cells associated with capillaries; folded nuclei with a finely granular chromatin pattern; wispy cytoplasm, hemosiderin	Positivity for desmin, EMA, CD99, and CD68 in approximately 50% of cases Negative for S100, CD34, and keratins	FNAC features are nonspecific and clinical correlation and ancillary studies are necessary to render the correct diagnosis
Epithelioid sarcoma	Small loosely cohesive clusters but predominantly dispersed epithelioid, polygonal and spindle-shaped cells with eccentrically placed nuclei, large nucleoli and dense cytoplasm; admixture of lymphocytes, plasma cells, histiocytes, granulomas, necrosis	Positive for EMA and low- and high-molecular keratins; more than 50% stain positively for CD34	Skin ulceration may be seen in subcutaneous tumors
Clear cell sarcoma	Smears with tigroid background; round, polygonal, or spindle-shaped cells with abundant clear to pale cytoplasm; round to ovoid nuclei with vesicular chromatin and often prominent nucleoli	Positive for S100, HBM45, melan A, and SOX10	t(12;22)(q13;q12) with EWSR1-ATF1 fusion is not present in malignant melanoma
Alveolar soft part sarcoma	Large, dyshesive epithelioid and polygonal cells with abundant granular cytoplasm and round nuclei with prominent nucleoli Bare nuclei and granular cytoplasmic background	50% stain positively for desmin and a small subset of cases for S100	Rhomboid or rod-shaped intracytoplasmic crystals staining on PAS after diastase digestion
Extrarenal rhabdoid tumor	Variable cellularity; large rhabdoid cells with eccentric nuclei, prominent nucleoli, and perinuclear density; smaller round, polygonal, and spindled cells; occasional binucleation and multinucleation	Positive for EMA, keratin, and vimentin; about 50% of cases are positive for CD99 and synaptophysin	PAS-positive diastase resistant

PAS, periodic acid-Schiff; NSE, neuron-specific endose; FNAC, fine-needle aspiration cytology; EMA, epithelial membrane antigen.

incidence of this is exceedingly low. As a precaution, the use of a single needle-insertion point even when performing several punctures is recommended when sampling a suspected sarcoma. Subsequent surgical removal of the needle tract can be facilitated by tattooing the site of needle insertion so that it can be identified later (Fig. 5).

References

1 Akerman M, Domanski HA: The cytology of soft tissue tumours. Monogr Clin Cytol 2003;16:1–112.

2 Domanski HA: Fine-needle aspiration cytology of soft tissue lesions: diagnostic challenges. Diagn Cytopathol 2007;35:768–773.

3 Garcia del Muro X, de Alava E, Artigas V, Bague S, Brana A, Cubedo R, Cruz J, Mulet-Margalef N, Narvaez JA, Martinez Tirado O, Valverde C, Verges R, Vinals J, Martin-Broto J: Clinical practice guidelines for the diagnosis and treatment of patients with soft tissue sarcoma by the Spanish Group for Research in Sarcomas (GEIS). Cancer Chemother Pharmacol 2016;77:133–146.

4 Siegel GW, Biermann JS, Chugh R, Jacobson JA, Lucas D, Feng M, Chang AC, Smith SR, Wong SL, Hasen J: The multidisciplinary management of bone and soft tissue sarcoma: an essential organizational framework. J Multidiscip Healthc 2015;8:109–115.

5 Pretell-Mazzini J, Barton MD Jr, Conway SA, Temple HT: Unplanned excision of soft-tissue sarcomas: current concepts for management and prognosis. J Bone Joint Surg Am 2015;97:597–603.

6 Davis LE, Ryan CW: Preoperative therapy for extremity soft tissue sarcomas. Curr Treat Options Oncol 2015;16:25.

7 Fleshman R, Mayerson J, Wakely PE Jr: Fine-needle aspiration biopsy of high-grade sarcoma: a report of 107 cases. Cancer 2007;111:491–498.

8 Traina F, Errani C, Toscano A, Pungetti C, Fabbri D, Mazzotti A, Donati D, Faldini C: Current concepts in the biopsy of musculoskeletal tumors. J Bone Joint Surg Am 2015;97:e7.

9 Domanski HA, Akerman M, Carlen B, Engellau J, Gustafson P, Jonsson K, Mertens F, Rydholm A: Core-needle biopsy performed by the cytopathologist: a technique to complement fine-needle aspiration of soft tissue and bone lesions. Cancer 2005;105:229–239.

10 Joudeh AA, Shareef SQ, Al-Abbadi MA: Fine-needle aspiration followed by core-needle biopsy in the same setting: modifying our approach. Acta Cytol 2016;60:1–13.

11 Ng VY, Thomas K, Crist M, Wakely PE Jr, Mayerson J: Fine needle aspiration for clinical triage of extremity soft tissue masses. Clin Orthop Relat Res 2010;468:1120–1128.

12 Kilpatrick SE, Ward WG, Cappellari JO, Bos GD: Fine-needle aspiration biopsy of soft tissue sarcomas: a cytomorphologic analysis with emphasis on histologic subtyping, grading, and therapeutic significance. Am J Clin Pathol 1999;112:179–188.

13 Panda KG, Hale MJ, Kruger D, Luvhengo TE: Comparison between preoperative biopsy and post-excision histology results in sarcoma: experience at Chris Hani Baragwanath Academic Hospital, Johannesburg, South Africa. S Afr J Surg 2014;52:45–48.

14 Verheijen P, Witjes H, van Gorp J, Hennipman A, van Dalen T: Current pathology work-up of extremity soft tissue sarcomas, evaluation of the validity of different techniques. Eur J Surg Oncol 2010;36:95–99.

15 Kumar S, Chowdhury N: Accuracy, limitations and pitfalls in the diagnosis of soft tissue tumors by fine needle aspiration cytology. Indian J Pathol Microbiol 2007;50:42–45.

16 Kubik MJ, Bovbel A, Goli H, Saremian J, Siddiqi A, Masood S: Diagnostic value and accuracy of imprint cytology evaluation during image-guided core needle biopsies: review of our experience at a large academic center. Diagn Cytopathol 2015;43:773–779.

17 Shield PW, Cosier J, Ellerby G, Gartrell M, Papadimos D: Rapid on-site evaluation of fine needle aspiration specimens by cytology scientists: a review of 3,032 specimens. Cytopathology 2014;25:322–329.

18 Olson MT, Novak A, Kirby J, Shahid H, Boonyaarunnate T, Ali SZ: Cytotechnologist-attended on-site evaluation of adequacy for metastatic disease involving bone and soft tissue. Acta Cytol 2013;57:550–556.

19 Mallik MK, Dey P, Gupta SK, Vasishta RK: Grading of soft tissue sarcomas on fine-needle aspiration cytology smear. Diagn Cytopathol 2010;38:109–112.

20 Mathur S, Kapila K, Verma K: Accuracy of cytological grading of spindle-cell sarcomas. Diagn Cytopathol 2003;29:79–83.

21 Palmer HE, Mukunyadzi P, Culbreth W, Thomas JR: Subgrouping and grading of soft-tissue sarcomas by fine-needle aspiration cytology: a histopathologic correlation study. Diagn Cytopathol 2001;24:307–316.

22 Weir MM, Rosenberg AE, Bell DA: Grading of spindle cell sarcomas in fine-needle aspiration biopsy specimens. Am J Clin Pathol 1999;112:784–790.

23 Singh HK, Kilpatrick SE, Silverman JF: Fine needle aspiration biopsy of soft tissue sarcomas: utility and diagnostic challenges. Adv Anat Pathol 2004;11:24–37.

24 Layfield LJ, Schmidt RL, Sangle N, Crim JR: Diagnostic accuracy and clinical utility of biopsy in musculoskeletal lesions: a comparison of fine-needle aspiration, core, and open biopsy techniques. Diagn Cytopathol 2014;42:476–486.

25 Kilpatrick SE, Geisinger KR: Soft tissue sarcomas: the usefulness and limitations of fine-needle aspiration biopsy. Am J Clin Pathol 1998;110:50–68.

26 Dey P, Mallik MK, Gupta SK, Vasishta RK: Role of fine needle aspiration cytology in the diagnosis of soft tissue tumours and tumour-like lesions. Cytopathology 2004;15:32–37.

FNA Cytology of Soft Tissue and Bone Tumors

Domanski HA, Walther CS: FNA Cytology of Soft Tissue and Bone Tumors. Monogr Clin Cytol.
Basel, Karger, 2017, vol 22, pp 13–14 (DOI: 10.1159/000475089)

Sampling and Preparation Techniques

Nonguided and Image-Guided Fine-Needle Aspiration

The technique for fine-needle aspiration (FNA) cytology of soft tissue tumors is the same as for other types of lesions. The length of the needle depends on the location of the lesion. Thorough palpation and estimation of size, site, and consistency of the tumor is essential. Since the surgeon may often want to decide where the needle should be inserted, close communication between the aspirator and surgeon is mandatory (Fig. 1). If the surgeon does not specifically indicate the insertion point/points, aspiration through the vertex is recommended [1, 2].

Percutaneous puncture of palpable lesions can be performed in outpatient clinics with or without local anesthesia and without radiologic guidance. Image-guided FNA is necessary for the examination of deep-seated and nonpalpable soft tissue lesions. Ultrasound guidance may be used in the FNA of superficial or deep lesions close to the muscle fascia, while CT is the best guidance modality for all deep-seated soft tissue lesions. A coaxial FNA technique is preferable in order to avoid multiple skin passages, and FNA may be followed directly by core needle biopsy. The on-site, immediate evaluation of smears stained by DiffQuick is an optimal way to ensure that an adequate sample for both routine examination and for ancillary studies has been taken (see Chapter 1, Fig. 2 and 3).

Direct Smears

The routine microscopic evaluation of FNA cytology specimens should be based on both wet-fixed, hematoxylin and eosin (HE)- or Papanicolaou (PAP)-stained smears, and air-dried, May-Grünwald-Giemsa- or DiffQuik-stained smears.

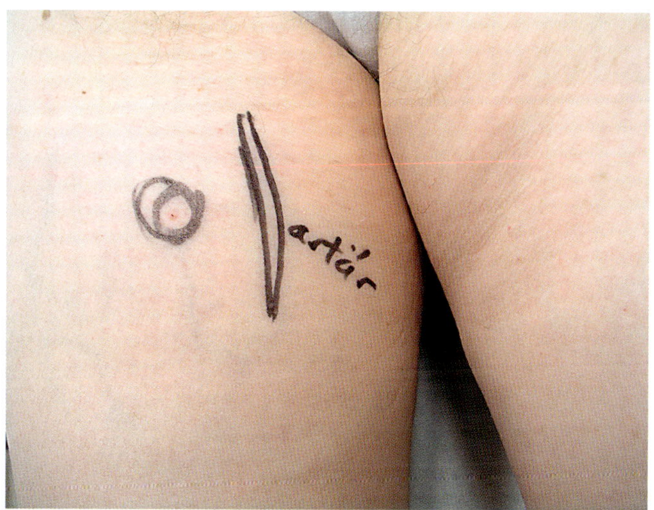

Fig. 1. Needle insertion area marked by the orthopedic surgeon.

Wet-fixed material is superior for the evaluation of nuclear details such as nucleoli or nuclear membrane and chromatin structure, while the cytoplasmic details and the background matrix are better elucidated in air-dried smears.

Liquid-Based Preparations

In addition to the liquid-based preparation of exudates or PAP smears, it has become popular to prepare even FNA specimens through a liquid medium. In our experience, cells and tissues obtained from epithelial neoplasms are usually better preserved than those of mesenchymal origin after liquid-based processing. The liquid-based preparation of FNA specimens from mesenchymal lesions has been problematic compared to those from epithelial neoplasms. The diagnostic criteria may be different in such specimens compared to regular smears. For example, an inflammatory or myxoid smear background, which is sometimes an important part of the diagnosis, is frequently lost after processing through Cytolyt. Nevertheless, in our clinic, we have found the liquid-based method to be useful, especially in the area of molecular biologic analyses (fluorescence in situ hybridization, FISH).

Cell Blocks

The preparation of cell blocks is superior to most other techniques devised to make the best use of aspirates. Since the original description by Koss [3] of the plasma thrombin method, several other methods for preparing cell blocks have been reported. Cell blocks provide multiple histologic sections and enable the performance of immunocytochemical and other special stains on slides of comparable quality. Another advantage of cell block preparation is better visualization of the tumor tissue pattern and architecture compared to FNA smears (see Chapter 1, Fig. 1–4).

References

1 Domanski HA: Fine-needle aspiration cytology of soft tissue lesions: diagnostic challenges. Diagn Cytopathol 2007;35:768–773.
2 Akerman M, Domanski HA: The cytology of soft tissue tumours. Monogr Clin Cytol 2003;16:1–112.
3 Koss L: Diagnostic Cytology and Its Histopathological Bases, ed 3. Philadelphia, Lippincott, 1979.

Chapter 3

Domanski HA, Walther CS: FNA Cytology of Soft Tissue and Bone Tumors. Monogr Clin Cytol.
Basel, Karger, 2017, vol 22, pp 15–21 (DOI: 10.1159/000475090)

Ancillary Techniques

Ancillary techniques are helpful when diagnosing soft tissue and bone tumors with fine-needle aspiration cytology (FNAC). The methods used on surgical tumor specimens are also applicable to cytologic material. Considering that FNA is minimally invasive, well tolerated by the patient, cost effective, and low risk, it is a valuable method for collecting material for ancillary as well as morphologic assessment [1]. This makes it possible to diagnose and classify mesenchymal lesions with high accuracy on cytologic material, which is usually collected prior to surgery and treatment [2]. Immunocytochemistry is the most commonly used technique and can be applied directly on aspirated material or on any of several types of preparations, including liquid-based techniques such as cytospin-preparation, or various "monolayer" techniques as well as cell blocks. This is, in many cases, sufficient to establish a diagnosis but the need for detailed genetic and molecular evaluation is steadily increasing in many soft tissue tumors, just as it is in other tumor types [2–5]. Molecular genetic methods can be used to verify or rule out a specific diagnosis and particular genetic changes have been described in many types of tumor, and these are steadily increasing (Table 1). However, they can also provide prognostic information and even determine treatment in gastrointestinal stromal tumors (GIST). Several genetic and cytogenetic molecular methods, including cytogenetics (chromosome banding), fluorescence in situ hybridization (FISH), polymerase chain reaction (PCR), single nucleotide polymorphism (SNP) array, and next-generation sequencing (NGS), can be applied to cytologic material [6–10]. However, since the amount of material provided by needle aspiration is often limited, it is important to choose the optimal method depending on what type of genetic information is required. A genetic overview of a tumor can be obtained with chromosome banding and SNP array, although the former needs fresh material for cell culturing. A targeted analysis searching for specific mutations and gene fusions can be obtained with FISH and PCR using both fresh and fixed material. NGS is a method that can deliver both an overview and detailed genetic information down to the nucleotide level. This can be performed on both fresh and fixed aspirates, but it is relatively expensive and the analysis is labor intensive due to the large amount of data it provides. Flow cytometry is mainly used to rule out soft tissue manifestations of lymphoma and leukemia. It is not used to diagnose soft tissue tumors, although it has been tested in a research setting and provided useful information in mesenchymal tumors [11, 12]. Electron microscopy can be used on cytologic specimens and deliver information concerning differentiation and submicroscopic cellular structures. This can help in determining tumor cell origin and differentiation.

Immunocytochemistry

Immunocytochemistry may be performed on any of several types of preparations; on direct smears, cytospin preparations, cell blocks, or liquid-based cytology. The results of immunolabeling of cytologic material can vary depending on the type of FNA specimen preparation and can be difficult to standardize. Cell blocks prepared from aspirated material provide an excellent means for processing an FNA specimen for immunohistochemical examinations. They permit the preparation of histologic sections of a quality similar to small core-needle biopsies. The processing of these slides for immunostaing follows the same procedure as for surgical biopsies with relevant controls and results comparable with open biopsies (see Chapter 1, Fig. 1–4).

Table 1. Fusion genes and mutations that can be used for clinical purposes in soft tissue and bone sarcomas

Diagnosis	Chromosome location	Genes (5′–3′)	Cellular function of mutation	Clinical use	Examples of methods used for detection
Ewing/primitive neuroectodermal tumor	t(11;22)(q24;q12) t(21;22)(q22;q12) t(7;22)(p22;q12) t(17;22)(q12;q12) t(2;22)(q33;q12) t(16;21)(p11;q22) t(2;16) inv(22)	*EWSR1-FLI1* *EWSR1-ERG* *EWSR1-ETV1* *EWSR1-ETV4* *EWSR1-FEV* *FUS-ERG* *FUS-FEV* *EWSR1-ZSG*	Overexpression of oncogenes including *MYC* and *IGF1*	Diagnostic	ICC (FLI1) Karyotype FISH (EWSR1 break apart probe) RT-PCR NGS
Desmoplastic small round cell tumor	t(11;22)(p13;q12) t(21;22)(q22;q12)	*EWSR1- WT1* *EWSR1-ERG*	Upregulates oncogenic factors including *PDGF* and *IL2Rβ*	Diagnostic, therapeutic	ICC (WT1) Cytogenetic karyotype FISH (EWSR1 split-apart probe) NGS
Clear cell sarcoma	t(12;22)(q13;q12) t(2;22)(q33;q12)	*EWSR1-ATF1* *EWSR1-CREB1*	Upregulation of *ARNT2, ATM, GPP34, MITF* genes	Diagnostic	FISH (EWSR1 split-apart probe) PCR NGS
Angiomatoid fibrous histiocytoma	t(12;16)(q13;p11) t(12;22)(q13;q12) t(2;22)(q33;q12)	*EWSR1-CREB1* *EWSR1-CREB1* *FUS-ATF1* *EWSR1-ATF1*	Transcription activation	Diagnostic	FISH RT-PCR NGS
Extraskeletal myxoid chondrosarcoma	t(9;22)(q22;q12) t(9;17)(q22;q11) t(9;15)(q22;q21) t(9;22)(q22;q15)	*EWSR1-NR4A3* *TAF2N-NR4A3* *TCF12-NR4A3* *TFG-NR4A3*	Probable transcription activation	Diagnostic	FISH RT-PCR NGS
Myxoid liposarcoma	t(12;16)(q13;p11) t(12;22)(q13;q12)	*FUS-DDIT3* *EWSR1-DDIT3*	Transcription activation	Diagnostic, potentially therapeutic	FISH (FUS split-apart probe) RT-PCR NGS
Low-grade fibromyxoid sarcoma	t(7;16)(q33;p11) t(11;16)(p11;p11)	*FUS-CREB3L2* *FUS-CREB3L1*	Transcription activation	Diagnostic	FISH (FUS split-apart probe) RT-PCR NGS
Congenital mesoblastic nephroma	t(12;15)(p13;q25)	*ETV6-NTRK3*	Aberrant tyrosine kinase activation	Diagnostic	FISH RT-PCR NGS
Infantile fibrosarcoma	t(12;15)(p13;q25)	*ETV6-NTRK3*	Aberrant tyrosine kinase activation	Diagnostic	FISH RT-PCR NGS
Inflammatory myofibroblastic tumor	t(1;2)(q25;q23) t(2;19)(q23;q13) t(2;17)(q23;q23) t(2;2)(p23;q13)	*TPM3-ALK* *TPM4-ALK* *CLTC-ALK* *RANBP2-ALK*	Overexpression of ALK C-terminal kinase regions	Diagnostic	ICC (ALK protein) FISH (ALK split-apart probe) RT-PCR NGS
Synovial sarcoma	t(X;18)(p11;q11) t(X;18)(p11;q11) t(X;18)(p11;q13) t(X;20)(p11;q13)	*SS18-SSX1* *SS18-SSX2* *SS18-SSX4* *SS18L1-SSX1*	Dysregulation of gene expression	Diagnostic, prognosis improved with *SS18-SSX2*	ICC (TLE1 protein) FISH (SYT probe) RT-PCR NGS
Endometrial stromal sarcoma	t(7;17)(p15;q21) t(6;7)(p21;p15) t(6;10)(p21;p11)	*JAZF1-SUZ12* *JAZF1-PHF1* *EPC1-PHF1*	Antiapoptotic effect	Diagnostic	RT-PCR NGS

Diagnosis	Chromosome location	Genes (5'–3')	Cellular function of mutation	Clinical use	Examples of methods used for detection
Dermatofibrosarcoma protuberans	t(17;22)(q22;q13)	*COL1A1-PDGFB*	*PDGFB* expression upregulated	Diagnostic, therapeutic (Gleevec responsive)	FISH RT-PCR NGS
Giant cell fibroblastoma	t(17;22)(q22;q13)	*COL1A1-PDGFB*	*PDGFB* expression upregulated	Diagnostic	FISH RT-PCR NGS
Alveolar rhabdomyosarcoma	t(2;13)(q35;q14) t(1;13)(q36;q14) t(2;X)(p35;q13) t(2;2)(q35;q23)	*PAX3-FOXO1A* *PAX7-FOXO1A* *PAX3-MLLT7* *PAX3-NCOAI*	Transcription activation	Diagnostic, better prognosis with *PAX7-FOXO1A* than *PAX3-FOXO1A*	Karyotype FISH (*FOXO1A* split-apart probe) RT-PCR
Alveolar soft part sarcoma	t(X;17)(p11;q25)	*ASPSL-TFE3*	Transcription activation	Diagnostic, potentially therapeutic (MET inhibition)	ICC (TFE3) RT-PCR
Aneurysmal bone cyst	t(16;17)(q22;p13) t(1;17)(p34;p13) t(3;17)(q21;p13) t(9;17)(q22;p13) t(17;17)(p13;q21)	*CDH11-USP6* *THRAP3-USP6* *CNBP-USP6* *OMD-USP6* *COL1A1-USP6*	*USP6* expression upregulated	Diagnostic	FISH, RT-PCR
Tenosynovial giant cell tumor	t(1;2)(p13;q37)	*CSF1-COL6A3*	Unclear *CSF1* expression upregulated in tumor cells	Diagnostic	Cytogenetic karyotype FISH RT-PCR
Pericytoma	t(7;12)(p22;q13)	*ACTB-GLI1*	Transcriptional activation	Diagnostic	FISH RT-PCR
Gastrointestinal stromal tumors	Point mutation 4q12	*KIT or PGDFRA*	Activation tyrosine kinase receptor	Diagnostic, therapeutic, imatinib responsive	ICC (c-Kit) PCR
Rhabdoid tumor	del 22q11.22	*SMARCB1*	Homozygous loss of tumor suppressor (*SMARCB*)	Diagnostic	ICC (INI1 lost)
Atypical lipomatous tumor/well differentiated liposarcoma	Ring chromosomes Giant marker chromosomes Amplification 12q15 region	*MDM2* amplification *CDK4, HMGA2* often coamplified	Overexpression downregulates tumor suppressor function (*TP53*)	Diagnostic	ICC (MDM2, CDK4) FISH
Desmoid-type fibromatosis	Trisomies chromosomes 8 and 20 5q deletion 3p21 point mutation	*APC* *CTNNB1*	Intranuclear accumulation of β-catenin	Diagnostic	ICC (β-catenin)

ICC, immunocytochemistry; FISH, fluorescent in situ hybridization; RT-PCR, reverse transcriptase-polymerase chain reaction; NGS, next-generation sequencing.

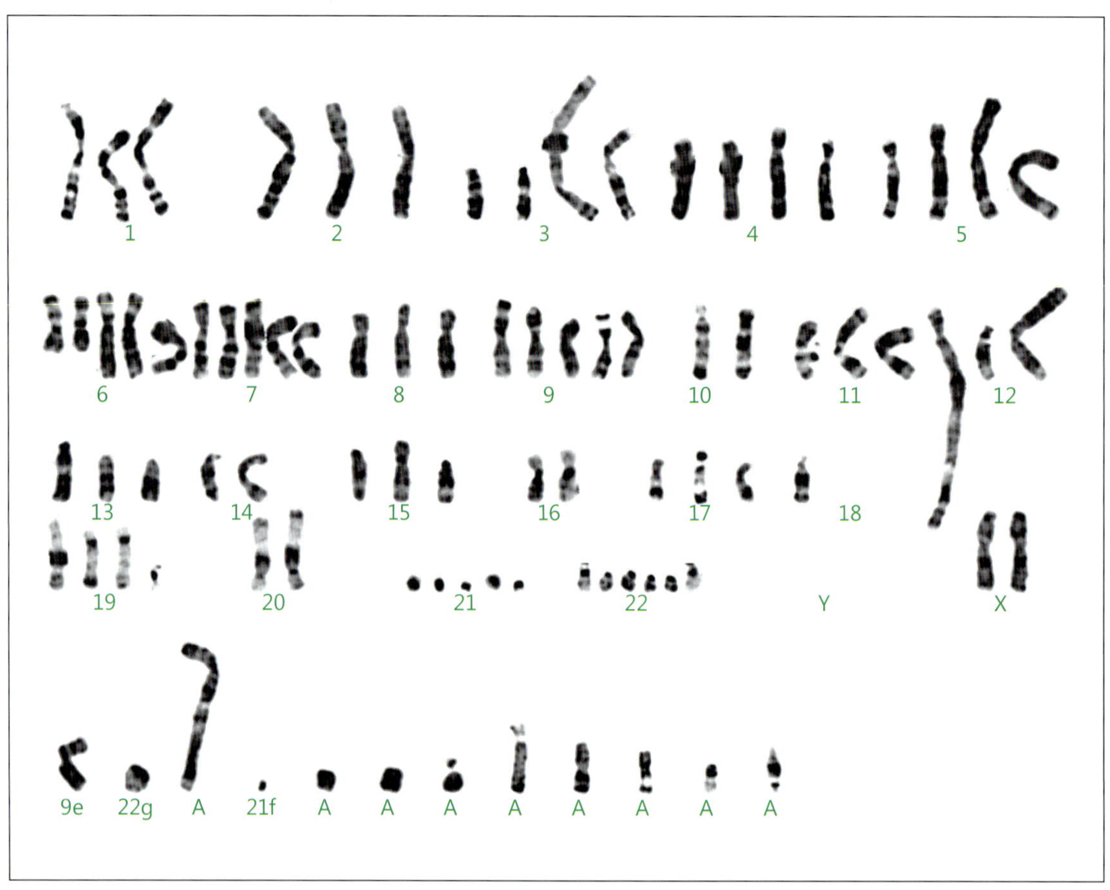

Fig. 1. A spindle cell liposarcoma displaying a complex karyotype with multiple chromosomal aberrations.

Molecular Techniques

Molecular techniques can provide useful information when diagnosing soft tissue and bone tumors. Mesenchymal neoplasms are often diagnostically challenging and the information derived from molecular techniques can be important to verify or rule out a specific diagnosis. The particular changes detected by these techniques are mainly used for diagnostic purposes, but can also be used to determine a prognosis, such as alveolar rhabdomyosarcoma [13]. In GIST, the specific mutations are used to direct treatment and predict responsiveness to tyrosine-kinase inhibitors [14]. The methods used to obtain genetic information are cytogenetics (chromosome banding; Fig. 1), FISH (Fig. 2), PCR (Fig. 3), SNP array (Fig. 4), and NGS.

Chromosome banding is a method that gives an overall view of the chromosomes in tumor cells through staining. The different chromosome regions are stained and appear

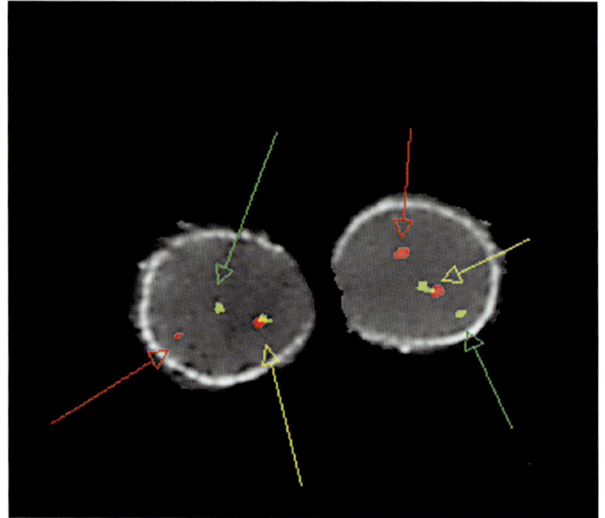

Fig. 2. Interphase FISH showing break-apart probes (BAP) for *EWSR1* rearrangement in an Ewing sarcoma.

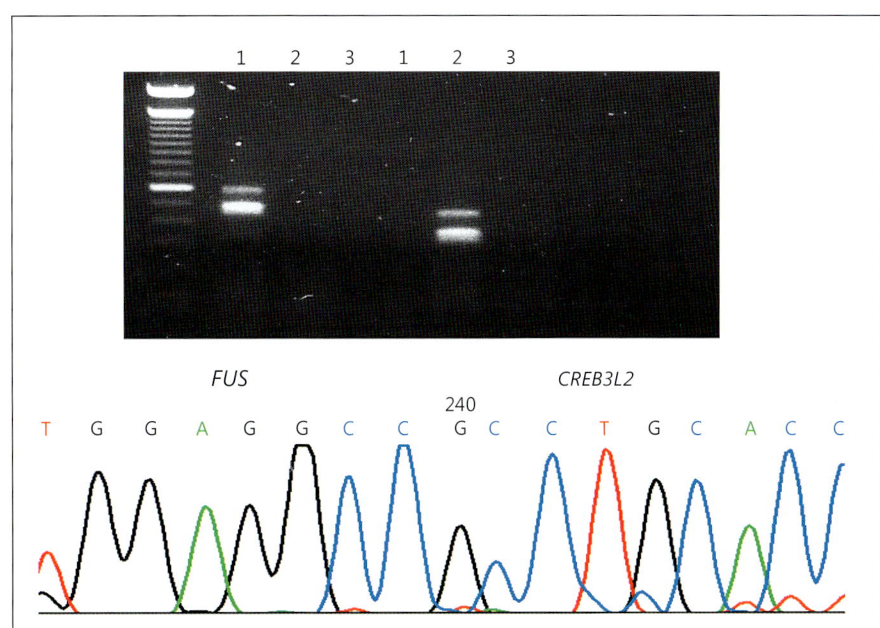

Fig. 3. RT-PCR demonstrating a *FUS/CREB3L2* fusion transcript in a low-grade fibromyxoid sarcoma and a chromatogram showing the nucleotide sequence of the fusion junction.

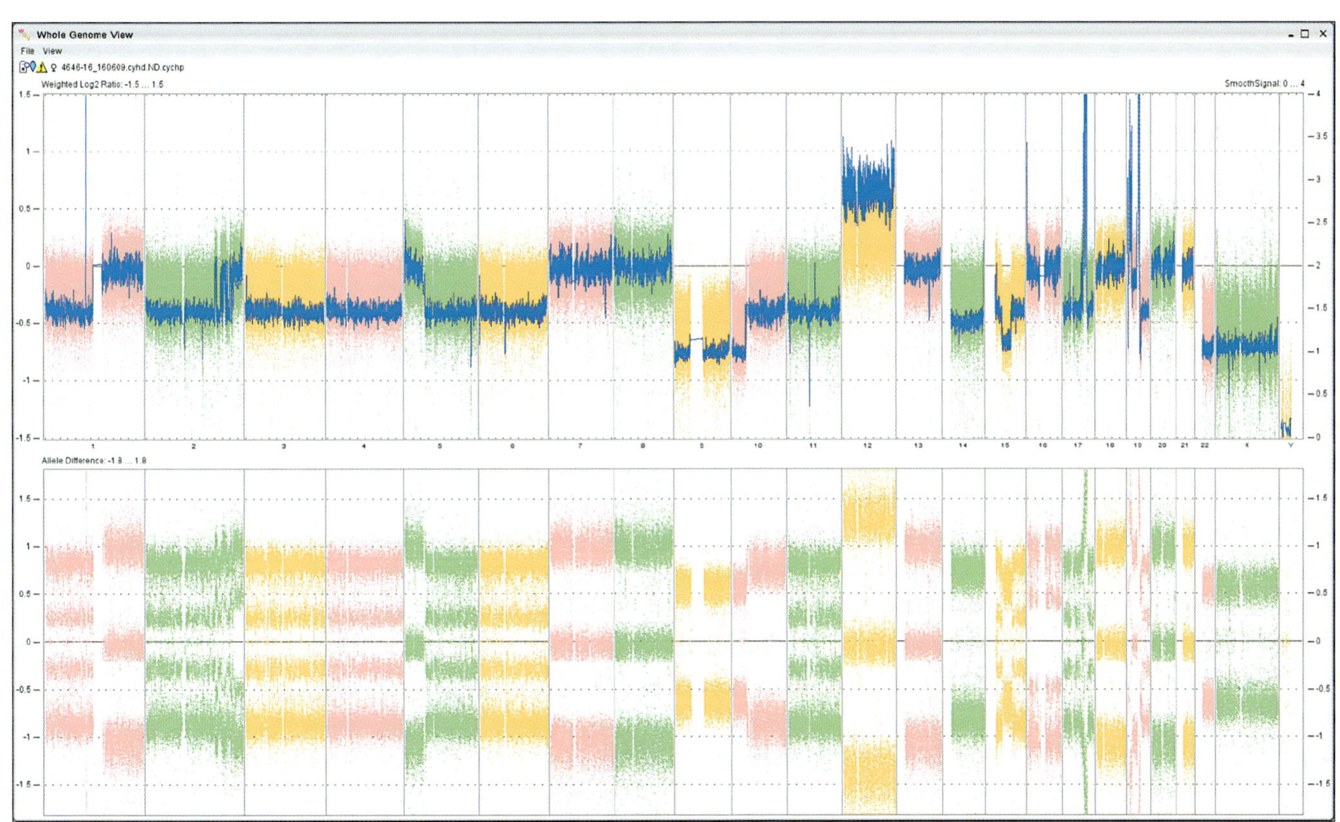

Fig. 4. SNP array results showing a GIST with chromosomal changes involving gains and losses (upper curve) as well as aberrant allele frequencies (lower curve).

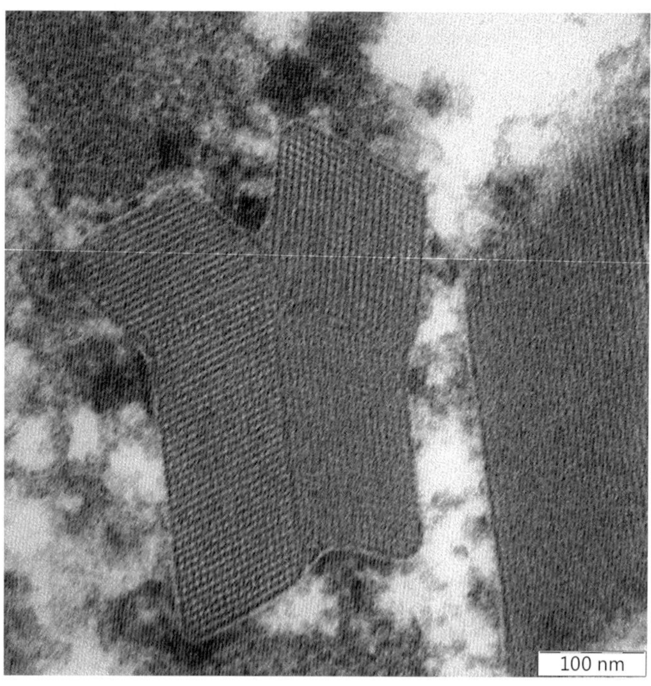

Fig. 5. Alveolar soft part sarcoma: cytoplasmic crystals that reveal periodic linear lamellar structures on ultrastructural examination.

as light or dark bands. It provides an overview of the chromosomes, permitting both structural and numerical changes to be detected. Producing a karyotype requires fresh material and the cells have to be cultured and arrested in mitosis in order to obtain the condensed chromosomes for analysis. The color used for staining the chromosomes is in most instances Giemsa. Drawbacks include that the technique has a relatively low resolution (5 million base pairs) and is labor intensive [15].

FISH is a method where fluorescence-tagged probes bind to complementary DNA sequences of interest. Numerical and structural rearrangements including chromosomal gains, amplifications, deletions, translocations, and gene fusions can be detected. The technique can be used on fresh or fixed cell material. The technique bridges the gap between chromosome banding and molecular genetics and has a resolution of approximately 5,000 base pairs. Drawbacks of the technique include that it requires knowledge of the chromosomal abnormalities beforehand, technical problems (i.e., imperfect hybridization, unspecific probe binding) and interobserver variability. These limitations can produce both false positive and false negative results. SNP array can be used to detect gains and losses as well as the allele frequency in the whole genome. Fresh/frozen material is needed for

the analyses but recently even fixed tissue has been used with success. The resolution of the method varies depending on the number of markers used, but is approximately 20,000 base pairs. Drawbacks of the technique include that it cannot detect balanced rearrangements and that contamination of normal cells could "mask" mutations.

PCR-based methods use DNA or RNA (reverse transcriptase-PCR) to detect translocations, gene breakpoints, point mutations, gene expression, and gene fusions. The technique is a reliable tool for detecting genetic changes in small amounts of material with a very low percentage of tumor cells, making it useful in FNAC material. Both fresh and fixed tumor material can be used. The method is highly sensitive and can be used for nucleotide segments of between 100 and 10,000 base pairs. The high sensitivity is also a drawback since contamination and procedure-generated artifacts can produce false results. NGS is a method for determining the order of nucleotides in a given DNA or RNA strand. This technique is highly effective and allows the detection of a number of genetic changes, including point mutations, insertions, deletions, copy number, translocations, fusion genes, and gene expression levels. Different types of material can be used for NGS, which makes the method versatile and useful. Fresh frozen tumor tissue, formalin-fixed tissue, and cytologic materials have all been shown to provide adequate material for analysis [16, 17].

NGS is performed by fragmenting DNA or RNA from a tumor sample and amplifying the fragments using PCR. This results in millions of copies of the fragmented sequences. Sequencing is then initiated by adding fluorescent-tagged nucleotides and reagents. The emission from each cluster of fragments is then imaged and recorded, resulting in the specific nucleotide sequence. The results are then aligned to the human reference genome. The technique can cover the whole genome, exons (exome sequencing), a selected gene panel (targeted sequencing), and RNA (transcriptome sequencing). Each nucleotide will be sequenced between 10 and 1,000 times. This is referred to as the depth of coverage and is the reason for the power of NGS to detect minor cell populations with mutations. The drawbacks of the NGS technology are that false positive results can arise from errors due to the many enhancement and alignment steps. False negative results can occur because certain sequences are difficult to map and, as in other techniques, mutations may go undetected due to contamination with normal cells. Finally, the analyses of the enormous volumes of data require both analytic skill and considerable computing power, which can be a limiting factor [18].

Electron Microscopy

Ultrastructural examination of aspiration smears can be useful in some areas of FNAC for the differentiation of epithelial and mesenchymal neoplasms and for revealing a specific histogenesis, which may be myogenic, neurogenic, or fibroblastic/myofibroblastic [19]. Electron microscopy may visualize ultrastructural hallmarks for some specific histologic types of neoplasm, such as Z-bands in rhabdomyosarcoma or intracytoplasmic periodic linear lamellar structures in alveolar soft part sarcoma [20] (Fig. 5).

References

1 Domanski HA: Fine-needle aspiration cytology of soft tissue lesions: diagnostic challenges. Diagn Cytopathol 2007;35:768–773.

2 Coley SM, Crapanzano JP, Saqi A: FNA, core biopsy, or both for the diagnosis of lung carcinoma: obtaining sufficient tissue for a specific diagnosis and molecular testing. Cancer Cytopathol 2015; 123:318–326.

3 Krane JF, Cibas ES, Alexander EK, Paschke R, Eszlinger M: Molecular analysis of residual Thin-Prep material from thyroid FNAs increases diagnostic sensitivity. Cancer Cytopathol 2015;123: 356–361.

4 Ryozawa S, Iwano H, Taba K, Sen-yo M, Uekitani T: Genetic diagnosis of pancreatic cancer using specimens obtained by EUS-FNA. Dig Endosc 2011;23(suppl 1):43–45.

5 Sanati S, Lu DW, Schmidt E, Perry A, Dehner LP, Pfeifer JD: Cytologic diagnosis of Ewing sarcoma/peripheral neuroectodermal tumor with paired prospective molecular genetic analysis. Cancer 2007;111:192–199.

6 Walther C, Domanski HA, von Steyern FV, Mandahl N, Mertens F: Chromosome banding analysis of cells from fine-needle aspiration biopsy samples from soft tissue and bone tumors: is it clinically meaningful? Cancer Genet 2011;204:203–206.

7 Ribeiro A, Peng J, Casas C, Fan YS: Endoscopic ultrasound guided fine needle aspiration with fluorescence in situ hybridization analysis in 104 patients with pancreatic mass. J Gastroenterol Hepatol 2014;29:1654–1658.

8 Wang Y, Liu Y, Zhao C, Li X, Wu C, Hou L, Zhang S, Jiang T, Chen X, Su C, Gao G, Li W, Wu F, Li A, Ren S, Zhou C, Zhang J: Feasibility of cytological specimens for ALK fusion detection in patients with advanced NSCLC using the method of RT-PCR. Lung Cancer 2016;94:28–34.

9 Young TA, Burgess BL, Rao NP, Gorin MB, Straatsma BR: High-density genome array is superior to fluorescence in-situ hybridization analysis of monosomy 3 in choroidal melanoma fine needle aspiration biopsy. Mol Vis 2007;13:2328–2333.

10 Vigliar E, Malapelle U, de Luca C, Bellevicine C, Troncone G: Challenges and opportunities of next-generation sequencing: a cytopathologist's perspective. Cytopathology 2015;26:271–283.

11 Wang H, Zhang J, Tao Q, Bian H, Shen Y, Li Y, Tao L, Wang C, Wang Y, Zhai Z: Flow cytometry used to identify histiocytic sarcoma: a case report. Cytometry B Clin Cytom 2016;90:546–550.

12 Hayashi Y, Bardsley MR, Toyomasu Y, Milosavljevic S, Gajdos GB, Choi KM, Reid-Lombardo KM, Kendrick ML, Bingener-Casey J, Tang CM, Sicklick JK, Gibbons SJ, Farrugia G, Taguchi T, Gupta A, Rubin BP, Fletcher JA, Ramachandran A, Ordog T: Platelet-derived growth factor receptor-alpha regulates proliferation of gastrointestinal stromal tumor cells with mutations in KIT by stabilizing ETV1. Gastroenterology 2015;149:420–432.e16.

13 Missiaglia E, Blaveri E, Terris B, Wang YH, Costello E, Neoptolemos JP, Crnogorac-Jurcevic T, Lemoine NR: Analysis of gene expression in cancer cell lines identifies candidate markers for pancreatic tumorigenesis and metastasis. Int J Cancer J Int Cancer 2004;112:100–112.

14 Nishida T, Goto O, Raut CP, Yahagi N: Diagnostic and treatment strategy for small gastrointestinal stromal tumors. Cancer 2016;122:3110–3118.

15 Smeets DF: Historical prospective of human cytogenetics: from microscope to microarray. Clin Biochem 2004;37:439–446.

16 Nikiforov YE, Ohori NP, Hodak SP, Carty SE, LeBeau SO, Ferris RL, Yip L, Seethala RR, Tublin ME, Stang MT, Coyne C, Johnson JT, Stewart AF, Nikiforova MN: Impact of mutational testing on the diagnosis and management of patients with cytologically indeterminate thyroid nodules: a prospective analysis of 1,056 FNA samples. J Clin Endocrinol Metab 2011;96:3390–3397.

17 Hedegaard J, Thorsen K, Lund MK, Hein AM, Hamilton-Dutoit SJ, Vang S, Nordentoft I, Birkenkamp-Demtroder K, Kruhoffer M, Hager H, Knudsen B, Andersen CL, Sorensen KD, Pedersen JS, Orntoft TF, Dyrskjot L: Next-generation sequencing of RNA and DNA isolated from paired fresh-frozen and formalin-fixed paraffin-embedded samples of human cancer and normal tissue. PLoS One 2014;9:e98187.

18 Meldrum C, Doyle MA, Tothill RW: Next-generation sequencing for cancer diagnostics: a practical perspective. Clin Biochem Rev 2011;32:177–195.

19 Turbat-Herrera EA, Herrera GA: Electron microscopy renders the diagnostic capabilities of cytopathology more precise: an approach to everyday practice. Ultrastruct Pathol 2005;29:475–482.

20 Machhi J, Kouzova M, Komorowski DJ, Asma Z, Chivukala M, Basir Z, Shidham VB: Crystals of alveolar soft part sarcoma in a fine needle aspiration biopsy cytology smear: a case report. Acta Cytol 2002;46:904–908.

Chapter 4

Domanski HA, Walther CS: FNA Cytology of Soft Tissue and Bone Tumors. Monogr Clin Cytol.
Basel, Karger, 2017, vol 22, pp 22–24 (DOI: 10.1159/000475091)

Normal Elements and the Cytologic Features of Reactive Changes in Soft Tissue

Adipocytic Tissue

Fine-needle aspiration smears of fat tissue show clusters of fat cells with an abundant univacuolated cytoplasm or empty space after the cytoplasm and peripherally situated small nuclei. Slender capillaries are frequent findings in the clusters. Smears from reactive fat tissue may show a myxoid background, multinucleated histiocytic cells, increasing numbers of fibroblasts and endothelial cells, and occasionally adipocytes with a multivacuolated cytoplasm resembling lipoblasts (Fig. 1).

Fibrotic Tissue

Fibroblasts are spindle-shaped cells with slender contours, containing ovoid or rounded nuclei with fine, evenly distributed chromatin distribution and inconspicuous nucleo-

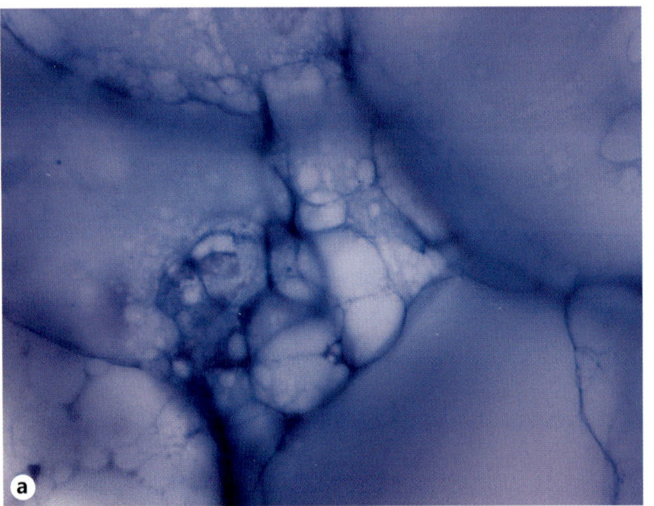
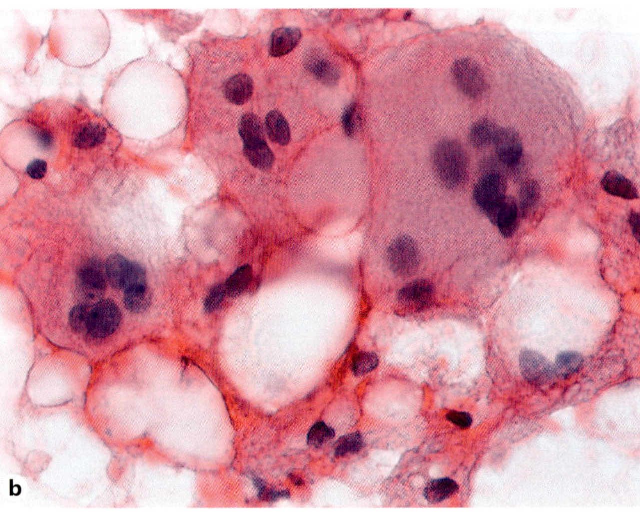

Fig. 1. Smears from reactive fat tissue may show adipocytes with a multivacuolated cytoplasm resembling lipoblasts (MGG stain; **a**) and multinucleated histiocytic cells (HE stain; **b**) that should not be misinterpreted as signs of malignancy.

li. Well-preserved fibroblasts show unipolar or bipolar cyto-plasmic processes but bare nuclei of fibroblasts are common findings in smears (Fig. 2). Reactive fibroblasts/myofibroblasts present as fusiform, rounded, or triangular, occasionally binucleated cells of variable sizes, with enlarged, irregular nuclei, and occasionally coarse chromatin and prominent macro nucleoli. These cells frequently contain an abundant cytoplasm with 1 to several processes or angulated cytoplasmic extensions (Fig. 2).

Striated Muscle

Muscle fibers are pink or amphophilic on Papanicolaou staining, eosinophilic in hematoxylin and eosin (HE) staining, and deep blue in May-Grünwald-Giemsa (MGG)-stained smears. Peripherally placed small nuclei and cross-striations may occasionally be observed (Fig. 3). Damaged and regenerating striated muscle fibers appear in smears as multinucleated "muscle giant cells" of varying shapes and within the cells the nuclei are often arranged in rows or eccentrically placed and have prominent nucleoli (Fig. 4).

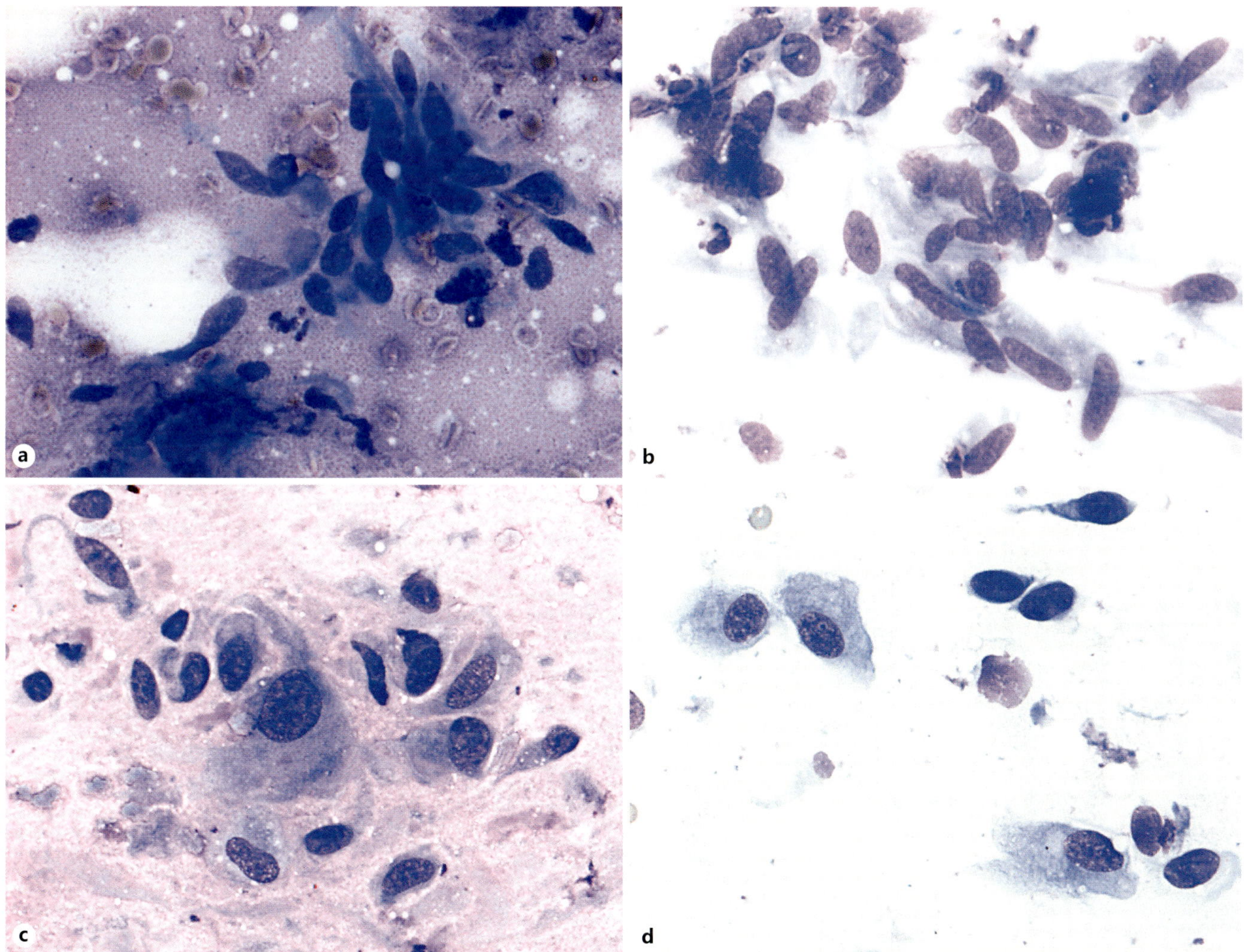

Fig. 2. a, **b** A loose cluster of uniform spindle-shaped fibroblasts with preserved cytoplasmic processes in some of these cells. MGG stain. **c**, **d** Reactive fibroblasts/myofibroblasts present as fusiform, rounded, or triangular cells of variable sizes, with enlarged nuclei showing occasional coarse chromatin. MGG stain.

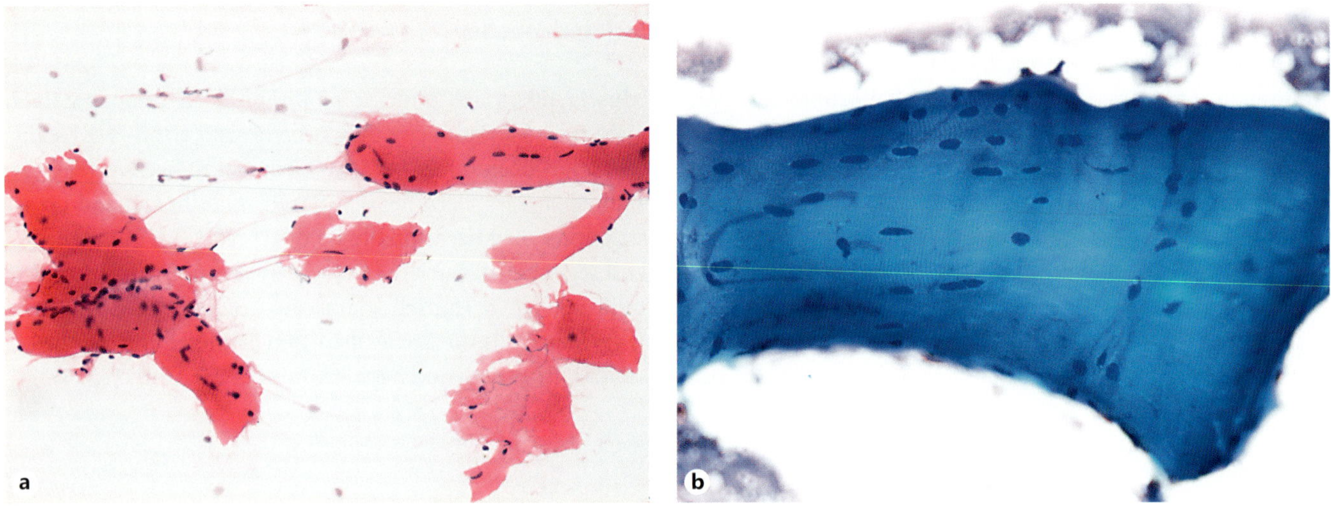

Fig. 3. Muscle fibers are eosinophilic (**a**) in HE- and deep blue in MGG-stained smears (**b**). Peripherally placed small nuclei and cross-striations may occasionally be observed.

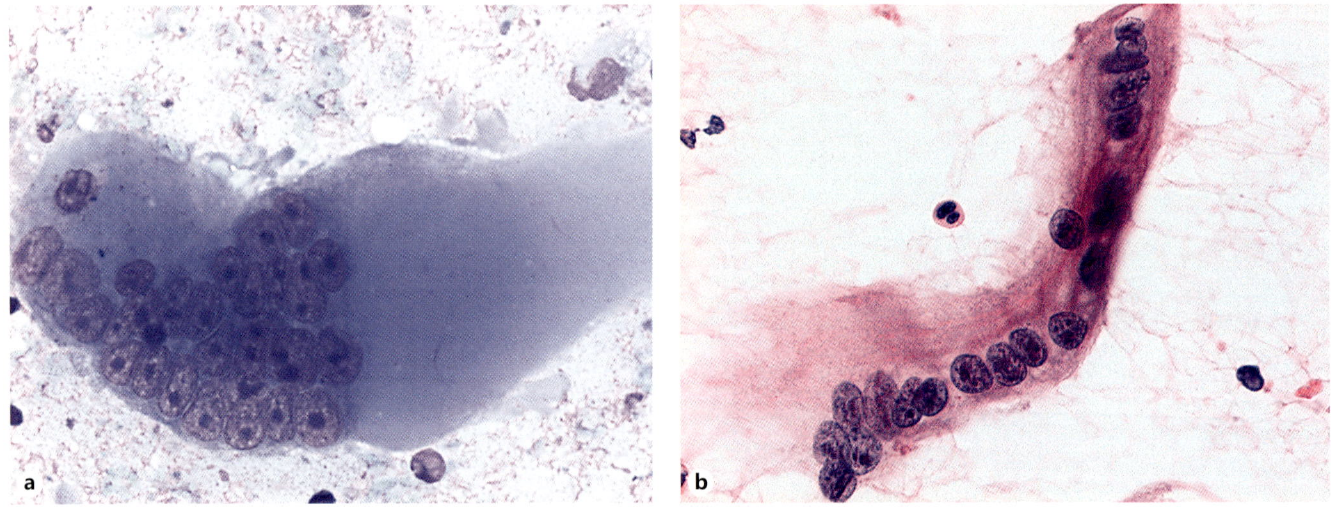

Fig. 4. Damaged and regenerating multinucleated "muscle giant cells" of varying shapes. Nuclei with prominent nucleoli (MGG stain; **a**) are often arranged in rows (HE stain; **b**).

Chapter 5

Domanski HA, Walther CS: FNA Cytology of Soft Tissue and Bone Tumors. Monogr Clin Cytol.
Basel, Karger, 2017, vol 22, pp 25–39 (DOI: 10.1159/000475092)

Adipocytic Tumors

Lipoma and Angiolipoma

Lipomas, the most common soft tissue tumor of adults, rarely present before the third decade of life. Lipomas usually appear as slowly growing, solitary or rarely multiple, subcutaneous, occasionally deeply seated (intramuscular or intermuscular lipoma) masses. Smears from lipoma are identical to those from normal adipose tissue (Fig. 1). The presence of other mesenchymal elements such as metaplastic bone and cartilage, fibrotic tissue (fibrolipoma), or degenerative/myxoid areas (myxolipoma) is very occasionally seen in fine-needle aspiration (FNA) smears. Angiolipomas occur commonly in young adults as small (usually smaller than 2 cm), well-delaminated, often multiple and tender subcutaneous nodules. FNA smears of angiolipomas do not differ from smears of regular lipomas.

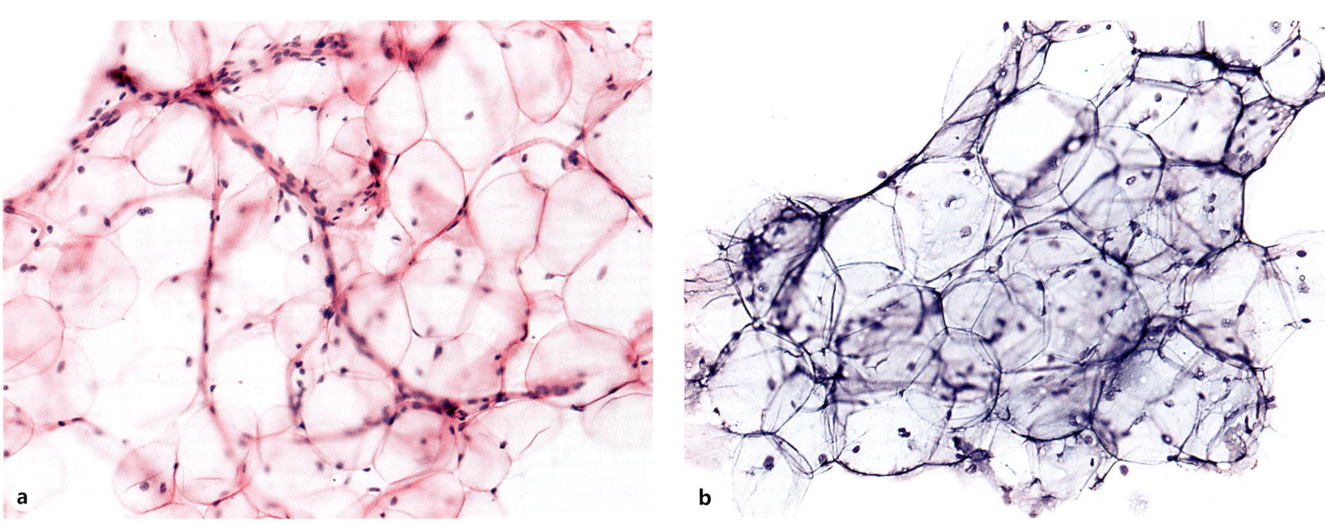

Fig. 1. Smears from lipoma show fatty tissue fragments with a variable number of capillaries, composed of cells containing a single fat vacuole (HE stain; **a**) and a small, uniform, peripheral nucleus (MGG stain; **b**).

Cytologic Features
- Fatty tissue fragments composed of cells containing a single fat vacuole and often a small, dark, peripheral nucleus
- Variable number of capillaries within the fatty tissue fragments
- Fragments of striated muscle mixed with fatty tissue fragments in inter/intramuscular lipoma
- Rarely with a myxoid matrix, collagenous tissue, or metaplastic cartilage/bone fragments

Ancillary Tests
Immunophenotype
In mature adipocytes: positive for S100, negative for MDM2.

Genetics
Lipomas are a heterogenous group of tumors from a genetic perspective. However, there are 3 major subgroups of genetic changes. The most common involves chromosome 12q13–15 and the pathogenetic important *HMGA2* gene. The exact tumorigenic mechanisms are not fully known but the dysregulation and truncation of the *HMGA2* gene is considered to be the decisive step and results in a strong expression of the gene, or part of it. This aberration is present in 65% of lipoma cases. The other 2 subgroups involve loss of material from chromosome 13q and changes in 6p21–23, and are present in 10 and 5% of lipomas, respectively [1, 2]. Angiolipomas show normal karyotypes but an abnormal expression of *HMGA2* can be seen [3]. The changes can be detected with cytogenetics on fresh material and with polymerase chain reaction (PCR), fluorescence in situ hybridization (FISH), single nucleotide polymorphism (SNP) array, and next-generation sequencing (NGS) on fixed material.

Differential Diagnosis
- Atypical lipomatous tumor
- Hibernoma
- Spindle cell lipoma
- Intramuscular hemangioma (with fatty involution)

Benign lipomas lack atypical stromal cells and the polymorphism of atypical lipomatous tumors. Compared to spindle cell lipoma, lipomas lack any spindle cell component and collagenous fibers. Smears from hibernomas commonly display an admixture of normal adipocytes resembling benign lipomas. In the vast majority of cases a predominant component of round to polygonal "brown fat" cells with an abundant finely vacuolated/granulated cytoplasm and small bland nuclei indicates the correct diagnosis. Smears from intramuscular hemangioma can occasionally mimic those from an intramuscular lipoma since muscle tissue adjacent to capillaries of hemangioma is frequently replaced by fat tissue.

Lipoblastoma and Lipoblastomatosis

Lipoblastoma is a tumor of early childhood and infancy that most commonly arises in the extremities, and rarely in the head and neck area, trunk, and retroperitoneum. Lipoblastoma may present either as a well-circumscribed subcutaneous tumor (lipoblastoma) or a deep-seated, diffusely infiltrative, ill-defined mass (lipoblastomatosis). Lipoblastomas are thought to be capable of maturation to a usual lipoma. Cytologic features include small to moderately sized adipocytes with a vacuolated cytoplasm and round uniform nuclei in a myxoid background matrix admixed with branching capillaries (Fig. 2). Smears may also be dominated by large ordinary univacuolated adipocytes [4–9]. Although FNA smears from a subset of lipoblastomas mimic myxoid liposarcoma, these 2 tumors occur in different age groups: lipoblastoma is most common in children younger than 3 years of age, while myxoid liposarcoma most often presents in young adults.

Cytologic Features
- Fatty tissue fragments usually within a myxoid background matrix
- Thin capillaries
- Few dissociated adipocytes
- Occasionally uni- or multivacuolated lipoblast-like cells and hibernoma-like cells

Ancillary Tests
Genetics
Genetic rearrangement of the chromosome region 8q11–13 involving the *PLAG1* gene has been reported in the majority of cases. Gene fusions *HAS2-PLAG1* and *COL1A2-PLAG1* result in upregulation of *PLAG1* that activates transcription. FISH, PCR, and NGS can detect these genetic changes on fresh or fixed material. Gain of chromosome 8 has also been noted and can be detected with cytogenetics [10].

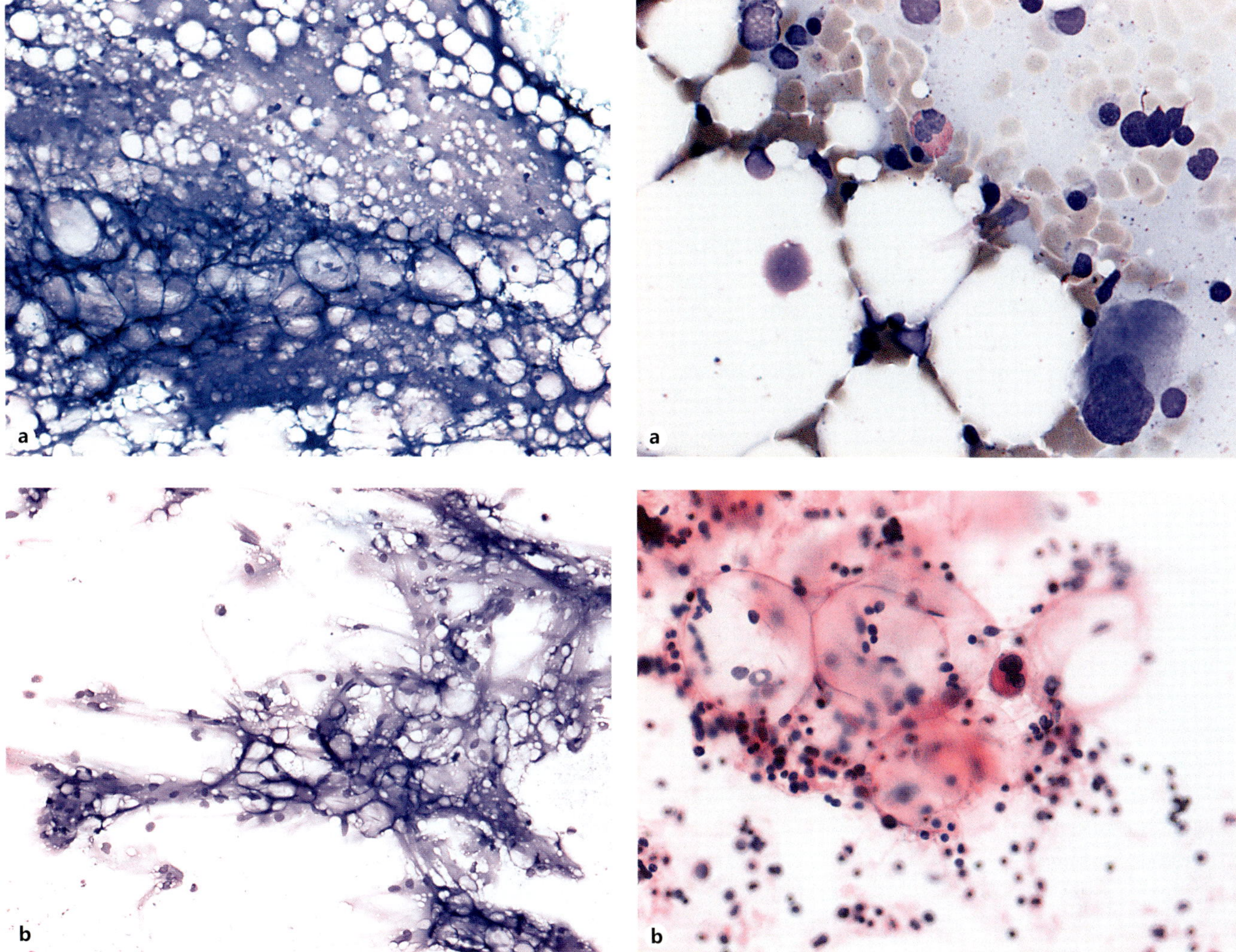

Fig. 2. a, **b** Smears from lipoblastoma show fatty tissue fragments within a myxoid background matrix and increased thin capillaries. MGG stain.

Fig. 3. a Smears from myelolipoma with a mixture of fat cells and normal hematopoietic elements. MGG stain. **b** Megakaryocytes should not be confused with malignant cells. HE stain.

Differential Diagnosis
- Myxoid liposarcoma
- Lipoma

The main differential diagnoses of lipoblastoma are myxoid liposarcoma and benign lipoma. Both myxoid liposarcoma and lipoma occur in the older patient population than lipoblastoma. Lipoblastomas lack the branching capillary network seen in smears from myxoid liposarcoma. Most lipomas lack the prominent myxoid background of a lipoblastoma.

Extra-Adrenal Myelolipoma

Myelolipoma is a benign tumor of older adults composed of mature fat and hematopoietic tissue. Myelolipomas usually occur in the adrenal gland and an extra-adrenal origin is very rare. In correctly sampled smears it is usually easy to recognize a mixture of fat cells or clusters of fat tissue and normal hematopoietic elements of all types, similar to what is seen in smears from bone marrow [11–16] (Fig. 3).

Cytologic Features
- Fatty tissue fragments and dispersed fat cells
- Mature hematopoietic elements (all 3 cell lines)

Ancillary Tests
Genetics
No recurrent genetic changes are known in this rare tumor.

Differential Diagnosis
- Conventional lipoma
- Extramedullary hematopoiesis

Conventional lipoma rarely occurs in the adrenals and lacks bone marrow elements. Extramedullary hematopoiesis is most often multifocal and associated with splenomegaly. Myelolipoma is most often an incidental finding on a CT scan or MRI scan of the abdomen/retroperitoneum. In FNA of myelolipoma, it is important to make sure that smears have been sampled from a soft tissue mass and not from the pelvic bones or vertebra.

Chondroid Lipoma

Chondroid lipoma is a very rare, benign lipomatous tumor occurring in both superficial and deep soft tissue of the proximal extremities, limb girdles, trunk, and head and neck region. FNA smears show clusters of mature adipocytes with an admixture of lipoblasts and small strands and clusters of chondroblast-like cells in a background of abundant myxochondroid matrix (Fig. 4).

Despite variation in size and shape, the nuclei of small chondroblast-like cells are bland in appearance. Lack of a branching capillary network is an important cytologic feature helpful in distinguishing chondroid lipoma from myxoid liposarcoma [17–20].

Cytologic Features
- Variable but often abundant myxochondroid background matrix
- Sheets and clusters of ordinary adipocytes
- Sheets and clusters of uni- or multivacuolated lipoblasts
- Small strands and clusters of chondroblasts with moderate granular cytoplasm and bland, occasionally coffee bean-shaped nuclei with irregular nuclear borders
- Lack of the plexiform capillary network seen in myxoid liposarcoma

Ancillary Tests
Immunophenotype
In lipoblast-like cells, positive for S100, rarely positive for focal keratin. Negative for smooth muscle actin (SMA) and epithelial membrane antigen (EMA).

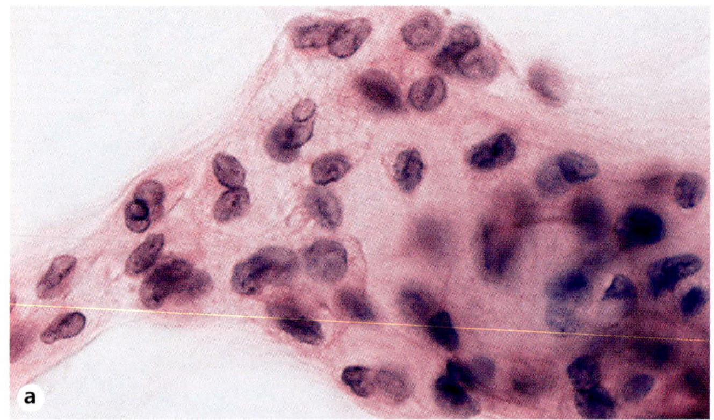

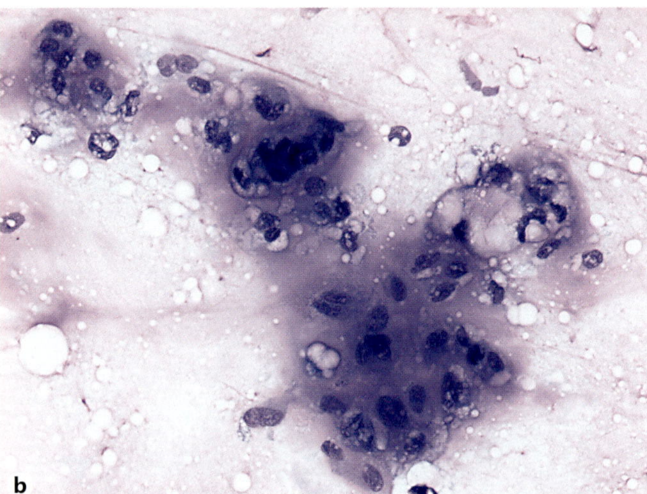

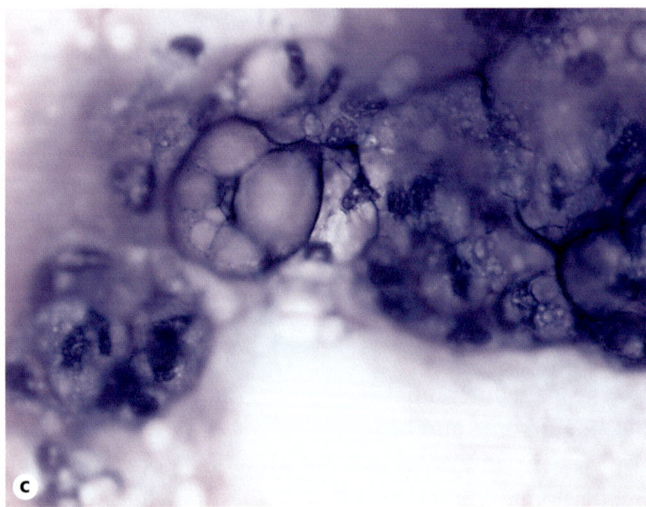

Fig. 4. Chondroid lipoma. **a** A cluster of chondroid cells in the myxochondroid matrix. HE stain. **b, c** Fragments of adipocytes with an admixture of chondroblast-like cells and lipoblasts, and an abundant myxochondroid background matrix. MGG stain.

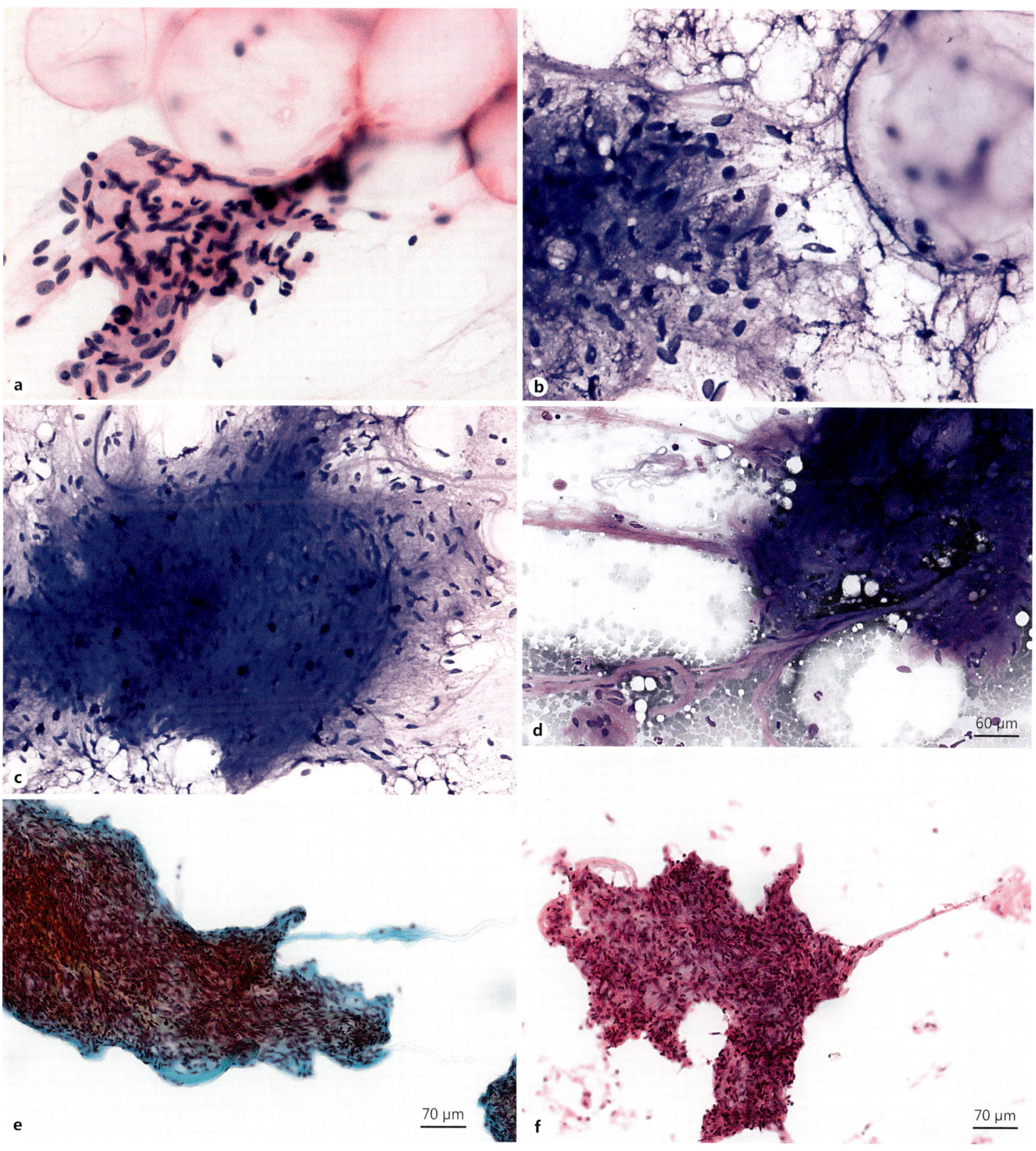

Fig. 5. a, **b** Spindle cell lipoma. A mixture of mature adipose tissue and loosely cohesive clusters of bland spindle cells with elongated, uniform nuclei. HE and MGG stains. **c** A myxoid background matrix and mast cells are common. MGG stain. **d–f** Long and narrow collagen-hyaline fibers attached to the edges of cell clusters of spindle cells is a diagnostically important but variable sign. MGG, PAP, and HE stains; **e**, **f** ThinPrep.

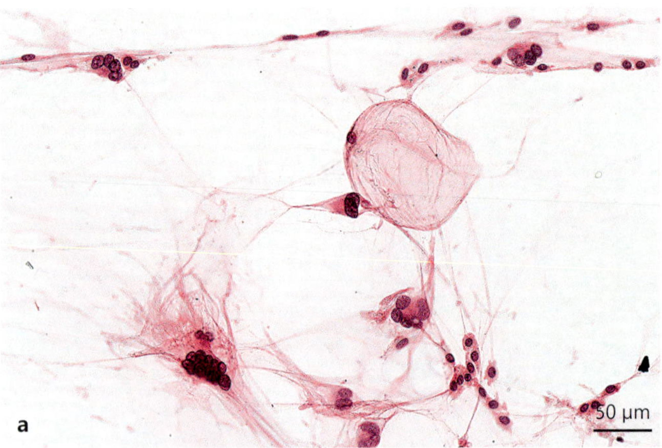

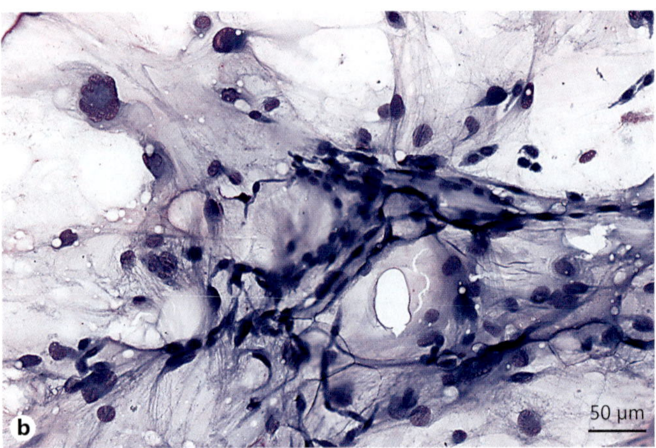

Fig. 6. Pleomorphic lipoma. **a** A mixture of mature fat, floret cells, and spindle cells. HE stain. **b** Occasionally prominent myxoid background matrix. MGG stain.

Genetics

A balanced chromosomal translocation, t(11;16)(q13; p12–13), has been reported in chondroid lipoma. The breakpoint at 11q13 has also been described in hibernomas [19, 20]. These changes can be detected by cytogenetics, FISH, SNP array, PCR, and NGS on fresh and fixed material.

Differential Diagnosis
- Myxoid liposarcoma
- Extraskeletal myxoid chondrosarcoma

Chondroid lipoma lacks the branching capillary network of myxoid liposarcoma. In addition, an abundance of multivacuolated lipoblasts and admixture of adipocytic tissue help to distinguish chondroid lipoma from myxoid liposarcoma and extraskeletal myxoid chondrosarcoma.

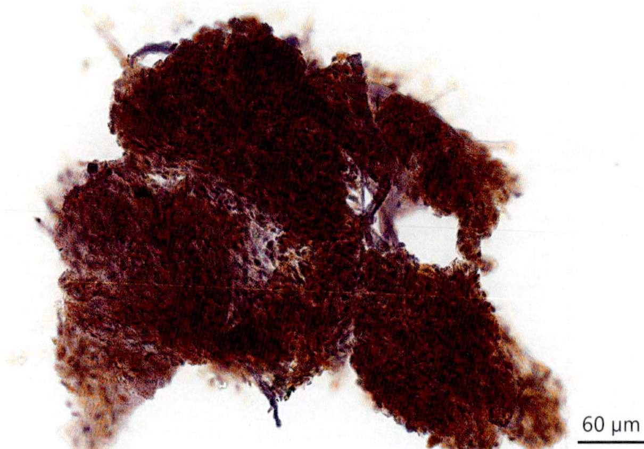

Fig. 7. Spindle cells show strong and diffuse reactivity for CD34 in both spindle cell lipoma and pleomorphic lipoma. CD34; ThinPrep.

Spindle Cell Lipoma and Pleomorphic Lipoma

These benign lipomatous tumors are variants of the same neoplasm, with a similar clinical presentation, cytogenetic features, and morphology. For both tumors, the typical clinical setting is a subcutaneous mass in the posterior neck region, upper back, and over the shoulders in middle-aged men. Head and mouth areas, including the tongue and orbit, are less common locations.

FNA smears of spindle cell lipoma show variable proportions of different elements in smears from different cases. Most contain fat fragments mixed with fascicles of uniform spindle cells with elongated, uniform nuclei and collagen fibers, occasionally in a myxoid background matrix (Fig. 5). Depending on the areas sampled, aspirates may show a predominance of fat tissue or of spindle cells, and smears occasionally show an abundant myxoid matrix [21–25]. A diagnostically important but variable sign in smears from spindle cell lipoma is the presence of fragments of brightly eosinophilic (in hematoxylin and eosin staining) collagen-hyaline fibers (Fig. 5) [23]. The presence of floret cells, which are multinucleated giant cells with hyperchromatic nuclei and a moderate amount of cytoplasm, is a characteristic finding in smears of pleomorphic lipoma [26] (Fig. 6). In addition to floret cells, smears from pleomorphic lipomas may contain collagen fibers and areas of myxoid background matrix similar to spindle cell lipoma. Hybrid forms with both spindle and pleomorphic lipoma features are not uncommon. Spindle cells typically express strong and uniform positivity for CD34 (Fig. 7).

Cytologic Features of Spindle Cell Lipoma
- A mixture of mature fat tissue and clustered or dispersed bland spindle cells
- Fragments of brightly eosinophilic (in HE staining) collagen-hyaline fibers
- An occasionally seen myxoid background matrix
- Mast cells (particularly in smears with the myxoid background)

Ancillary Tests
Immunophenotype
Spindle cells are positive for CD34; commonly BCL-2 positive. Negative for SMA and S100.

Genetics
These variants of lipomatous tumors show more complex karyotypes compared to ordinary lipomas, and complete or partial loss of chromosomes 13 and/or 16 has been reported. Cytogenetics, FISH, SNP array, and NGS can visualize the changes on available material [27].

Differential Diagnosis
- Schwannoma
- Myxoid liposarcoma
- Dermatofibrosarcoma protuberans
- Low-grade myxofibrosarcoma
- Lipomatous "fat forming" solitary fibrous tumor

Cytologic Features of Pleomorphic Lipoma
- Fragments of mature fat
- Variable number of floret cells
- Variable number of spindle cells
- Occasionally myxoid background matrix
- Occasionally mast cells

Differential Diagnosis
- Well-differentiated liposarcoma/atypical lipomatous tumor

Due to the variable proportions of spindle cells, fatty and collagenous tissue, and occasional myxoid background, smears of spindle cell lipoma may be misinterpreted as other types of spindle cell or myxoid soft tissue tumors [28, 29]. Positivity for CD34 and negativity for S100 helps to exclude schwannoma. The clinical presentation of dermatofibrosarcoma protuberans differs from that of spindle cell lipoma and there is a lack of collagen fibers of spindle cell lipoma in smears from these neoplasms. Smears from the myxoid variant of spindle cell lipoma lacks the branching network of thin capillaries of myxoid liposarcoma and thick-walled vessels of myxofibrosarcoma. Smears from atypical lipomatous tumor/well-differentiated liposarcoma most often contain atypical stromal cells with enlarged hyperchromatic nuclei and occasional floret cells similar to pleomorphic lipoma. Pleomorphic lipomas are distinguished from liposarcoma by their superficial location and anatomic distribution in the head and neck area, as well as by CD34 positivity in spindle cells and their cytogenetic findings.

Hibernoma

Hibernoma is a rare, benign lipomatous tumor of brown fat derivation. It is commonly situated subcutaneously in the interscapular region, on the back or chest wall (sites of normal deposits of brown fat), but can also be intramuscular, most often in the thigh and back. FNA of hibernomas yield moderately to highly cellular smears containing clusters or fragments of round to oval and polygonal "hibernoma cells" of variable sizes, with vacuolated or granular cytoplasm and centrally placed small uniform nuclei [30–32] (Fig. 8). Regular large adipocytes are often intermingled with "hibernoma cells" and areas of regular fat tissue may be seen in cell clusters of hibernoma [33]. The tumor tissue fragments often contain numerous capillary vessels. Ordinary lipoma-like fat cells may dominate the smears and the typical hibernoma cells may be in a minority, thus posing diagnostic challenges in small samples.

Cytologic Features
- Clusters and sheets of polygonal and oval cells with abundant microvacuolated and granular cytoplasm and small, uniform nuclei
- Mixture of areas of regular adipocytes and "hibernoma cells"/brown fat cells
- Numerous capillaries
- Rare lipoblast-like cells

Ancillary Tests
Immunophenotype
Variable S100 positivity, occasionally focal CD34 positive.

Genetics
A recurrent genetic change involving structural rearrangements of 11q13 can be seen. It can be visualized with cytogenetics or FISH on fresh or fixed material [34].

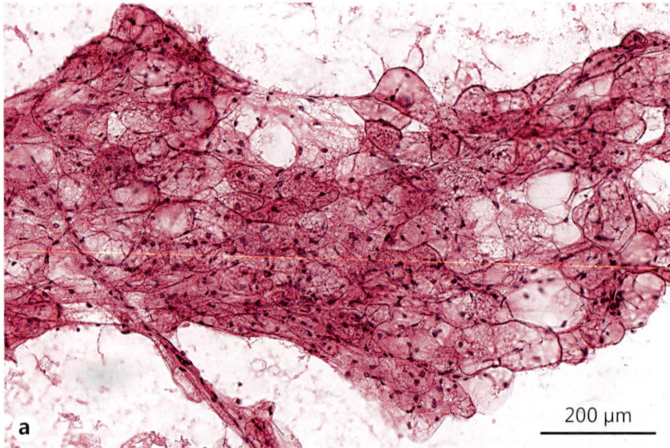

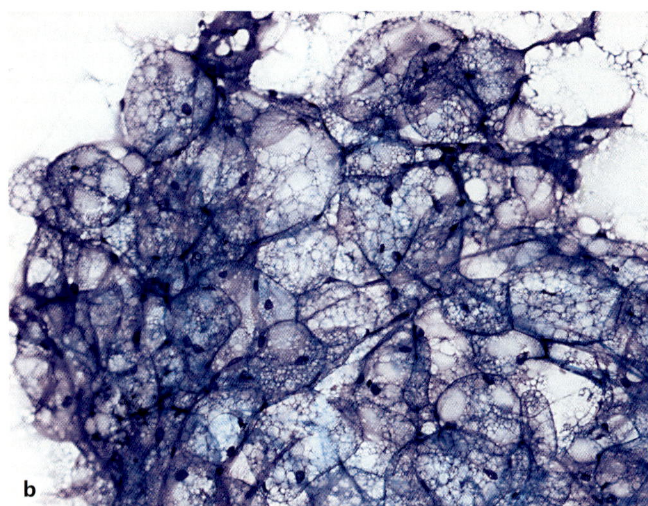

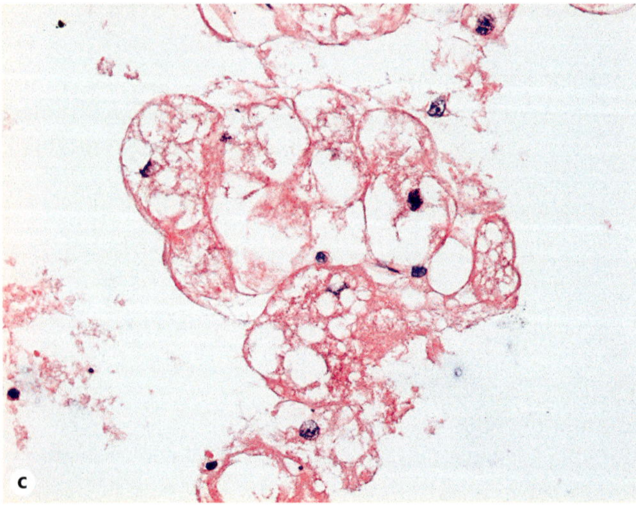

Fig. 8. Hibernoma. **a**, **b** Clusters of round to oval and polygonal cells with abundant vacuolated and granulated cytoplasm and small uniform nuclei. Cell clusters contain delicate capillaries. HE and MGG stains. **c** Micromorphology of hibernoma preserved in cell block sections. HE stain.

Differential Diagnosis
- Well-differentiated liposarcoma/atypical lipomatous tumor
- Lipoma with fat necrosis
- Granular cell tumor
- Lipoblastoma
- Adult rhabdomyoma

Hibernomas with a large proportion of mature adipocytes in smears can be wrongly diagnosed as common lipoma. Granular cell tumor and adult rhabdomyoma lack adipocytic differentiation and cells of these neoplasms display a granular rather than microvacuolated cytoplasm. In addition, granular cell tumor shows immunoreactivity for S100 and stains positive for periodic acid-Schiff staining. Adult rhabdomyoma shows positive immunostaining for muscle-specific actin, desmin, myogenin, and MyoD1. Hibernoma cells may be misinterpreted as lipoblasts, but nuclei in these cells are neither hyperchromatic/atypical nor scalloped.

Atypical Lipomatous Tumor/Well-Differentiated Liposarcoma

Well-differentiated liposarcoma is a locally aggressive, non-metastasizing adipocytic neoplasm of adults occurring predominantly in the retroperitoneum or mediastinum. When the tumor of identical morphology arises at surgically curable sites such as superficial soft tissues and the lower limbs, the term "atypical lipomatous tumor" is preferred. Cytologic findings in these tumors include the mixture of ordinary lipoma-like tissue fragments and atypical stromal cells with enlarged, irregular hyperchromatic nuclei [9, 35–37]. Bare atypical nuclei and floret cells are common findings in the background of the smears (Fig. 9). Atypical lipoblasts with cytoplasmic vacuoles and scalloped nuclei are rare findings of the smears and are not necessary for the cytologic diagnosis of liposarcoma.

Cytologic Features
- Clusters and sheets of regular fat cells
- Large atypical stromal cells with irregular, hyperchromatic nuclei
- Bare atypical nuclei in the background of the smears
- Rare, multivacuolated atypical lipoblasts
- Occasional floret cells

Ancillary Tests
Immunophenotype
Positive for nuclear MDM2 and CDK4; adipocytes and lipo-
blasts are S100 positive.

Genetics
Atypical lipomatous tumor/well-differentiated liposarcoma are characterized by ring or giant marker chromosomes derived from 12q13–15, which are present in
most cases. They contain an amplification of regions
12q14–15 and the *MDM2* and *CDK4* genes. Amplifications of these genes can be used for differential diagnostic
purposes and are readily detected by FISH and PCR [38].
Other amplified regions originating from 10p11–14 and
12q12–21 can also be found and used for diagnostic purposes using FISH and PCR [39]. NGS can be used for detection of all the mentioned aberrations. Both fresh and
fixed material can be used depending on availability and
the chosen method.

Differential Diagnosis
- Lipoma
- Dedifferentiated liposarcoma
- Hibernoma
- Pleomorphic lipoma
- Chondroid lipoma
- Fat necrosis
- Any other mesenchymal tumor with nuclear atypia and
  a fat component

Extensive sampling of large atypical lipomatous tumors/
well-differentiated liposarcoma is necessary as the majority
of these neoplasms include large areas of lipoma-like tissue
and diagnostic areas containing atypical cells and lipoblasts
may be very limited. The cytoplasm of lipophages in fat necrosis is foamy and filled with small vacuoles. Unlike those
in atypical lipoblasts, the nuclei are neither hyperchromatic
nor scalloped. Smears from atypical lipomatous tumors/
well-differentiated liposarcoma may contain floret cells.
Lack of an atypical stromal component and lipoblasts as well
as immunoreactivity for CD34 in the spindle cell component helps to distinguish pleomorphic lipoma from liposarcoma. Atypical lipomatous tumors/well-differentiated liposarcoma lack a chondromyxoid matrix and chondrocyte-
like cells of chondroid lipoma.

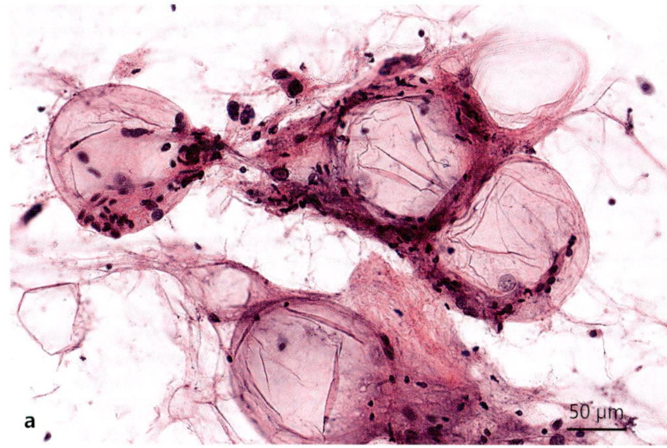
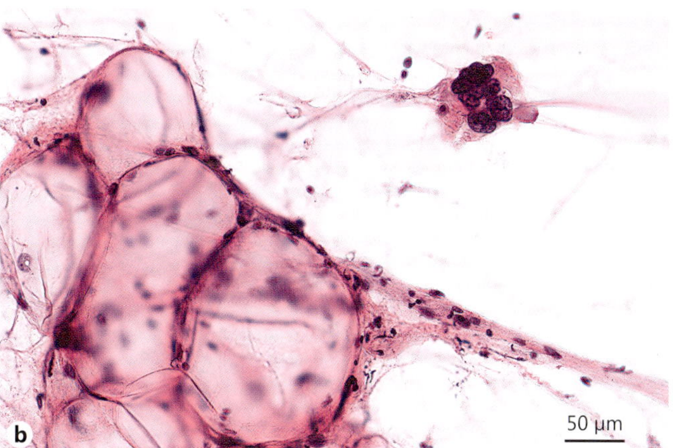
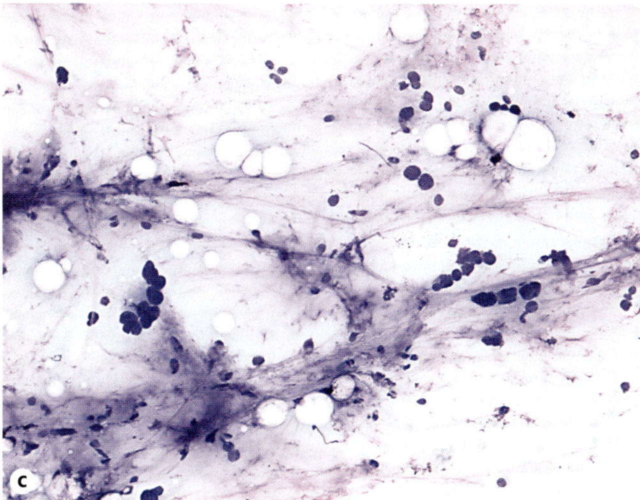

Fig. 9. Atypical lipomatous tumor/well-differentiated liposarcoma.
a Clusters and sheets of fat cells with occasional variation in size and
admixture of large atypical stromal cells with irregular, hyperchromatic nuclei. HE stain. **b**, **c** Bare atypical nuclei and atypical multinucleated "floret-like" cells and occasional myxoid background are other findings in smears. HE and MGG stains.

Dedifferentiated Liposarcoma

Dedifferentiated liposarcoma is a nonlipogenic sarcoma containing a component of atypical lipomatous tumor/well-differentiated liposarcoma. Dedifferentiation occurs in approximately 10% of atypical lipomatous tumor/well-differentiated liposarcoma, while the majority of dedifferentiated liposarcomas arise de novo. Dedifferentiated liposarcomas occur in middle-aged and elderly adults, and the most common location is retroperitoneal/abdominal followed by the spermatic cord, trunk, extremities, and head and neck area.

Cytologic Features
- Clusters and sheets of atypical spindle cells of variable size and with irregular, hyperchromatic nuclei
- Bare atypical nuclei
- Occasional well-differentiated lipogenic elements
- Occasional inflammatory cells
- Rare atypical lipoblasts

Ancillary Tests
Immunophenotype
Positive for nuclear MDM2 and CDK4; variable desmin, SMA, and CD34 positivity. Negative for S100 and keratins.

Genetics
Supernumerary ring and giant marker chromosomes containing the 12q13–15 regions with an amplification of 12q14 including *MDM2* and *CDK4* can be seen with FISH, PCR, and NGS on fresh or fixed material [40].

Differential Diagnosis
- Undifferentiated pleomorphic sarcoma
- Myxofibrosarcoma
- Leiomyosarcoma
- Malignant peripheral nerve sheath tumor
- Fibroblastic/myofibroblastic soft tissue tumors

The cytologic diagnosis of dedifferentiated liposarcoma is difficult. It is based on the clinical presentation, radiographic data, the presence of well-differentiated liposarcomatous, high-grade sarcomatous components in smears, and ancillary studies [41].

Myxoid Liposarcoma and Round Cell Liposarcoma

Myxoid Liposarcoma
Myxoid/round-cell liposarcoma accounts for 15–20% of liposarcomas. It occurs in young adults and the most common site of involvement is in the deep soft tissue, preferably of the thigh. Rarely, myxoid/round cell liposarcoma arises in the subcutaneous tissue.

In optimal aspirates diagnostic features include clusters of tumor tissue with an abundant myxoid matrix with round to ovoid primitive cells, and a branching network of thin capillaries. Slightly atypical lipoblasts within clusters of the tumor tissue can occasionally be noted [37, 42, 43] (Fig. 10).

Cytologic Features
- Clusters and sheets of small, round to ovoid, occasionally spindled and stellate nonlipogenic primitive mesenchymal cells with a scant cytoplasm embedded in the myxoid matrix
- Tumor cells with bland nuclei with fine chromatin, and inconspicuous nucleoli
- Generally monotonous appearance with minimal pleomorphism and few dispersed tumor cells
- Usually a prominent branching, delicate capillary network within the tumor clusters and sheets
- Uni- or multivacuolated lipoblasts, some with signet-ring features
- No or very few mitoses

Ancillary Tests
Immunophenotype
Variable S100 positivity. Negative for MDM2, CDK4, CD34, keratins, desmin, and SMA.

Genetics
In 95% of the cases a recurrent t(12:16)(q13;p11) translocation is present. This results in a *FUS-DDIT3* fusion gene which induces transcriptional activation [44, 45]. The fusion is sensitive for myxoid liposarcoma and is not found in morphologically similar tumors, including well-differentiated/dedifferentiated liposarcoma of the retroperitoneum and myxofibrosarcoma [46]. The mutation can be detected by cytogenetics, FISH, RT-PCR, and NGS on fresh or fixed material. FISH for *DDIT3* rearrangement is very helpful in difficult cases, especially the round cell variant.

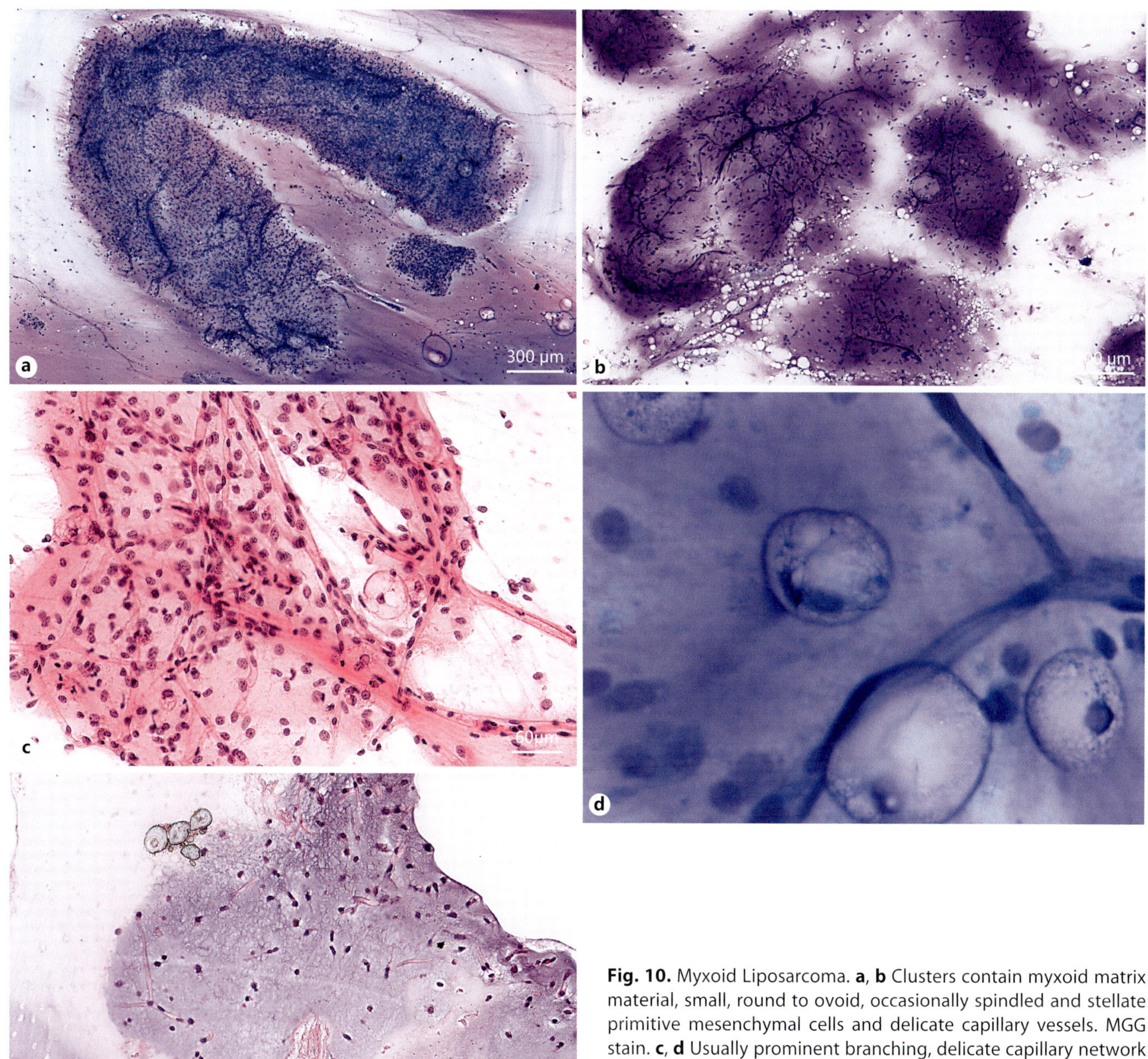

Fig. 10. Myxoid Liposarcoma. **a**, **b** Clusters contain myxoid matrix material, small, round to ovoid, occasionally spindled and stellate primitive mesenchymal cells and delicate capillary vessels. MGG stain. **c**, **d** Usually prominent branching, delicate capillary network "chicken-wire" and lipoblasts within are seen in the tumor clusters and sheets. HE and MGG stains. **e** Cell block sections with discrete myxoid tissue fragments contain delicate "chicken-wire" capillaries and small uniform tumor cells. HE stain.

Differential Diagnosis

- Spindle-cell lipoma with an abundant myxoid matrix
- Intramuscular cellular myxoma
- Low-grade myxofibrosarcoma

Most smears from myxoid liposarcomas contain clusters of round to oval bland cells in an abundant myxoid matrix and a branching network of thin capillaries. In addition to a prominent myxoid background of smears, slightly atypical, often univacuolate or bivacuolate lipoblasts resembling signet-ring cells and scattered mast cells are other findings in FNA smears. The size and architectural pattern of capillary vessels in smears are important diagnostic criteria. Capillaries in smears from myxofibrosarcoma most often appear as short segments of capillaries of variable size, but are usually

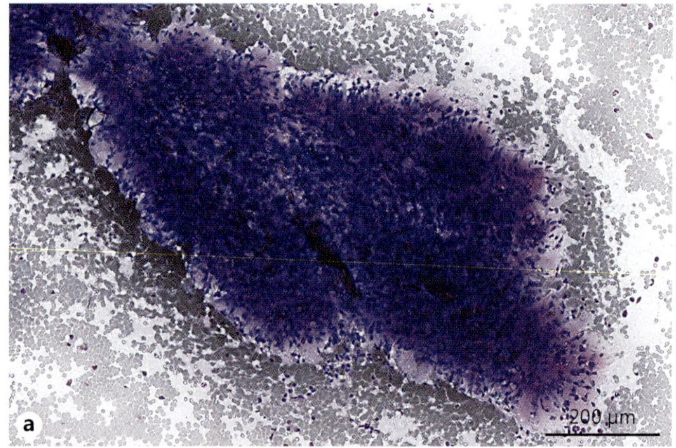

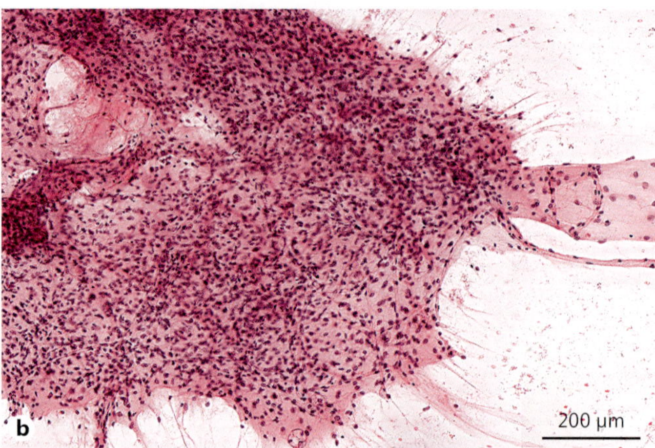

Fig. 11. a, **b** Round cell liposarcoma (hypercellular myxoid liposarcoma). A rich yield of tight (crowded) clusters and clumps of round or ovoid cells, embedded in a slightly myxoid matrix. The capillary network is less prominent, obscured by clusters of tumor cells. MGG and HE stains.

thicker than tiny branching capillaries of myxoid liposarcoma. In intramuscular myxoma, only rare scattered fragments of small capillaries may be found in the background of smears.

Round Cell Liposarcoma (Hypercellular Myxoid Liposarcoma)
A subset of myxoid liposarcomas have hypercellular areas containing numerous round to ovoid cells with a scant cytoplasm, mixed with few to no lipoblasts. The myxoid matrix is limited and the capillary network less prominent, often obscured by clusters of tumor cells (Fig. 11).

Cytologic Features
- A rich yield of tight (crowded) clusters and clumps of round or ovoid tumor cells with somewhat hyperchromatic nuclei, embedded in slightly myxoid matrix
- Many tumor cells show a high nuclear/cytoplasmic ratio and round nuclei with vesicular chromatin
- Less conspicuous myxoid matrix and capillaries compared to myxoid liposarcoma
- Few or absent lipoblasts

Ancillary Tests
Immunophenotype
Variable S100 positivity. Negative for MDM2, CDK4, CD34, keratins, desmin, and SMA.

Genetics
Characterized by the same recurrent translocation t(12;16) (q13;p11) with fusion of the *DDIT3* gene on chromosome 12 and the *FUS* gene on chromosome 16 seen in myxoid liposarcoma. In the round cell variant, detection of the *DDIT3* rearrangement with FISH can be very helpful in difficult cases.

Differential Diagnosis
- Other types of round cell sarcoma infiltrating adipose tissue
- Soft tissue metastasis of renal cell carcinoma

Pleomorphic Liposarcoma

Pleomorphic liposarcoma is a rare, high-grade pleomorphic sarcoma with lipoblastic differentiation. Most cases occur in the extremities and retroperitoneum in elderly patients. The most important clue to the diagnosis is the presence of highly atypical uni- or multinucleated lipoblasts. However, pleomorphic liposarcomas most frequently yield smears representative of pleomorphic sarcoma without evidence of atypical lipoblasts. Smears contain markedly pleomorphic spindle, polygonal, and epithelioid cells with an admixture of anaplastic multinucleated tumor cells. Mitoses and necrosis are common [9, 35, 37] (Fig. 12).

Cytologic Features
- Dispersed cells and cell clusters
- Pleomorphic tumor cells including multinucleated giant tumor cells
- Variable presence of highly atypical, uni- or multinucleated lipoblasts

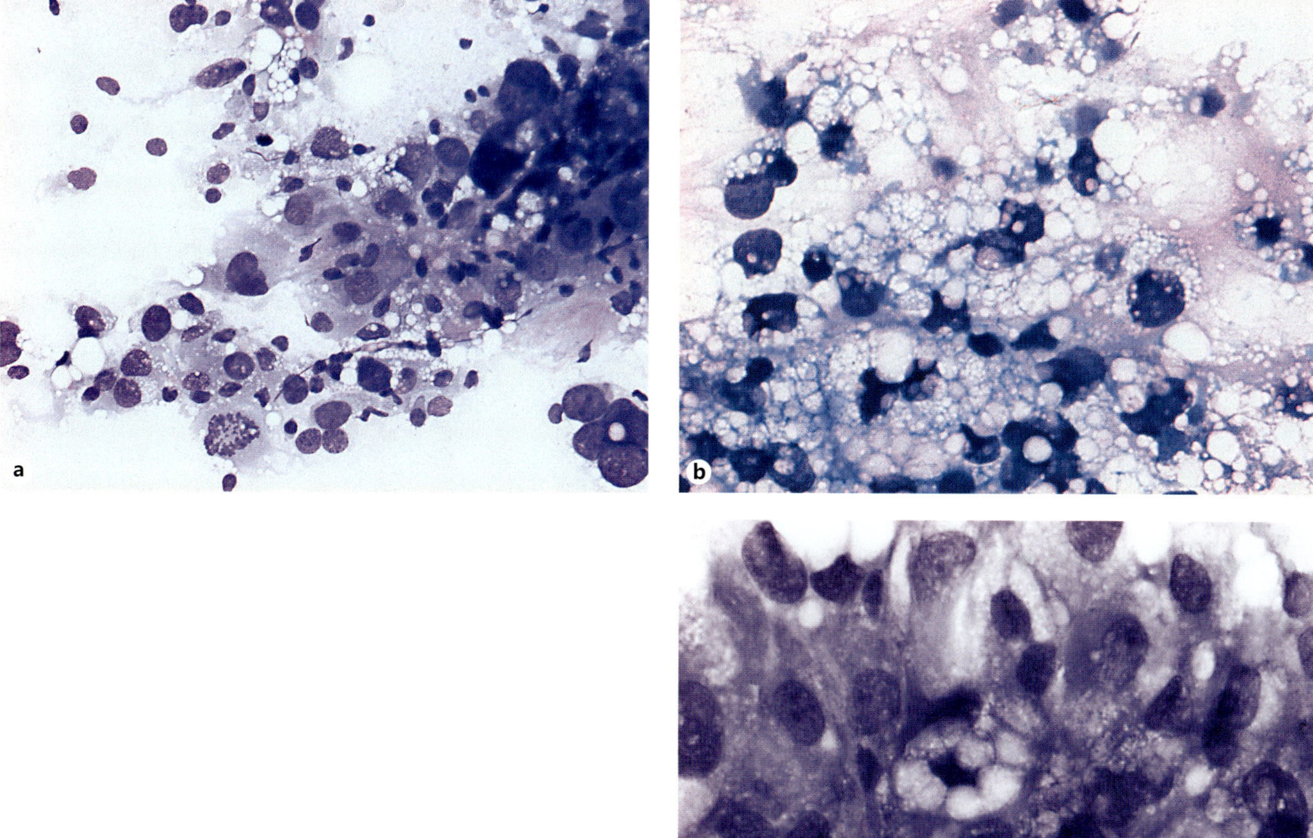

Fig. 12. a–c Pleomorphic liposarcoma. Dispersed cells and cell clusters of pleomorphic cells including mitoses and atypical lipoblasts. MGG stain.

- Cells with hyaline cytoplasmic droplets are occasionally present
- Necrosis

Ancillary Tests
Immunophenotype
Lipoblasts are S100 positive; occasionally focal positive for EMA and keratins. Negative for MDM2 and CDK4.

Genetics
The genetic profile resembles those of other pleomorphic sarcomas and often displays a complex karyotype [47]. Cytogenetics, SNP array, and NGS can provide an overview of the often complex genetic profile.

Differential Diagnosis
- Pleomorphic high-grade sarcoma of another lineage
- Poorly differentiated carcinoma

Most smears from pleomorphic liposarcoma display the same pleomorphic findings as can be seen in pleomorphic sarcomas derived from other cell types. The presence of unequivocal atypical lipoblasts in smears is required for the specific diagnosis of pleomorphic liposarcoma.

References

1 Bartuma H, Hallor KH, Panagopoulos I, Collin A, Rydholm A, Gustafson P, Bauer HC, Brosjo O, Domanski HA, Mandahl N, Mertens F: Assessment of the clinical and molecular impact of different cytogenetic subgroups in a series of 272 lipomas with abnormal karyotype. Genes Chromosomes Cancer 2007;46:594–606.

2 Ashar HR, Fejzo MS, Tkachenko A, Zhou X, Fletcher JA, Weremowicz S, Morton CC, Chada K: Disruption of the architectural factor HMGI-C: DNA-binding AT hook motifs fused in lipomas to distinct transcriptional regulatory domains. Cell 1995;82:57–65.

3 Bartuma H, Panagopoulos I, Collin A, Trombetta D, Domanski HA, Mandahl N, Mertens F: Expression levels of HMGA2 in adipocytic tumors correlate with morphologic and cytogenetic subgroups. Mol Cancer 2009;8:36.

4 Kalaivani Selvi S, Pradhan P, Rajesh NG, Gochhait D, Barwad A: Lipoblastoma presenting as a rapidly growing paravertebral mass and masquerading as myxoid liposarcoma on fine needle aspiration cytology. Diagn Cytopathol 2016;44:426–429.

5 Verma S, Bansal K, Manchanda V, Gupta R: Aspiration cytology diagnosis of lipoblastoma of the back. APSP J Case Rep 2014;5:21.

6 Hong R, Choi DY, Do NY, Lim SC: Fine-needle aspiration cytology of a lipoblastoma: a case report. Diagn Cytopathol 2008;36:508–511.

7 Kloboves-Prevodnik VV, Us-Krasovec M, Gale N, Lamovec J: Cytological features of lipoblastoma: a report of three cases. Diagn Cytopathol 2005;33: 195–200.

8 Lopez-Ferrer P, Jimenez-Heffernan JA, Yebenes L, Vicandi B, Viguer JM: Fine-needle aspiration cytology of lipoblastoma: a report of two cases. Diagn Cytopathol 2005;32:32–34.

9 Walaas L, Kindblom LG: Lipomatous tumors: a correlative cytologic and histologic study of 27 tumors examined by fine needle aspiration cytology. Hum Pathol 1985;16:6–18.

10 Bartuma H, Domanski HA, Von Steyern FV, Kullendorff CM, Mandahl N, Mertens F: Cytogenetic and molecular cytogenetic findings in lipoblastoma. Cancer Genet Cytogenet 2008;183:60–63.

11 Hernandez-Amate A, Rios-Martin JJ, Diaz-Delgado M, Garcia-Escudero A, Otal-Salaverri C, Gonzalez-Campora R: Cytological diagnosis of a presacral myelolipoma: a case report diagnosed by fine-needle aspiration. Diagn Cytopathol 2008;36: 921–922.

12 Skorpil M, Tani E, Blomqvist L: Presacral myelolipoma in a patient with rectal cancer: diagnosis by magnetic resonance imaging and aspiration cytology. Acta Radiol 2007;48:1049–1051.

13 Rossi M, Ravizza D, Fiori G, Trovato C, Renne G, Miller MJ, Tamayo D, Crosta C: Thoracic myelolipoma diagnosed by endoscopic ultrasonography and fine-needle aspiration cytology. Endoscopy 2007;39(suppl 1):E114–E115.

14 Gong Y, Sun X: Fine-needle aspiration of a presacral myelolipoma. Diagn Cytopathol 2006;34:29–30.

15 Varone V, Ciancia G, Bracale U, Merola G, Vetrani A, Pettinato G, Cozzolino I: Multidisciplinary diagnostic approach combining fine needle aspiration, core needle biopsy and imaging features of a presacral myelolipoma in a patient with concurrent breast cancer. Pathol Res Pract 2015;211: 261–263.

16 Chakrabarti I, Bhowmik S, Sinha MG, Bera P: Ultrasound-guided aspiration cytology of retroperitoneal masses with histopathological corroboration: a study of 71 cases. J Cytol 2014;31:15–19.

17 Jimenez-Heffernan JA, Gonzalez-Peramato P, Perna C: Diagnosis of chondroid lipoma by fine-needle aspiration biopsy. Arch Pathol Lab Med 2002; 126:774.

18 Yang YJ, Damron TA, Ambrose JL: Diagnosis of chondroid lipoma by fine-needle aspiration biopsy. Arch Pathol Lab Med 2001;125:1224–1226.

19 Gisselsson D, Domanski HA, Hoglund M, Carlen B, Mertens F, Willen H, Mandahl N: Unique cytological features and chromosome aberrations in chondroid lipoma: a case report based on fine-needle aspiration cytology, histopathology, electron microscopy, chromosome banding, and molecular cytogenetics. Am J Surg Pathol 1999;23: 1300–1304.

20 Thomson TA, Horsman D, Bainbridge TC: Cytogenetic and cytologic features of chondroid lipoma of soft tissue. Mod Pathol 1999;12:88–91.

21 D'Antonio A, Baldi C, Memoli D, Caleo A, Rosamilio R, Zeppa P: Fine needle aspiration biopsy of intraparotid spindle cell lipoma: a case report. Diagn Cytopathol 2013;41:171–173.

22 Fasig JH, Robinson RA, McCulloch TM, Fletcher MS, Miller CK: Spindle cell lipoma of the parotid: fine-needle aspiration and histologic findings. Arch Pathol Lab Med 2001;125:820–821.

23 Domanski HA, Carlen B, Jonsson K, Mertens F, Akerman M: Distinct cytologic features of spindle cell lipoma: a cytologic-histologic study with clinical, radiologic, electron microscopic, and cytogenetic correlations. Cancer 2001;93:381–389.

24 Agoff SN, Folpe AL, Grieco VS, Garcia RL: Spindle cell lipoma of the oral cavity: report of a rare intramuscular case with fine needle aspiration findings. Acta Cytol 2001;45:93–98.

25 Guo Z, Voytovich M, Kurtycz DF, Hoerl HD: Fine-needle aspiration diagnosis of spindle-cell lipoma: a case report and review of the literature. Diagn Cytopathol 2000;23:362–365.

26 Chen X, Yu K, Tong GX, Hood M, Storper I, Hamele-Bena D: Fine needle aspiration of pleomorphic lipoma of the neck: report of two cases. Diagn Cytopathol 2010;38:184–187.

27 Dal Cin P, Sciot R, Polito P, Stas M, de Wever I, Cornelis A, Van den Berghe H: Lesions of 13q may occur independently of deletion of 16q in spindle cell/pleomorphic lipomas. Histopathology 1997; 31:222–225.

28 Gupta S, Gupta R, Sodhani P: Spindle cell lipoma with predominant nerve sheath tumor-like areas: a potential diagnostic pitfall on aspiration cytology. Diagn Cytopathol 2015;43:1017–1019.

29 Agarwal S, Nangia A, Jyotsna PL, Pujani M: Spindle cell lipoma masquerading as lipomatous pleomorphic adenoma: a diagnostic dilemma on fine needle aspiration cytology. J Cytol 2013;30:55–57.

30 Prendes BL, Kohli C, Brooks JS, Newman JG: Cervical hibernoma, a rare, benign tumor: case report. Ear Nose Throat J 2011;90:E19–E21.

31 Saqi A, Yu GH, Marshall MB: Fine-needle aspiration of hibernoma. Diagn Cytopathol 2003;29: 44–45.

32 Lemos MM, Kindblom LG, Meis-Kindblom JM, Remotti F, Ryd W, Gunterberg B, Willen H: Fine-needle aspiration characteristics of hibernoma. Cancer 2001;93:206–210.

33 Thejasvi K, Niveditha SR, Suguna BV, Hemalata M, Kusuma V: Cytomorphology of hibernoma: a report of 2 cases. Acta Cytol 2010;54:875–878.

34 Maire G, Forus A, Foa C, Bjerkehagen B, Mainguene C, Kresse SH, Myklebost O, Pedeutour F: 11q13 alterations in two cases of hibernoma: large heterozygous deletions and rearrangement breakpoints near GARP in 11q13.5. Genes Chromosomes Cancer 2003;37:389–395.

35 Kapila K, Ghosal N, Gill SS, Verma K: Cytomorphology of lipomatous tumors of soft tissue. Acta Cytol 2003;47:555–562.

36 Collins BT, Gossner G, Martin DS, Boyd JH: Fine needle aspiration biopsy of well-differentiated liposarcoma of the neck in a young female: a case report. Acta Cytol 1999;43:452–456.

37 Klijanienko J, Caillaud JM, Lagace R: Fine-needle aspiration in liposarcoma: cytohistologic correlative study including well-differentiated, myxoid, and pleomorphic variants. Diagn Cytopathol 2004;30:307–312.

38 Shimada S, Ishizawa T, Ishizawa K, Matsumura T, Hasegawa T, Hirose T: The value of MDM2 and CDK4 amplification levels using real-time polymerase chain reaction for the differential diagnosis of liposarcomas and their histologic mimickers. Hum Pathol 2006;37:1123–1129.

39 Pedeutour F, Maire G, Pierron A, Thomas DM, Garsed DW, Bianchini L, Duranton-Tanneur V, Cortes-Maurel A, Italiano A, Squire JA, Coindre JM: A newly characterized human well-differentiated liposarcoma cell line contains amplifications of the 12q12-21 and 10p11-14 regions. Virchows Arch 2012;461:67–78.

40 Macarenco RS, Erickson-Johnson M, Wang X, Jenkins RB, Nascimento AG, Oliveira AM: Cytogenetic and molecular genetic findings in dedifferentiated liposarcoma with neural-like whorling pattern and metaplastic bone formation. Cancer Genet Cytogenet 2006;171:126–129.

41 Marino-Enriquez A, Hornick JL, Dal Cin P, Cibas ES, Qian X: Dedifferentiated liposarcoma and pleomorphic liposarcoma: a comparative study of cytomorphology and MDM2/CDK4 expression on fine-needle aspiration. Cancer Cytopathol 2014; 122:128–137.

42 Kilpatrick SE, Ward WG, Bos GD: The value of fine-needle aspiration biopsy in the differential diagnosis of adult myxoid sarcoma. Cancer 2000; 90:167–177.

43 Nemanqani D, Mourad WA: Cytomorphologic features of fine-needle aspiration of liposarcoma. Diagn Cytopathol 1999;20:67–69.

44 Perez-Losada J, Sanchez-Martin M, Rodriguez-Garcia MA, Perez-Mancera PA, Pintado B, Flores T, Battaner E, Sanchez-Garcia I: Liposarcoma initiated by FUS/TLS-CHOP: the FUS/TLS domain plays a critical role in the pathogenesis of liposarcoma. Oncogene 2000;19:6015–6022.

45 Goransson M, Andersson MK, Forni C, Stahlberg A, Andersson C, Olofsson A, Mantovani R, Aman P: The myxoid liposarcoma FUS-DDIT3 fusion oncoprotein deregulates NF-κB target genes by interaction with NFKBIZ. Oncogene 2009;28:270–278.

46 Antonescu CR, Elahi A, Humphrey M, Lui MY, Healey JH, Brennan MF, Woodruff JM, Jhanwar SC, Ladanyi M: Specificity of TLS-CHOP rearrangement for classic myxoid/round cell liposarcoma: absence in predominantly myxoid well-differentiated liposarcomas. J Mol Diagn 2000;2: 132–138.

47 Mertens F, Fletcher CD, Dal Cin P, De Wever I, Mandahl N, Mitelman F, Rosai J, Rydholm A, Sciot R, Tallini G, Van den Berghe H, Vanni R, Willen H: Cytogenetic analysis of 46 pleomorphic soft tissue sarcomas and correlation with morphologic and clinical features: a report of the CHAMP Study Group. Chromosomes and morphology. Genes Chromosomes Cancer 1998;22:16–25.

Domanski HA, Walther CS: FNA Cytology of Soft Tissue and Bone Tumors. Monogr Clin Cytol.
Basel, Karger, 2017, vol 22, pp 40–60 (DOI: 10.1159/000475094)

Fibroblastic/Myofibroblastic Tumors

Nodular Fasciitis

Nodular fasciitis is a relatively common self-limited benign fibroblastic-myofibroblastic lesion, which can mimic malignant spindle-cell and pleomorphic sarcomas. Nodular fasciitis can occur in any age group, but is most common in young adults as a small, rapidly growing, painful, or tender mass in the subcutaneous tissue in the upper extremities, trunk, and head and neck region. Variants of nodular fasciitis include intravascular fasciitis arising in small- and medium-sized blood vessels and cranial fasciitis occurring in infants and young children in the periosteum of the skull, often with extensions to the adjacent soft tissue and bone [1].

Nodular fasciitis may cause considerable diagnostic difficulties in cytologic examination, as fine-needle aspiration (FNA) smears are usually cellular, containing proliferating fibroblasts and myofibroblasts with a wide variation in size and shape of the nuclei [2–4]. Spindle-shaped cells with cytoplasmic processes and fusiform nuclei are the most common cell type, but plump cells with ovoid, rounded, or irregular nuclei are also present. Another typical finding is the presence of polyhedral or triangular myofibroblasts with abundant cytoplasm and occasionally 1 or 2 rounded nuclei at the periphery near the cytoplasmic membrane, resembling ganglion cells (Fig. 1). Despite hypercellularity and nuclear pleomorphism throughout the smears, the chromatin in all cells is finely granular.

A myxoid matrix is common in FNA smears of nodular fasciitis at its early, growing phase, giving the impression of a myxoid sarcoma such as myxofibrosarcoma (MFS). Persistent nodular fasciitis often yields smears containing relatively uniform, haphazardly arranged myofibroblasts with a "cell culture" appearance. A collagenous matrix is often present. The vast majority of nodular fasciitis regress spontaneously and a "wait and see" treatment option is indicated in cases with a typical clinical presentation and characteristic cytomorphology in FNA smears [2, 5–16].

Cytologic Features
- Cellular aspirates
- Often myxoid background matrix
- Dispersed spindle cells mixed with small- and medium-sized clusters and sheets of spindle cells
- Variable anisocytosis and anisokaryosis
- Ganglion-like cells
- Cell culture-like appearance
- Admixture of inflammatory cells and histiocytes
- Occasional multinucleated giant cells
- Mitoses

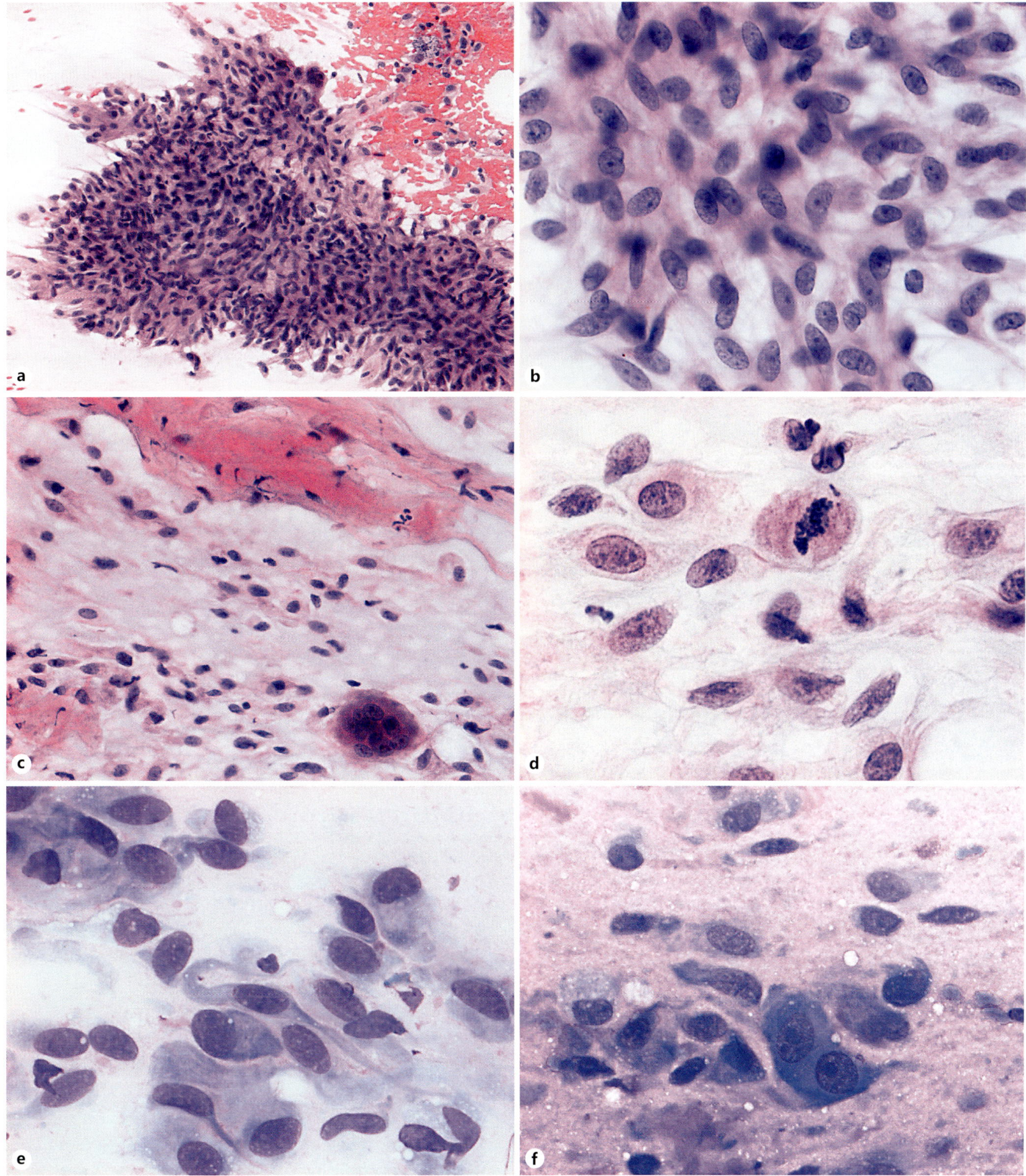

Fig. 1. Nodular fasciitis. Smears show clusters and sheets of spindle cells (**a**), occasionally with a cell-culture appearance (**b**), osteoclast-like giant cells, fragments of collagenous matrix (**c**), and mitoses (**d**). HE stain. **e**, **f** Spindle cells with cytoplasmic processes and plump cells with ovoid, rounded, or irregular nuclei with an admixture of ganglion-like cells are further common findings in smears from nodular fasciitis. MGG stain.

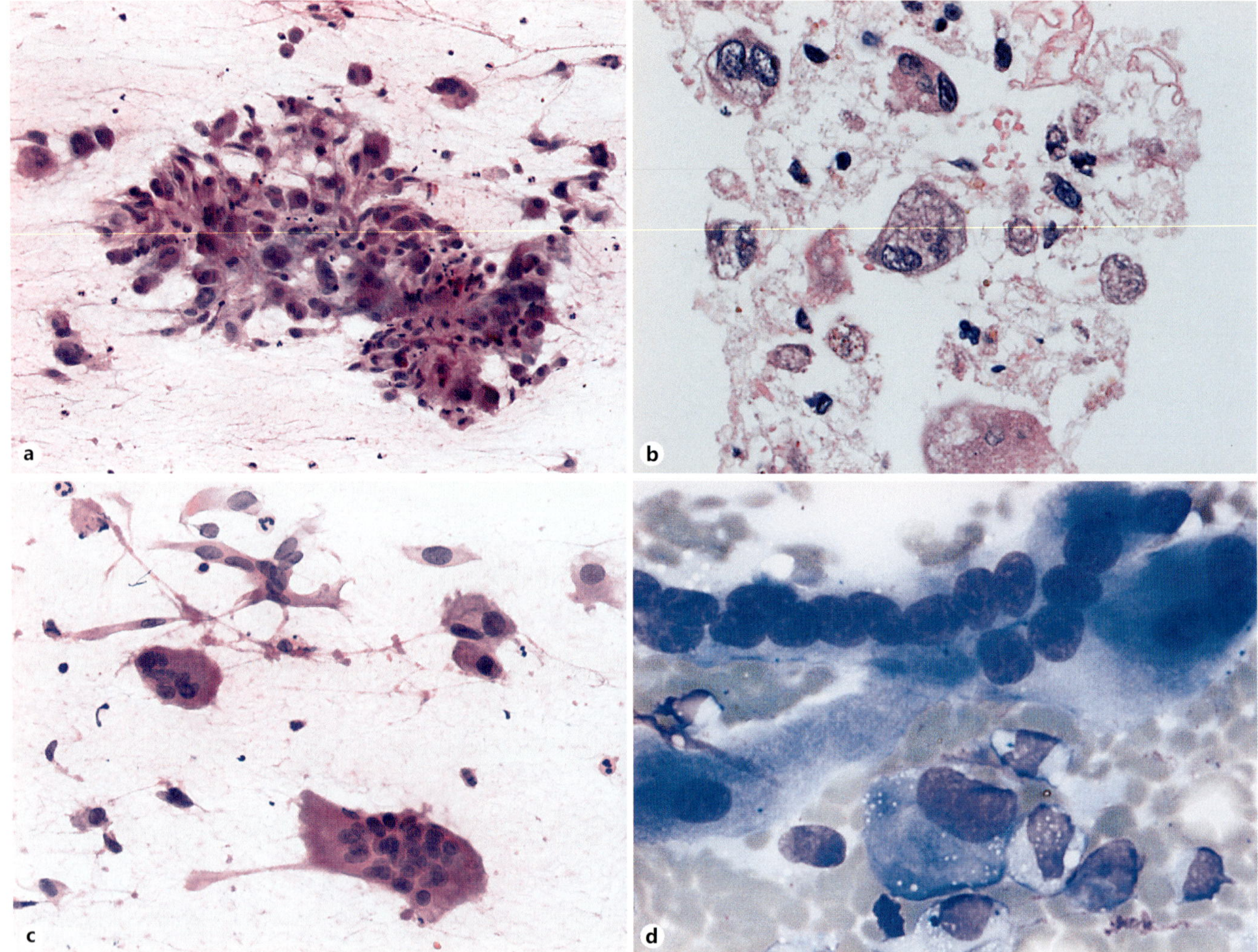

Fig. 2. a–c Smears from proliferative fasciitis show loosely cohesive sheets of spindle cells with numerous "ganglion-like" cells and occasional multinucleated osteoclast-like cells. HE stain; cell block section (**b**). **d** Smears from proliferative myositis contain multinucleated regenerating muscle fibers in addition to the fibroblastic-myofibroblastic cells. MGG stain.

Ancillary Tests
Immunophenotype
Diffusely positive for smooth muscle actin (SMA), occasionally focal desmin, and CD68. Negative for keratins, CD34, β-catenin, and S100.

Genetics
A balanced translocation t(17;22)(p13;q13) resulting in an *MYH9-USP6* gene fusion can be found and is highly indicative of the diagnosis [17]. The fusion leads to the upregulation of *USP6*, which is involved in cell signaling and movement [18]. The fusion can be detected in both fresh and fixed material using cytogenetics, fluorescence in situ hybridization (FISH), polymerase chain reaction (PCR), and next-generation sequencing (NGS).

Differential Diagnosis
- Pleomorphic, spindle-cell, and myxoid sarcomas
- Desmoid fibromatosis

Cellular smears from cases of nodular fasciitis, showing nuclear pleomorphism, prominent nucleoli, mitoses, and occasionally a myxoid background, may suggest a variety of pleomorphic or myxoid sarcomas but the bland nuclear chromatin favors a benign process. One of the important differentials in the examination of FNA smears of nodular fasciitis, especially deeply seated fasciitis, is leiomyosarcoma. Fasciitis

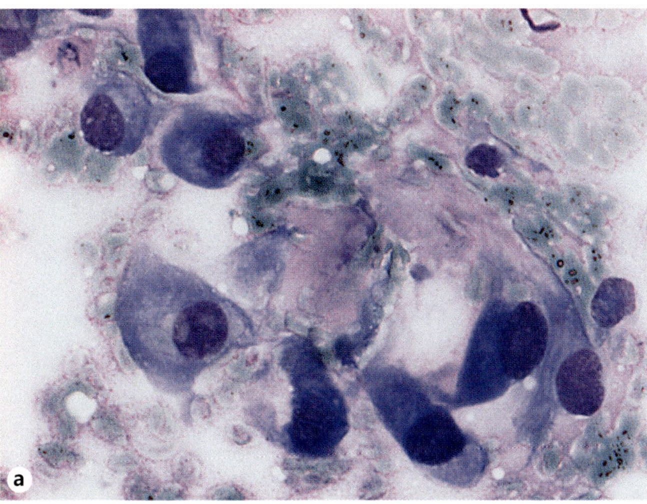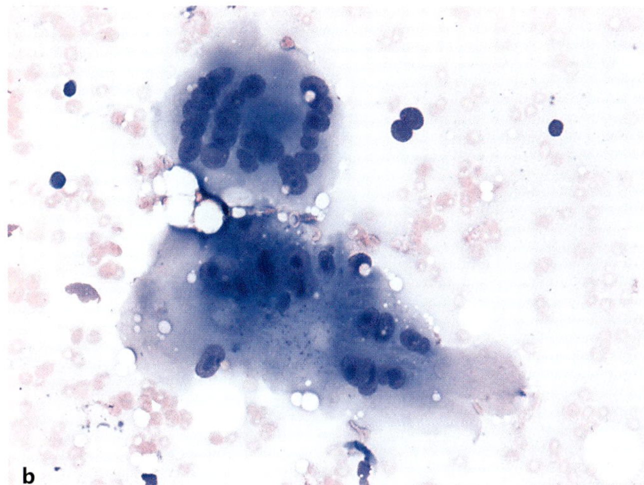

Fig. 3. a, **b** Smears from myositis ossificans show a mixture of proliferating myofibroblasts, osteoblasts, and occasionally regenerating muscle fibers ("muscle giant cells"). MGG stain.

may show very focal immunoreactivity for desmin. Distinct positive staining for desmin favors leiomyosarcoma [19].

Proliferative fasciitis and proliferative myositis, which are related pseudosarcomatous lesions, share many cytologic features with nodular fasciitis. However, the myxoid background matrix is less prominent and the ganglion cell-like cells are more numerous. Smears from pseudosarcomatous proliferations lack immunoreactivity for β-catenin, which helps to exclude desmoid-type fibromatosis. When the clinical history is typical (a rapidly growing, tender tumor) and the cytologic features are typical, an attitude of "wait and see" is justifiable as the vast majority of nodular fasciitis regress considerably or disappear within weeks or months.

Proliferative Fasciitis and Proliferative Myositis

Pseudosarcomatous lesions related to nodular fasciitis include proliferative fasciitis and proliferative myositis, which develop predominantly in adults. Proliferative myositis commonly arises in the trunk, whereas proliferative fasciitis is more common in the extremities [9, 15, 20, 21]. Both proliferative fasciitis and myositis share many cytologic features with nodular fasciitis. However, the myxoid background matrix is less prominent and the ganglion-like cells are usually numerous and often exhibit large nucleoli in proliferative fasciitis. In proliferative myositis, smears contain mul-

tinucleated regenerating muscle fibers in addition to the fibroblastic-myofibroblastic cells (Fig. 2). Mitotic figures can be found in FNA smears from both lesions.

Ancillary Tests
Immunophenotype
Positive for SMA. Negative for keratins, CD34, desmin, myogenin, MYOD1, and S100.

Genetics
One case has displayed a trisomy of chromosome 2, but the significance of this remains to be confirmed [22].

Myositis Ossificans

Myositis ossificans is a rapidly growing soft tissue lesion, arising most often in the musculature of the extremities, buttock, and shoulder in young adults. Myositis ossificans may be mistaken clinically as being soft tissue sarcoma, especially extraskeletal osteosarcoma. The mass is often tender and presents ossification in a zonal pattern. The characteristic cytologic findings are the mixture of proliferating fibroblasts/myofibroblasts, osteoblasts, osteoclast giant cells, occasionally regenerating muscle fibers ("muscle giant cells"), and rarely small bone fragments (Fig. 3). Myositis ossificans is typically a self-limiting lesion and may resolve spontaneously some weeks/months after presentation.

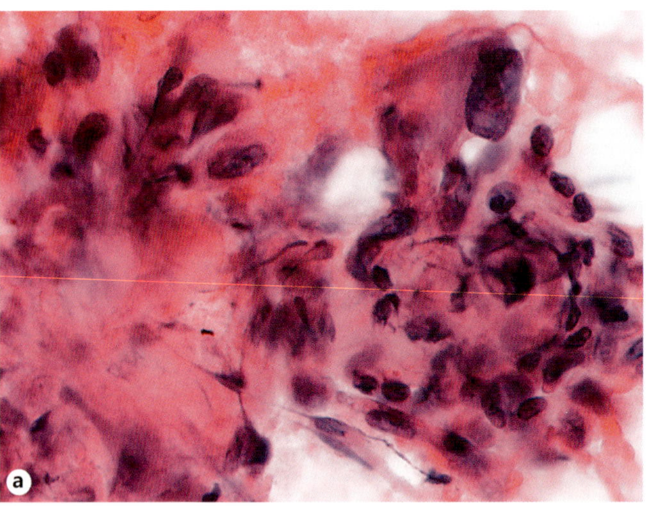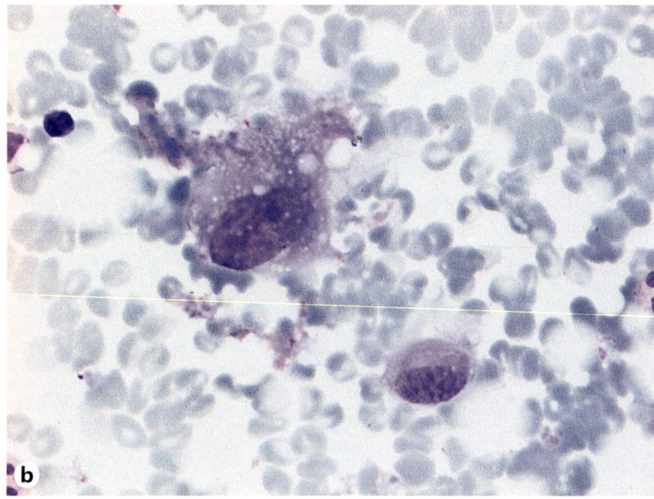

Fig. 4. Ischemic fasciitis. **a** Aspiration smears are composed of proliferating fibroblasts and myofibroblasts. HE stain. **b** Occasionally with atypical features with large, irregular nuclei and dense, smudged chromatin. MGG stain.

Cytologic Features
- Proliferating spindle cells – fibroblasts/myofibroblasts with variable anisocytosis and anisokaryosis
- Osteoblasts, often with reactive changes
- Osteoclasts
- "Muscle giant cells"
- Occasionally small calcifications
- Rare mitoses

Ancillary tests
Genetics
There are no known recurrent genetic aberrations.

Differential Diagnosis
- Pleomorphic sarcoma
- Extraskeletal osteosarcoma

Ischemic Fasciitis (Atypical Decubital Fibroplasia)

Ischemic fasciitis is a reactive process arising as a poorly circumscribed, nonulcerated mass in the deep subcutaneous tissue overlying bony prominences, and is usually associated with chronic pressure of these areas in immobilized patients. Ischemic fasciitis is composed of zones of proliferating fibroblasts-myofibroblasts alternated with fat tissue and necrosis. Aspiration smears are composed of fibroblasts and myofibroblasts, occasionally with atypical features of prolif-

erating myofibroblasts with large, irregular nuclei, and dense and smudged chromatin (Fig. 4). In addition, smears may contain inflammatory cells, necrotic debris, and occasionally myxoid stroma and rare ganglion-like cells.

Ancillary Tests
Immunophenotype
Positive for variable SMA, CD34, and occasionally focal desmin. Negative for keratins and S100.

Genetics
There are no known recurrent genetic aberrations.

Elastofibroma

Elastofibroma dorsi is a relatively rare reactive soft tissue proliferation in elderly individuals, particularly women. It commonly presents as a slowly growing deep-seated unilateral or occasional bilateral mass located near the inferior margin of the scapula or between the inferior part of the scapula and the chest wall. This typical location together with the age/sex of the patients and imaging findings is often suggestive of the diagnosis. Elastofibroma dorsi is composed of abundant hypocellular collagenous stroma with an admixture of bland fibroblasts, mature adipose tissue, and numerous disrupted elastic fibers within collagenous stroma. FNA smears show small sheets or clusters of uniform

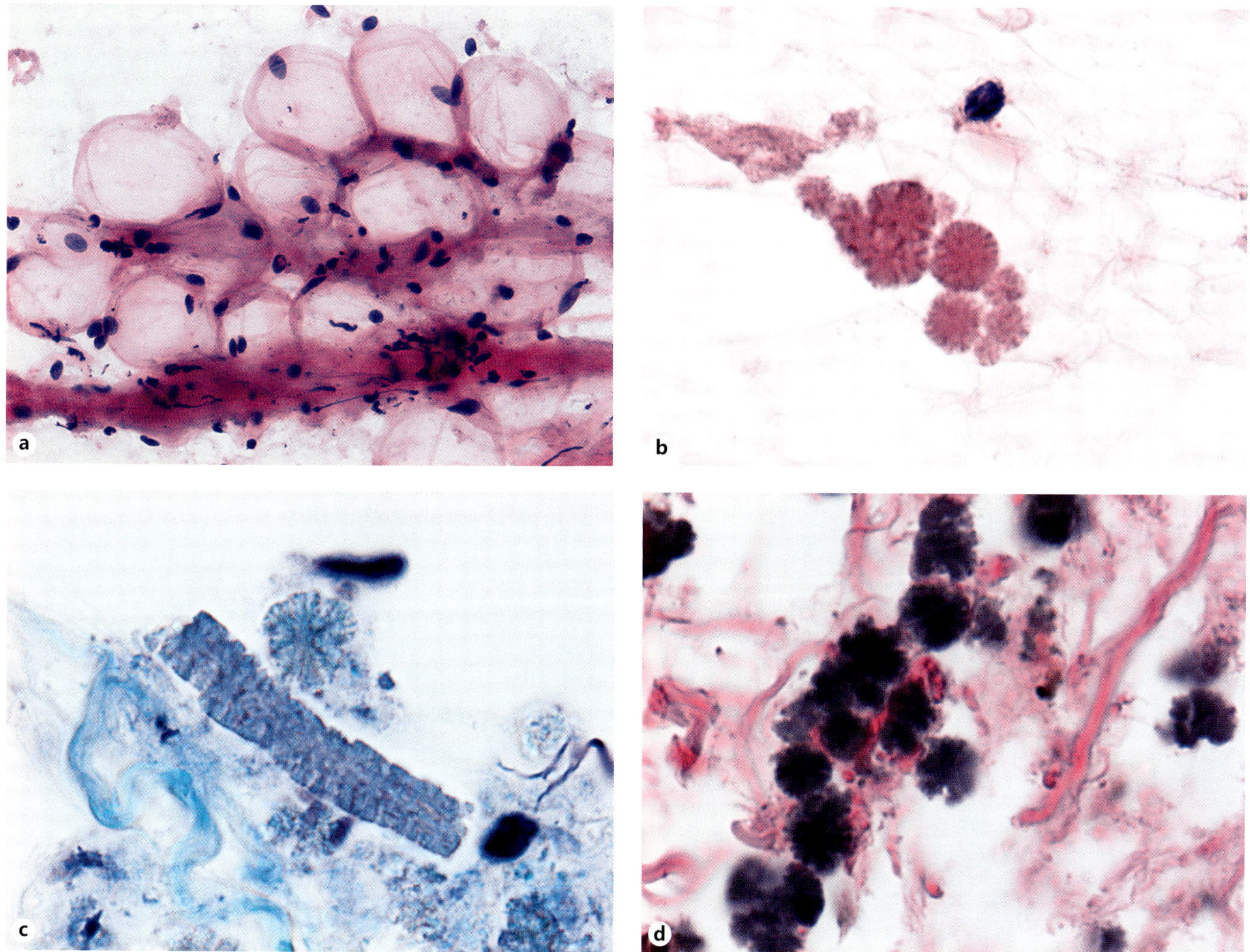

Fig. 5. Elastofibroma. **a** Mature adipocyte mixture with hypocellular collagenous stroma and spindle cells. HE stain. The presence of elastic fibers that appear as linear "braid-like," globular, and stellate structures with serrated edges is best appreciated on alcohol-fixed and HE- (**b**) or PAP-stained (**c**) smears, and in elastin stain on cell block sections (**d**).

spindle cells, clusters or dispersed mature adipocytes, and fragments of acellular collagen matrix. The main diagnostic feature is the presence of elastic fibers with serrated borders, corresponding to faulty elastin fibrillogenesis. Elastic fibers appearing as linear ("braid-like"), globular, and stellate structures with serrated edges [23–30] are usually easy to find in wet-fixed, Papanicolaou (PAP)- or hematoxylin and eosin (HE)-stained smears examined with high-power magnification (Fig. 5). These structures are very subtle in air-dried smears [26]. Diagnostic difficulties arise when the typical serrated elastic fibers are missing.

Cytologic Features
- Variably cellular smears – often moderate to scanty
- Fat tissue intermingled with collagen fragments/collagen fibers and uniform spindle cells in small loosely cohesive groups or dispersed
- Elastic fibers present as linear ("braid-like") and globular bodies with a shell-like and stellate appearance and the characteristic serrated "moth-eaten" edges

Ancillary Tests
Cytochemistry
Elastic stains.

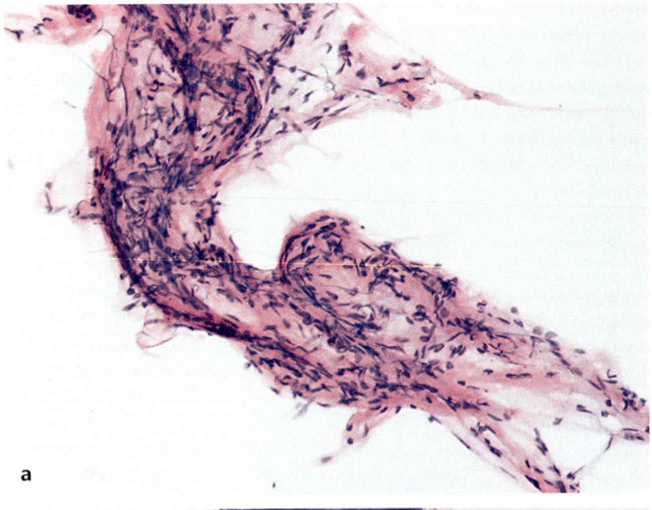

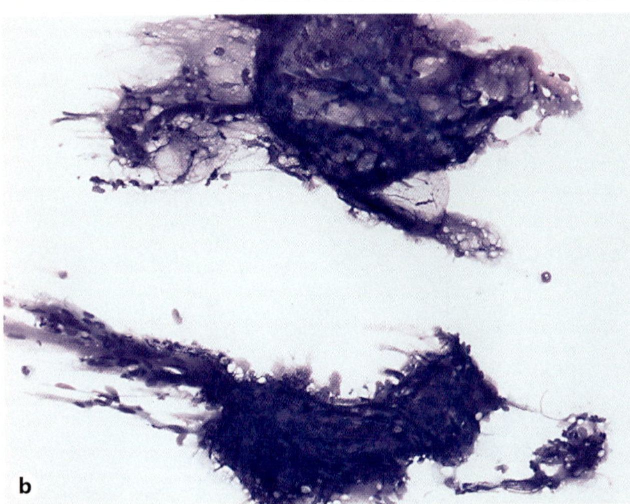

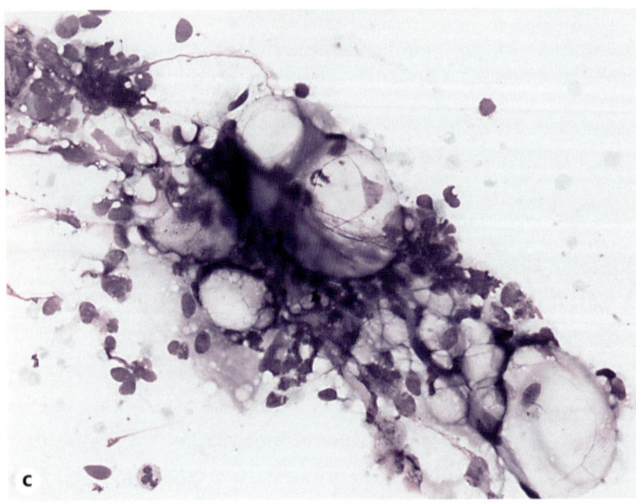

Fig. 6. Fibrous hamartoma of infancy. **a** A loosely cohesive cluster of bland spindle cells and capillaries. HE stain. **b** Clusters of bland spindle cells with capillaries in a fatty background. MGG stain. **c** Bland spindle cells and bare nuclei with an admixture of mature fat. MGG stain.

Genetics

Recurrent gains at chromosomal locations Xq12-q22 and 19 have been reported in 30% of cases. Cytogenetics, FISH, single nucleotide polymorphism (SNP) array, and NGS can detect these changes on fresh or fixed material [31].

Differential Diagnoses

- Extra-abdominal desmoid
- Lipoma

The cytologic diagnosis of elastofibroma can be difficult, especially when the FNA specimen is limited and lacks characteristic elastin fibers, which are the main diagnostic feature of elastofibroma.

Fibrous Hamartoma of Infancy

Fibrous hamartoma of infancy is a rare, benign, usually solitary tumor composed of a mixture of mature adipose tissue, septa, and bands of fibrous tissue with hypocellular areas alternating with fascicles of fibroblasts/myofibroblasts and nests of small primitive round to ovoid and spindled cells in a basophilic, myxoid matrix. Fibrous hamartoma of infancy occurs in infants and children up to 2 years of age, but approximately 25% of cases are congenital. Typical sites include deep dermis and subcutaneous tissue of the trunk (axilla, upper back), shoulders, and groin/perineum. Smears of fibrous hamartoma of infancy show variable cellularity and are composed of small sheets and clusters of bland spindle cells with an admixture of dispersed spindle cells and fragments of mature adipose tissue (Fig. 6) [32–34].

Cytologic Features

- A mixture of normal fatty tissue and bland spindle cells, dispersed or in sheets and clusters
- Variable amounts of myxoid matrix

Ancillary Tests
Immunophenotype
Positive for SMA, focal CD34. Positive for S100 in the lipomatous component. Negative for β-catenin.

Genetics
Very few cases have been analyzed but complex translocations have been described and illustrated with FISH [35]. Cytogenetics, SNP array, and NGS can also be utilized on fresh and fixed material to detect any changes.

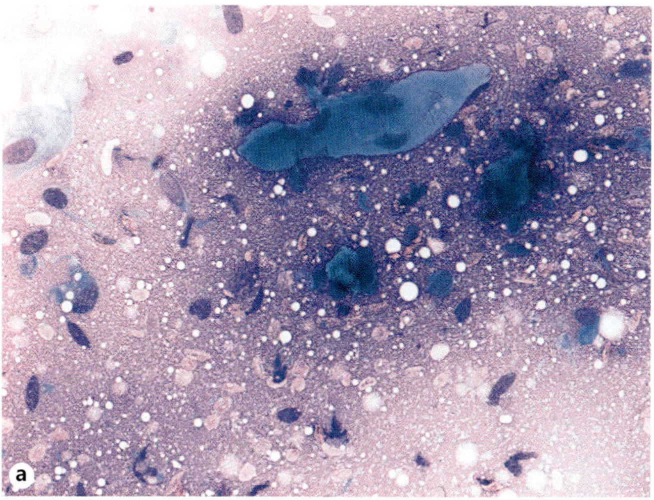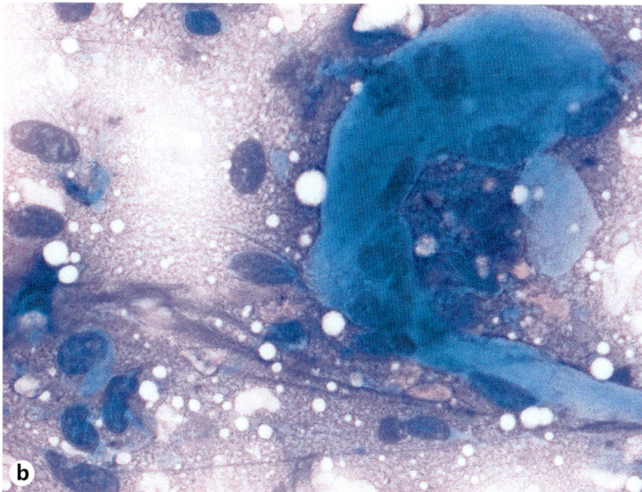

Fig. 7. Fibromatosis colli. **a**, **b** Hypocellular smears with bland spindle cells, bare nuclei, and "muscle giant cells." MGG stain.

Differential Diagnosis
- Infantile fibrosarcoma

Occasionally, smears of fibrous hamartoma of infancy contain tight clusters of spindle cells resembling those in infantile fibrosarcoma. However, most infantile fibrosarcomas arise in the extremities and yield hypercellular smears of primitive spindle cells without a fatty component, compared to the paucity of the spindle cell component seen in fibrous hamartoma of infancy.

Fibromatosis Colli (Torticollis)

Fibromatosis colli is a diffuse proliferation of fibroblasts within the muscle tissue arising in the mid to lower portion of sternocleidomastoid muscle. The involved muscle fibers are atrophic and contain regenerating "muscle giant cells." Most cases of those uncommon tumor-like lesions occur in newborn infants, typically presenting between the second and fourth weeks of life. Smears of fibromatosis colli contain a double population of bland spindle cells and disrupted fragments of striated muscle/"muscle giant cells" with nuclei showing prominent nucleoli [36] (Fig. 7). There is a risk of misinterpreting "muscle giant cells" as malignant cells. The vast majority of fibromatoses colli is self-limited and regresses spontaneously; the primary therapy is expectancy and clinical symptom control.

Cytologic Features
- Bland fibroblasts and myofibroblasts, dispersed or clustered
- "Muscle giant cells" and tadpole cells
- Occasionally small tufts of myxoid matrix
- Stripped nuclei

Ancillary Tests
Immunophenotype
Positive for SMA. Negative for β-catenin.

Genetics
There are no known recurrent genetic aberrations.

Differential Diagnosis
- Pleomorphic sarcoma

Desmoid-Type Fibromatosis

Fibromatoses represent a broad spectrum of infiltrative (locally aggressive) and nonmetastasizing myofibroblastic neoplasms. Extra-abdominal deep fibromatosis usually arises in the proximal parts of extremities, and in the pelvic girdle and shoulder region, most commonly in young adults and teenagers. Abdominal wall fibromatosis is often associated with pregnancy. These 2 subtypes of fibromatoses are commonly examined by FNA while plantar, palmar, and mesenteric fibromatoses rarely undergo FNA. Because of

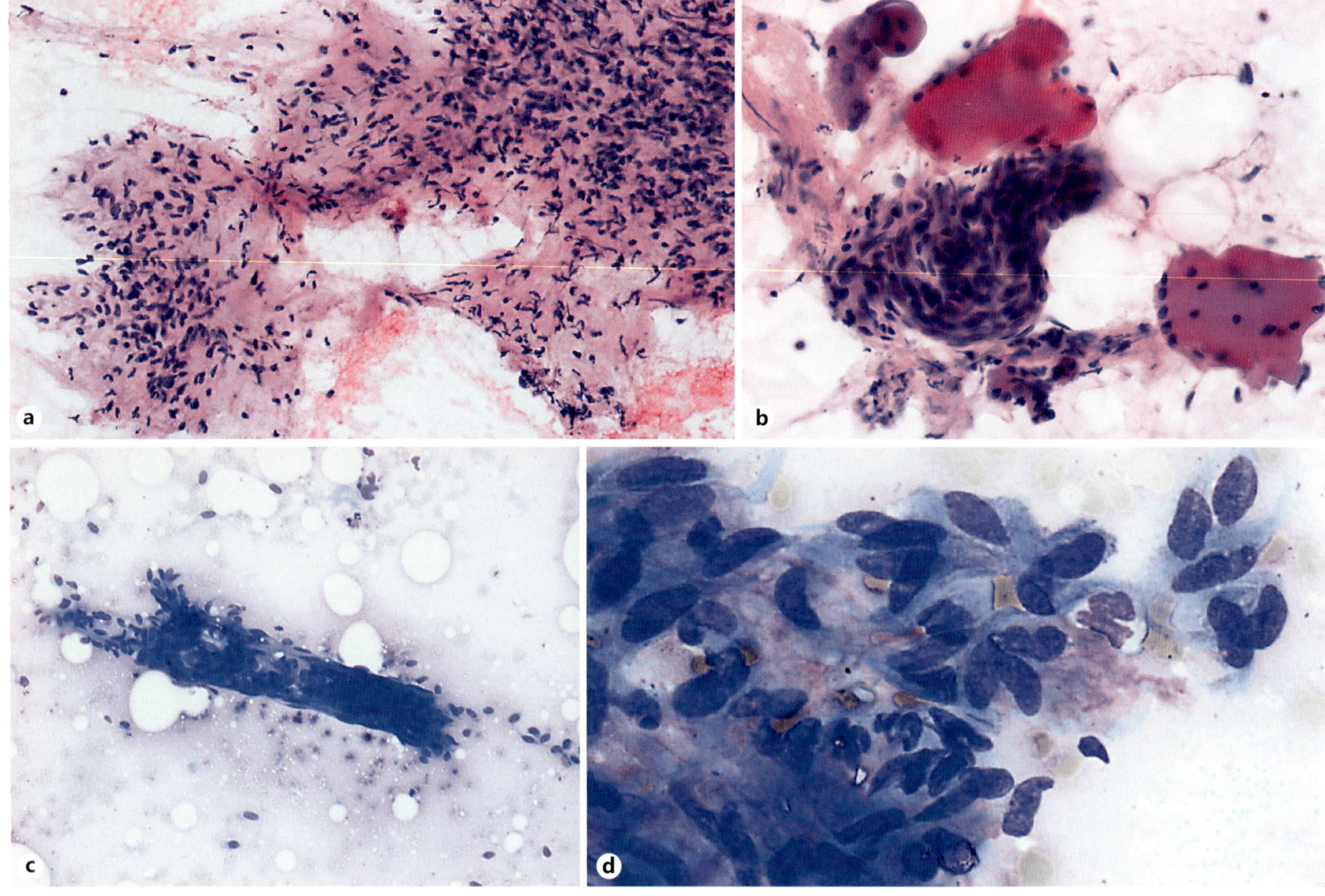

Fig. 8. Desmoid fibromatosis. **a** Loosely cohesive clusters of bland or slightly pleomorphic spindle cells, many of these with crush artifacts, embedded in a collagenous matrix. HE stain. **b** A cohesive cluster of spindle cells with fragments of paucicellular collagenous stroma and damaged striated muscle cells. HE stain. **c** Bland spindle cells in long fascicles, a useful clue in the cytologic diagnosis of desmoid fibromatosis. MGG stain. **d** Fibroblasts with elongated fusiform nuclei, insignificant nucleoli, and slight anisokaryosis embedded in a collagenous matrix. MGG stain.

abundant collagenous stroma, vigorous aspiration using larger needles is often necessary in order to obtain material sufficient for diagnosis. Smears are most often of low to moderate cellularity and contain a mixture of uniform, occasional slightly atypical spindle cells and fragments of paucicellular collagenous stroma [12, 37, 38]. Bland spindle cells arranged in long fascicles is an additional important cytologic feature suggestive of desmoid [39] (Fig. 8).

Cytologic Features
- Variable yield, but often moderate/scanty cellularity
- Clustered or dispersed fibroblasts
- Fibroblasts with elongated fusiform nuclei, insignificant nucleoli, and slight anisokaryosis
- Bland or slightly atypical spindle cells in collagenous stroma arranged in long, slender fascicles
- Cytoplasmic processes are seen in preserved cells but stripped nuclei and crush artifact are a common finding
- Fragments of paucicellular collagenous stroma
- Occasional regenerating striated muscle fibers (muscle giant cells)

Ancillary Tests
Immunophenotype
Positive for SMA, MSA, focal desmin, and β-catenin. Negative for CD34, h-caldesmon, S100, and CD117.

Genetics

Trisomies for chromosomes 8 and/or 20 can be found in the tumor cells [40]. Cytogenetics, FISH, SNP array, and NGS can used for evaluation on fresh or fixed material, depending on what is available.

Differential Diagnosis
- Nodular fasciitis
- Low-grade fibromyxoid sarcoma (LGFMS)
- Deep-seated leiomyoma
- Solitary fibrous tumor (SFT)
- Low-grade malignant peripheral nerve sheath tumor
- Monophasic synovial sarcoma
- Fibrosarcoma

Smears from desmoids may show a myxoid matrix, evoking the differential diagnosis of low-grade myxoid spindle-cell lesions, such as nodular fasciitis or LGFMS. Cells in smears from a desmoid are less pleomorphic than those of nodular fasciitis and the ganglion cell-like cells are not presented. When the yield is poor and the characteristic mixture of collagen fragments and fibroblasts is missing, differential diagnosis regarding the spindle cell tumors noted above is difficult. Demonstration of the aberrant nuclear expression of β-catenin is helpful to confirm the diagnosis.

Dermatofibrosarcoma Protuberans

Dermatofibrosarcoma protuberans (DFSP) is a low-grade, locally aggressive fibroblastic neoplasm that most frequently affects the dermis and subcutis. This rare tumor tends to recur locally but has no metastatic potential. However, similar to some other sarcomas, recurrent and primary DFSP can progress to fibrosarcomatous (high-grade) DFSP with increased metastatic risk. FNA smears from DFSP are characterized by tight, often 3-dimensional clusters of bland spindle cells embedded in a collagenous/fibrillar and, occasionally, metachromatic matrix. The tumor cells show poorly defined cytoplasmic borders and relatively uniform or slightly atypical, spindle-shaped or oval nuclei with finely dispersed chromatin. Naked nuclei are commonly seen in smears while tissue fragments showing a storiform pattern and entrapped fat tissue are less characteristic [41–50]. The FNA cytomorphology alone is not sufficiently characteristic to permit a confident diagnosis of DFSP (Fig. 9). A definitive diagnosis requires the confirmatory CD34 positivity by immunocytochemistry [44, 46, 51].

Cytologic Features of DFSP
- Variable yield
- Tight clusters or fascicles of spindle cells embedded in a collagen matrix
- Dispersed spindle cells and stripped nuclei
- Slight to moderate cellular and nuclear atypia but bland nuclear chromatin and inconspicuous nucleoli
- Pale and poorly defined cytoplasm, better-preserved cells with bipolar cytoplasmic extensions
- Occasionally fat fragments with an admixture of spindle cells

Ancillary Tests

Immunophenotype

Positive for CD34. Negative for S100, SMA, desmin, and S100.

Genetics

Cytogenetically supernumerary ring chromosomes with material derived from chromosomes 17 and 22 are often found [52]. A translocation t(17,22)(q21;q13) can be found in the majority of cases using FISH and PCR [53]. Both the translocation and the ring chromosome result in a fusion gene *COL1A1-PDGFB*, which stimulates cell growth and tumor development. FISH, SNP array, and NGS can be used for evaluation on fresh or fixed material.

Differential Diagnosis
- Cellular benign fibrous histiocytoma
- Neurofibroma
- Schwannoma
- Nodular fasciitis
- SFT
- Other spindle-cell sarcomas arising in skin and subcutaneous tissue

Cellular smears from DFSP are most often considered low-grade malignant spindle cell sarcoma. The most important differential diagnosis is cellular benign fibrous histiocytoma. The presence of histiocytes and/or giant cells favors histiocytoma. Furthermore, the spindle cells in fibrous histiocytoma are negative or only focally positive for CD34.

Extrapleural Solitary Fibrous Tumor

SFT is a fibroblastic tumor initially described in the pleura but can occur practically in any extrapleural location of the body. The common sites include deep soft tissue of the

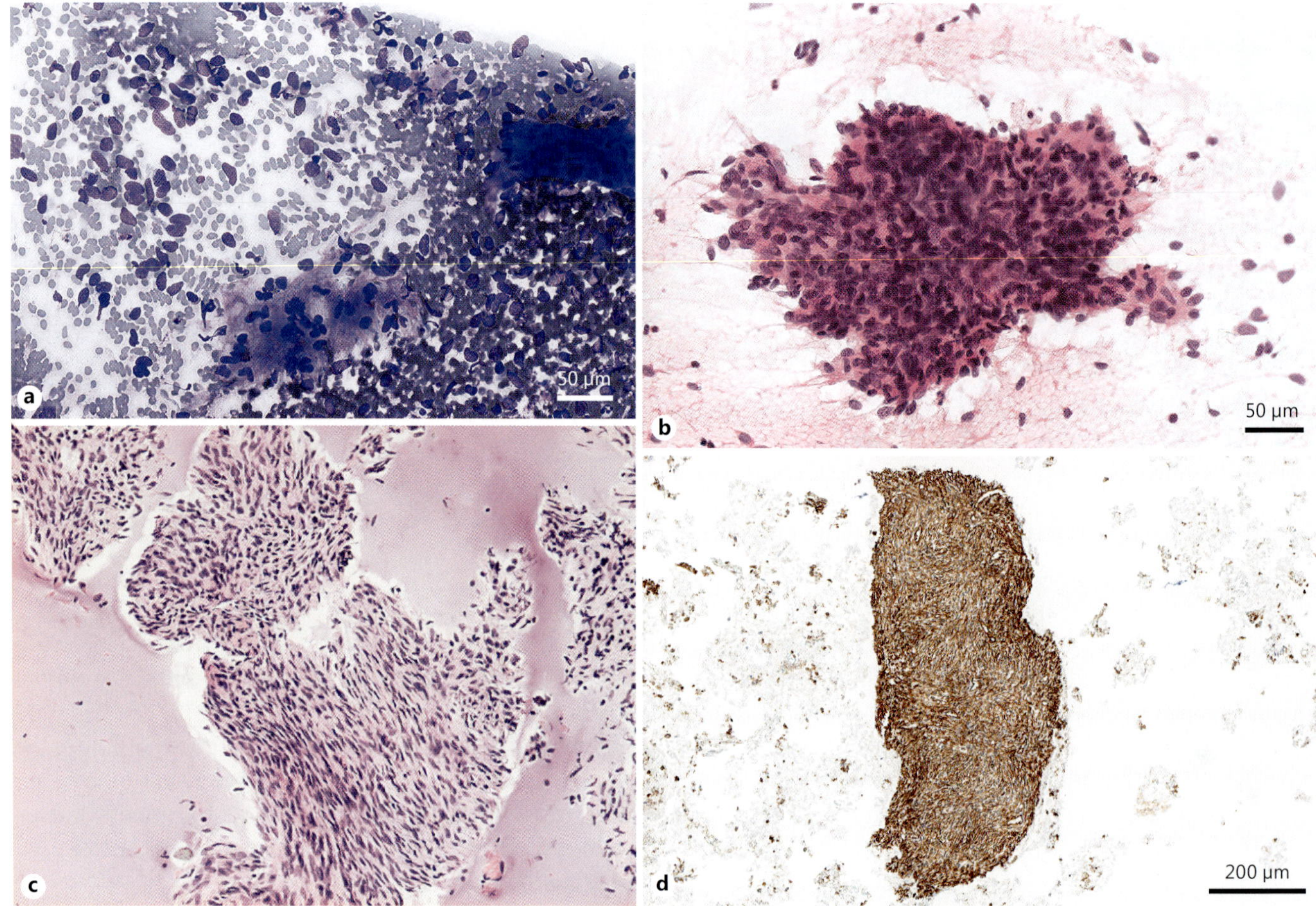

Fig. 9. DFSP. **a** Numerous dispersed naked nuclei with slight to moderate nuclear atypia but bland nuclear chromatin and inconspicuous nucleoli. MGG stain. **b** Tight cluster of spindle cells embedded in a collagen matrix and some dispersed bland spindle cells. HE stain. **c** The cell block section shows a microscopic pattern suggestive of DFSP. HE stain. **d** Diffuse positivity for CD34 on the cell block section confirms the diagnosis of DFSP.

lower extremities, head and neck region, mediastinum, and retroperitoneum. Tumors previously labeled as hemangiopericytoma and the rare lipomatous hemangiopericytoma are now classified as SFT and lipomatous "fatforming" SFT. The majority of SFT are benign but approximately 5–10% behave in a malignant fashion, and both malignant and dedifferentiated forms of SFT have been reported.

The aspirate yields variably cellular smears containing bland "fibroblast-like" spindle cells, either dispersed and in loosely cohesive or tight clusters and fascicles. The tumor cells contain spindle or ovoid nuclei and scanty cytoplasm and bland nuclei with finely dispersed chromatin. Naked nuclei, ropy collagen fibers, and mast cells are common [54–65]. The prominent "staghorn" vascular pattern seen in histology is rarely appreciated in FNA smears, but can be seen in cell block sections (Fig. 10).

Cytologic Features

- Variable cellularity
- A mixture of dispersed cells and tight, fascicle-like clusters
- Uniform population of bland spindle cells with inconspicuous nucleoli
- Stripped nuclei
- Ropy collagen fibers
- Mast cells
- Three-dimensional clusters of uniform spindle cells mixed with mature fat in the fat-forming variant

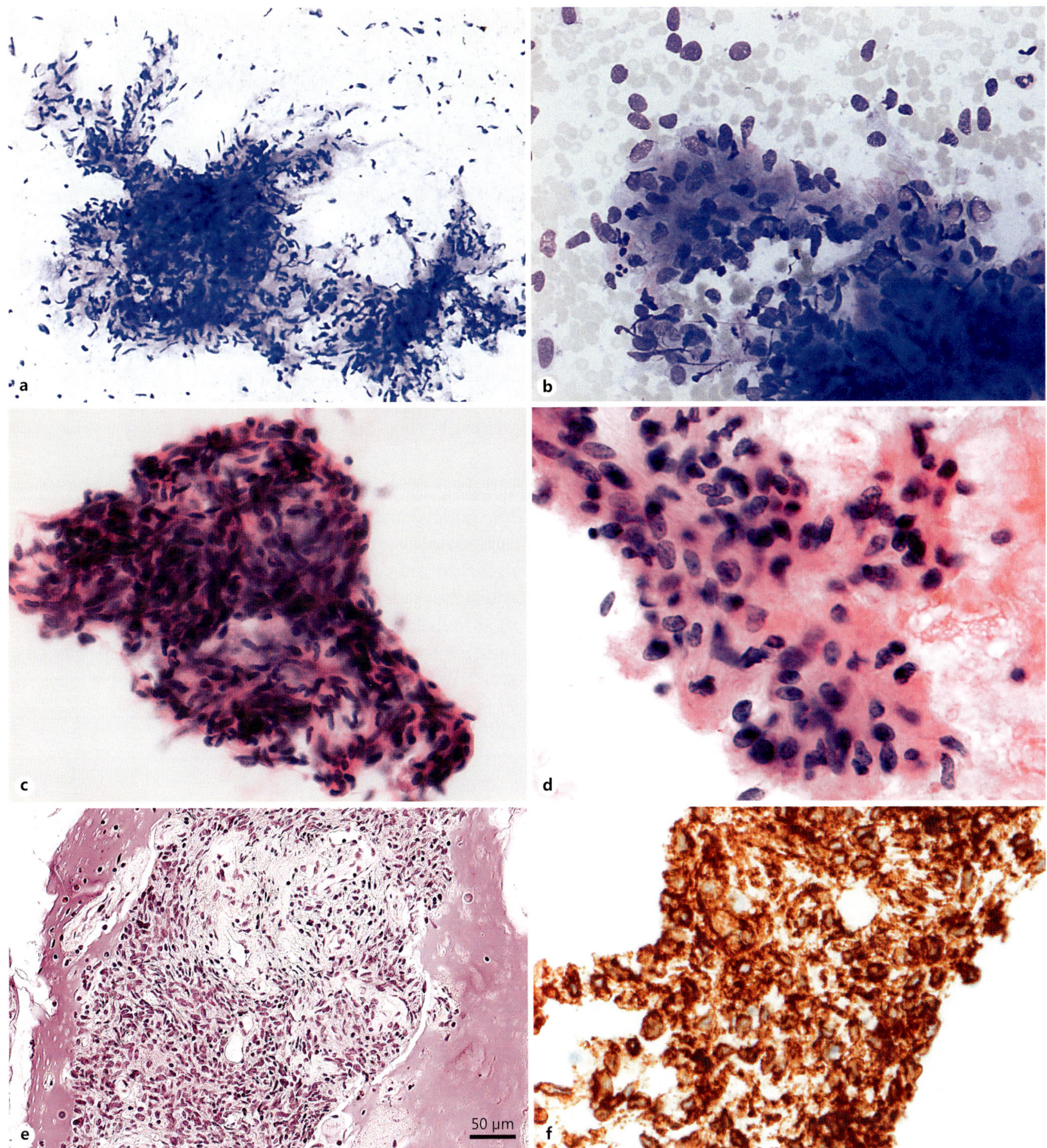

Fig. 10. SFT. **a**, **b** A mixture of dispersed cells and loosely cohesive or tight clusters of bland spindle cells in a collagenous/myxoid background. MGG stain. **c**, **d** Clusters of "fibroblast-like" tumor cells containing spindle or ovoid nuclei and scanty cytoplasm is a common finding in FNA smears. HE stain. **e** The "staghorn" vascular pattern and alternating cellular and collagenous areas can be appreciated in cell block sections. HE stain. **f** Diffuse and strong expression of CD34 support with diagnosis SFT. Cell block; CD34.

Ancillary Tests
Immunophenotype
Positive for CD34, which may be decreased or lost in malignant SFT, nuclear STAT6, and occasionally focal positivity for SMA and epithelial membrane antigen (EMA). Negative for CD117, DOG1, S100, desmin, and keratins.

Genetics
There are no recurrent genetic changes but tumors exceeding 10 cm in size display abnormal karyotypes involving both structural and numerical aberrations [66].

Differential Diagnosis
- Monophasic synovial sarcoma
- Desmoid-type fibromatosis
- LGFMS
- Low-grade malignant peripheral nerve sheath tumor
- Benign or malignant lipomatous tumors versus the fat-forming variant of SFT

A correct diagnosis of SFT is difficult based on cytomorphology alone, due to its morphologic overlapping with other benign and malignant spindle cell neoplasms. The smears from the fat-forming variant SFT show clusters of uniform spindle cells admixed with mature adipose tissue and display variably prominent myxoid changes, capillaries, and lipoblast-like cells, which can lead to the misinterpretation of an SFT as myxoid liposarcoma or spindle cell lipoma [67]. Immunocytochemistry is often diagnostically helpful as the spindle cells of SFT display distinctive immunoreactivities for CD34, CD99, STAT6, and Bcl-2, and limited reactivities for EMA and keratins; the profile distinguishes it from other spindle cell tumors.

Inflammatory Myofibroblastic Tumor

Inflammatory myofibroblastic tumor (IMT) once belonged to the spectrum of lesions termed "inflammatory pseudotumor," but over the last 2 decades IMT has been recognized as a low-grade neoplasm with distinctive clinical, pathologic, and molecular features. IMT shows a predilection for the visceral soft tissue and lung of children and adolescents. IMT has a relatively high recurrence rate (up to 25%) and approximately 5% of cases have the potential to metastasize. The FNA features of IMT are variable, and often impose a benign, reactive impression. The smears show a mixture of plump and slightly pleomorphic spindle cells (myofibroblasts) either in cohesive sheets or scattered in a background of inflammatory cells (mainly plasma cells and lymphocytes), and occasional large ganglion-like cells.

Cytologic Features
- Variable but often hypercellular smears
- Mixture of plump and slightly atypical myofibroblasts which are dispersed or arranged in tight sheets
- Inflammatory infiltrate including plasma cells, lymphocytes, and histiocytes
- Occasional ganglion-like cells

Ancillary Tests
Immunophenotype
Positive for SMA, variable desmin, ALK1 in up to 60% of cases, and occasionally focal keratins. Negative for S100, EMA, CD117, and myogenin.

Genetics
In young patients rearrangement of chromosome band 2p23 involving the *ALK* gene, resulting in ALK protein overexpression, is seen in 50–70% of cases [68]. However, in adult cases over the age of 40 years the aberration is uncommon [69]. A FISH with an *ALK* split probe on fresh and/or fixed material can be diagnostically useful. Cytogenetics, SNP array, and NGS can also be used on available material.

Differential Diagnosis
- Reactive myofibroblastic proliferation
- Angiomatoid fibrous histiocytoma
- Follicular dendritic cell sarcoma
- Desmoid-type fibromatosis
- Gastrointestinal stromal tumor
- Inflammatory leiomyosarcoma

Morphologic mimics can be distinguished from IMT by the positive immunoreactivity for specific markers such as CD117, DOG1 and CD34 in GIST, β-catenin in desmoid fibromatosis, CD21, CD35, and D2-40 in dendritic cell sarcoma, and SMA, desmin, and caldesmon in leiomyosarcoma. Positivity for desmin and EMA and the demonstration of *EWSR1* gene rearrangement helps to distinguish angiomatoid fibrous histiocytoma from IMT.

Myxoinflammatory Fibroblastic Sarcoma

Myxoinflammatory fibroblastic sarcoma is a rare, locally aggressive and rarely metastasizing fibroblastic/myofibroblastic neoplasm of adults, typically arising in the subcutaneous

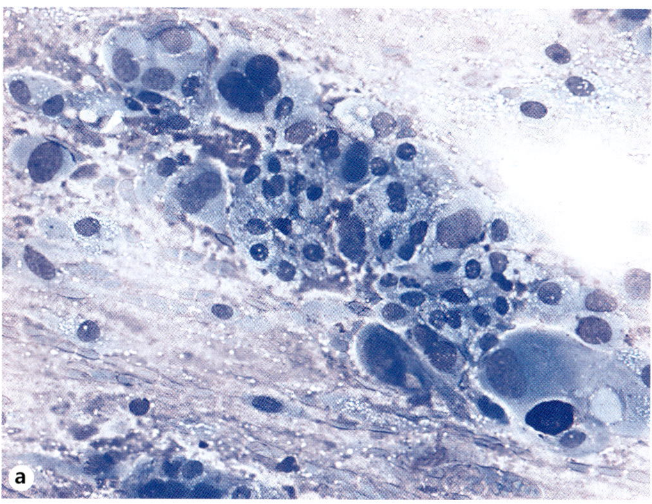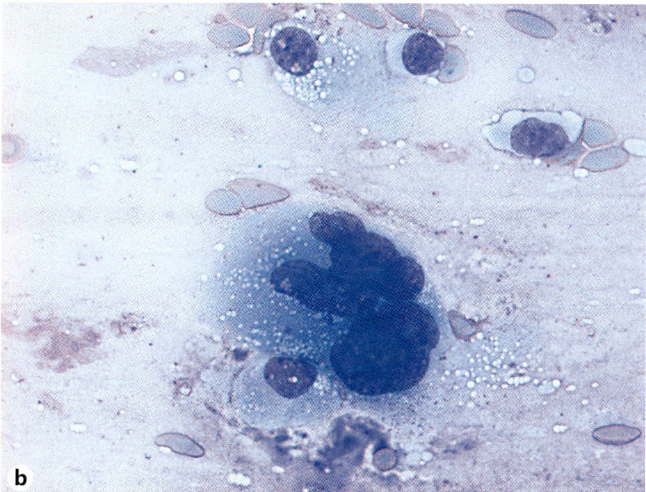

Fig. 11. Myxoinflammatory fibroblastic sarcoma. **a**, **b** FNA smears consist of plump epithelioid cells with abundant cytoplasm and occasional macronucleoli mixed with bizarre virocyte or ganglion-like giant cells and sheets of bland spindle cells in a myxoid matrix. MGG stain.

tissue of the distal (acral) extremities. FNA smears consist of plump epithelioid cells with occasional macronucleoli mixed with sheets and clusters of bland spindle cells in a myxoid matrix with an admixture of inflammatory cells [70–76] (Fig. 11).

Cytologic Features
- Spindled to epithelioid cells with variably prominent nucleoli, nuclear pseudoinclusions
- Bipolar cytoplasmic extensions
- Myxoid background material
- Bizarre virocyte or ganglion-like giant cells
- Large epithelioid cells with occasional lipoblast-like features
- Inflammatory infiltrate with hemosiderin and macrophages

Ancillary Tests
Immunophenotype
Variable positivity for CD34, EMA, CD117, CD68, nuclear INI1, and rare focal keratins.

Genetics
The karyotypes are often complex, heterogeneous, and display a translocation t(1;10)(p22–31;q24–25) with simultaneous loss of 3p material. The functional result of the t(1;10) translocation is the upregulation of the *FGF8* gene, which has oncogenic properties [77]. Theses mutations can be detected by cytogenetics, FISH, and NGS on fresh or fixed material.

Differential Diagnosis
- MFS
- Nodular/proliferative fasciitis

Myxoinflammatory fibroblastic sarcoma should not be confused with benign pseudosarcomatous proliferations such as nodular and proliferative fasciitis or with myxoid sarcomas such as MFS. Immunocytochemical examinations are of limited value while clinical presentation and cytomorphologic features of potential mimics helps in the rendering of a correct diagnosis. The majority of MFS arise in the subcutaneous tissues versus deep soft tissues of limbs and limb girdles, and rarely on the trunk and head and neck region of older adults. Smears from MFS lack bizarre virocytes or a prominent inflammatory infiltrate. Nodular and proliferative fasciitis present most often as a rapidly growing, self-limited proliferation that typically arises in the subcutaneous tissues of the upper extremities, trunk, and head and neck.

Infantile Fibrosarcoma

Infantile fibrosarcoma is a rarely metastasizing, locally infiltrative fibroblastic sarcoma of intermediate malignancy arising in infants before the age of 3 years and in approximately 50% of cases as a congenital neoplasm. The most common location is in the superficial and deep soft tissue of extremities (especially distal extremities) followed by the trunk and head and neck area. The clinical presentation is

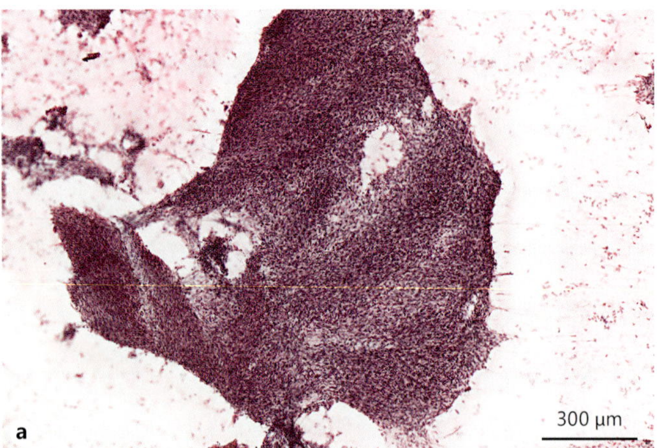 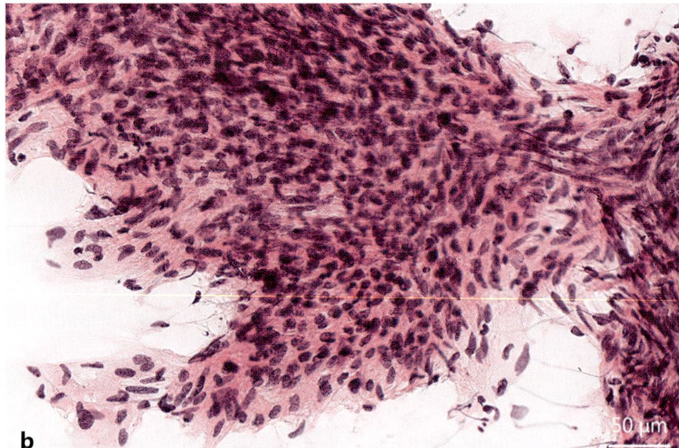

Fig. 12. Infantile fibrosarcoma. **a**, **b** Tight 3-dimensional clusters and fascicles of slight to moderate pleomorphic spindle cells.

usually of a solitary, fast-growing, nontender, and large mass. The main histologic features are fibroblast-like cells with moderate atypia arranged in tight fascicles and often numerous mitoses. Foci of myxoid stroma, areas of round cells, and a hemangiopericytoma-like vascular pattern may be seen. FNA smears show tight clusters and fascicles of slight to moderate pleomorphic spindle cells (Fig. 12).

Cytologic Features
- Cellular aspirate
- Tight clusters and fascicles of slightly to moderate pleomorphic spindle cells
- Spindle cells with bland nuclei
- Numerous mitoses

Ancillary Tests
Immunophenotype
Variable focal positivity for CD34 and SMA. Negative for desmin, myogenin, S100, and keratins.

Genetics
The majority of infantile fibrosarcomas display a t(12;15)(p13;q25) chromosomal translocation resulting in the *ETV6-NTRK3* gene fusion, which produces an oncogenic protein acting as a tyrosine kinase and influencing signaling cascades [78]. This can be readily detected by cytogenetics, FISH, PCR, and NGS on fresh or fixed material.

Differential Diagnosis
- Fibrous hamartoma of infancy
- Embryonal rhabdomyosarcoma

The spindle cell population in smears from infantile fibrosarcoma and from fibrous hamartoma of infancy may show similar features. In addition, an occasionally seen mixture of spindle and round cells in aspirates may give a false impression of embryonal rhabdomyosarcoma. A distinctive *ETV6-NTRK3* gene fusion and negative reactivity for desmin, myogenin, and MyoD-1 helps to establish the correct diagnosis.

Adult Fibrosarcoma

Adult fibrosarcoma, once considered the most common sarcoma in adults, is now a rare diagnosis of exclusion. Cases of monophasic synovial sarcoma and malignant peripheral nerve sheath tumor were notoriously labelled fibrosarcoma before the era of ancillary techniques. Adult fibrosarcoma arises commonly in the deep soft tissue of the proximal extremities, trunk, and head and neck region of adults. The neoplastic cells are often arranged in tightly cohesive clusters and fascicles resemble fibroblasts with a slight to moderate degree of atypia. Smears usually contain a minor component of dispersed spindle cells and naked spindle-shaped nuclei.

Cytologic Features
- Spindle cells arranged in tight clusters, fascicles, or as dispersed cells
- Slight to moderate cellular and nuclear atypia
- Stripped nuclei are common findings

Ancillary Tests
Immunophenotype
Positive for vimentin and focal SMA. Negative for other markers.

Genetics
Genetically, adult fibrosarcoma display both structural and numerical chromosomal changes but no specific characteristic abnormalities [79]. However, a small subset of superficial fibrosarcomas show the same genetic alternations (*PDGRFB1-COL1AI* fusion gene transcripts) as DFSP [80]. These genetic changes can be detected with cytogenetics, FISH, SNP array, PCR, and NGS on available material.

Differential Diagnosis
- Desmoid fibromatosis
- SFT
- Synovial sarcoma
- Malignant peripheral nerve sheath tumor
- Fibrosarcomatous dermatofibrosarcoma protuberans
- Nodular fasciitis
- Dedifferentiated liposarcoma

Adult fibrosarcoma is currently a vanishingly rare entity. It is a diagnosis of exclusion that should be made with extreme caution. Dedifferentiated sarcoma and fibrosarcomatous progression from DFSP should be excluded. Subsets of superficial fibrosarcomas, however, show the same genetic alternations (*PDGRFB1-COL1AI* fusion gene transcripts) as DFSP, indicating the fibrosarcoma variant which arises in DFSP in adults. Adult fibrosarcoma is often diagnosed as a low- or high-grade spindle-cell sarcoma not otherwise specified in FNA smears.

Myxofibrosarcoma

Myxofibrosarcoma (MFS), previously known as myxoid malignant fibrous histiocytoma, is a malignant fibroblastic neoplasm with a variable cellular pleomorphism, myxoid stroma, and prominent curvilinear vascularity. MFS commonly arises in the subcutaneous tissue in the extremities and limb girdles, and rarely in the trunk and head and neck region of elderly patients, but may also arise in the deep, subfascial/intramuscular tissues. Smears of low-grade MFS show variable cellularity but are often hypocellular and characterized by noncohesive slightly to moderately pleomorphic spindled and stellate cells and a prominent myxoid background. It can be difficult to distinguish low-grade MFS from benign myx-

oid lesions such as intramuscular myxoma and myxoid nodular fasciitis. The presence of a moderate nuclear pleomorphism and fragments of curved capillaries in the myxoid matrix are the most important clues to the diagnosis of MFS in FNA smears [81–86] (Fig. 13). High-grade MFS presents a marked cellular and nuclear pleomorphism, including multinucleated bizarre tumor cells. Cells with vacuolated cytoplasm resembling lipoblasts may be observed in smears from both low-grade and high-grade tumors.

Cytologic Features
- Dispersed cells and cell clusters
- Abundant myxoid background
- Fragments of curved vessels embedded in the myxoid matrix
- Slightly to moderately atypical spindle cells in a low-grade neoplasm
- Marked cellular and nuclear pleomorphism in high-grade neoplasm
- Occasional pseudolipoblasts

Ancillary Tests
Immunophenotype
Focally positive for SMA, MSA, and CD34. Negative for MDM2, CDK4, desmin, S100, and keratins.

Genetics
Genetic evaluation display highly complex karyotypes but no specific recurrent mutation has been described [87].

Differential Diagnosis
- Intramuscular myxoma
- Myxoid liposarcoma
- Nodular fasciitis
- LGFMS
- Spindle cell lipoma

Smears from intramuscular myxomas are hypocellular with a predominance of myxoid matrix and scattered small loosely adhesive sheets of bland spindle cells with small uniform nuclei and long cytoplasmic extensions. The nuclear pleomorphism and atypia seen in MFS are absent in smears from intramuscular myxoma. One important cytologic feature which helps to distinguish intramuscular myxoma and nodular fasciitis from MFS is a lack of vessels or only rare single fragments of coarse vessels in the myxoid background. The vascular component of MFS, when present, appears as short segments or curved coarser vessel fragments. Immunocytochemistry is of limited value. S100 protein positivity

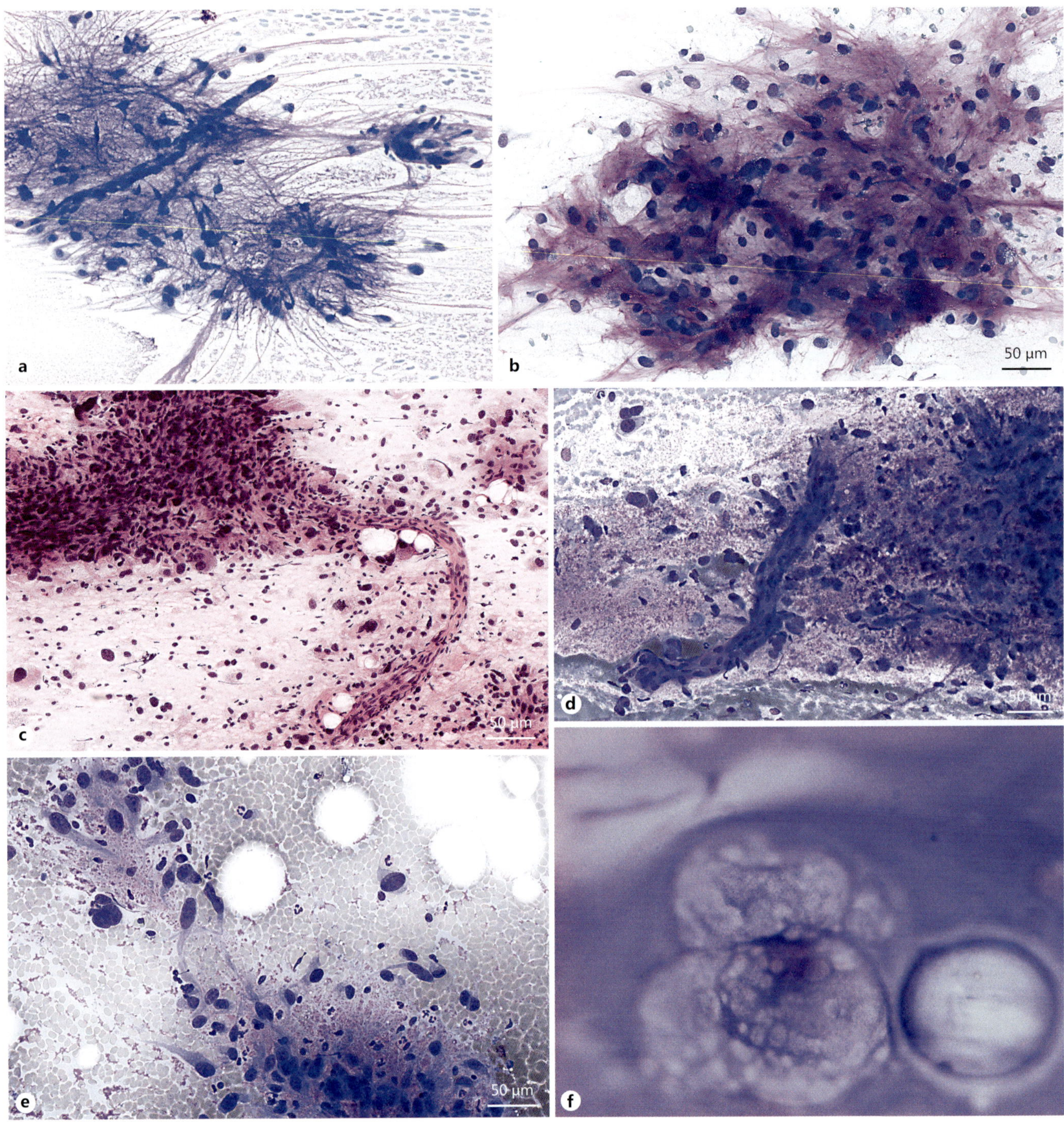

Fig. 13. MFS. **a**, **b** FNA smears from low-grade MFS is characterized by slightly and moderately atypical spindle cells and can be difficult to distinguish from benign myxoid lesions such as intramuscular myxoma and myxoid nodular fasciitis. MGG stain. **c**, **d** The presence of moderate nuclear pleomorphism and fragments of curved capillaries in the myxoid matrix are the most important clues to the diagnosis of MFS in FNA smears. HE and MGG stains. **e**, **f** Marked cellular and nuclear pleomorphism and occasional "pseudolipoblasts" in high-grade MFS.

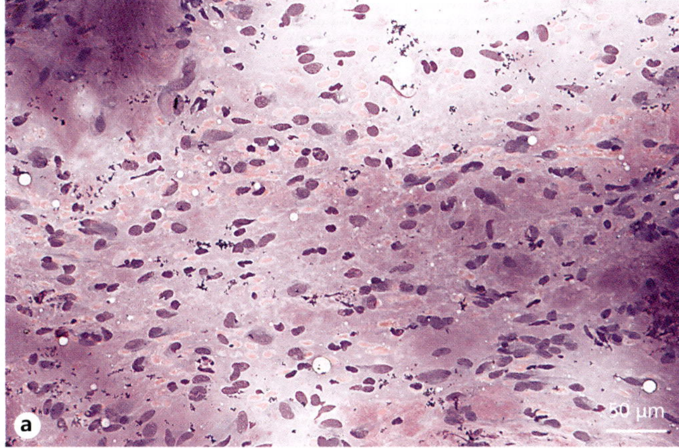

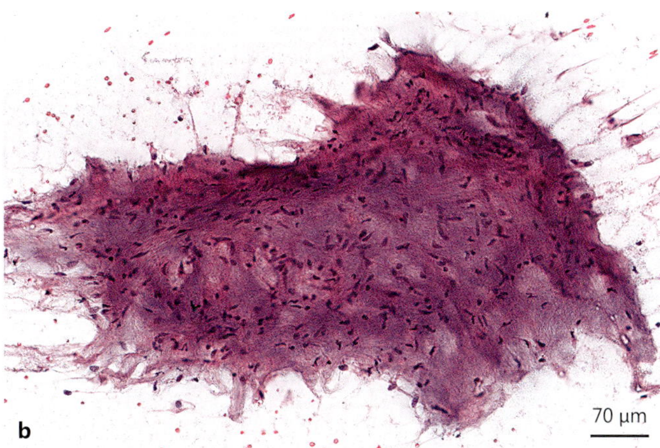

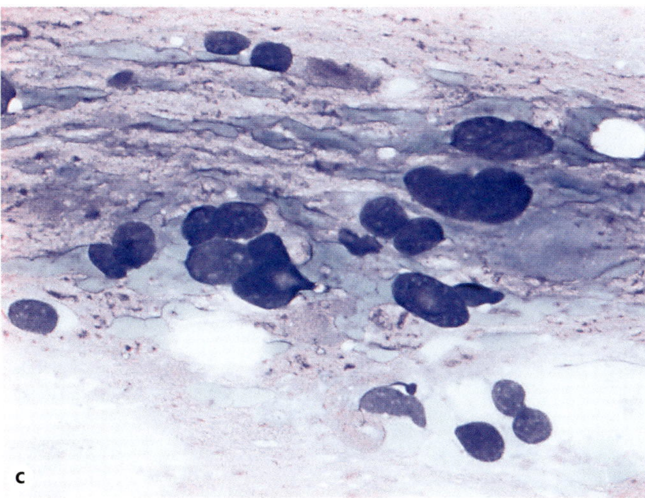

Fig. 14. Low-grade fibromyxoid sarcoma. **a** FNA smears show dispersed slightly/moderately pleomorphic spindle and round/polygonal cells, bare nuclei, and fragments of collagenous matrix in the myxoid background. HE stain. **b** Cluster of loosely cohesive bland spindle cells embedded in the collagenous/myxoid matrix. HE stain. **c** Occasional moderately pleomorphic cells and naked nuclei in the myxoid background. MGG stain.

in lipoblast-like cells is a feature of myxoid liposarcoma. The tumor cells in MFS are focally actin positive and consistently vimentin positive.

Low-Grade Fibromyxoid Sarcoma

Low-grade fibromyxoid sarcoma (LGFMS) is an uncommon, slowly growing, malignant fibroblastic neoplasm related genetically to a subset of sclerosing epithelioid fibrosarcoma. Most LGFMS arise in the deep soft tissues of the extremities and trunk in young adults, but may also occur in other age groups and locations. In both histologic sections and FNA smears, the bland appearance of tumor cells may lead to the misperception of a benign spindle cell or a myxoid lesion. A minority of cases contain foci of increased cellularity with epithelioid morphology and moderate nuclear pleomorphism. Scattered rosette-like structures with a central hyalinized core surrounded by fibroblast-like cells are seen in histologic sections in a subset of cases. FNA smears usually show clusters of bland spindle and round/polygonal cells embedded in a collagenous and myxoid matrix with an admixture of uniform or slightly/moderately pleomorphic spindle cells, bare nuclei, and fragments of collagen and myxoid tissue in varying proportions. [88–90] (Fig. 14). It is very difficult to render a diagnosis of LGFMS based on FNA cytology alone due to the morphologic overlapping with other spindle cell and myxoid lesions. The cytologic features of LGFMS have been described in case reports and in a series of 8 cases [91].

Cytologic Features
- Fascicles/clusters and dispersed cells
- Fibroblast-like spindle cells with slightly atypical nuclei
- Monotonous appearance with occasional mild anisokaryosis
- Naked nuclei are common
- Often abundant myxoid matrix
- Fragments of collagen-rich tissue in the background
- Occasional cells with an epithelioid morphology and moderately pleomorphic nuclei
- Occasional fragments of curvilinear vessels in the myxoid areas

Ancillary Tests
Immunophenotype
Positive for cytoplasmic MUC4, variable positivity for EMA, CD34, SMA, and claudin-1. Negative for β-catenin, desmin, S100, and keratins.

Genetics

In two-thirds of cases, these tumors present a specific t(7;16) (q33;p11) translocation as the only chromosomal change. In another 25% of cases, they display a supernumerary ring chromosome [92, 93]. Both anomalies result in a *FUS-CREB3L2* fusion gene acting as an oncogenic transcription factor [94]. FISH and PCR can detect these anomalies and can be very helpful in diagnosing difficult myxoid tumors. However, cytogenetics, SNP array, and NGS can also be utilized depending on the available material.

Differential Diagnosis
- Intramuscular myxoma
- Schwannoma
- Desmoid-type fibromatosis
- Low-grade MFS
- Soft tissue perineurioma
- DFSP (myxoid variant)

Intramuscular myxoma is usually less cellular in FNA than LGFMS. Positive staining for S100 helps to distinguish schwannoma and positivity for CD34 DFSP from LGFMS. Smears from perineurioma show cytomorphology overlapping LGFMS and molecular genetic techniques are very useful in rendering the correct diagnosis. Due to the myxoid background and the slightly atypical spindle cells in smears, LGFMS may be misdiagnosed as a low-grade MFS. From a clinical point of view this is not a serious pitfall as the treatment (primary wide surgery) is the same in both sarcomas.

References

1 Oh CK, Whang SM, Kim BG, Ko HC, Lee CH, Kim HJ, Kim YW, Kwon KS: Congenital cranial fasciitis – "watch and wait" or early intervention. Pediatr Dermatol 2007;24:263–266.

2 Allison DB, Wakely PE Jr, Siddiqui MT, Ali SZ: Nodular fasciitis: a frequent diagnostic pitfall on fine-needle aspiration. Cancer Cytopathol 2017;125:20–29.

3 Sinhasan SP, Bharathi KV, Bhat RV, Hartimath BC: Intra-muscular nodular fasciitis presenting as swelling in neck: challenging entity for diagnosis. J Clin Diagn Res 2014;8:155–157.

4 Reitzen SD, Dogan S, Har-El G: Nodular fasciitis: a case series. J Laryngol Otol 2009;123:541–544.

5 Kumaran A, Puthenparambath S: Fine-needle aspiration diagnosis of nodular fasciitis: a case report. J Cytol 2016;33:172–174.

6 Kang A, Kumar JB, Thomas A, Bourke AG: A spontaneously resolving breast lesion: imaging and cytological findings of nodular fasciitis of the breast with FISH showing USP6 gene rearrangement. BMJ Case Rep 2015;2015:213076.

7 Gibson TC, Bishop JA, Thompson LD: Parotid gland nodular fasciitis: a clinicopathologic series of 12 cases with a review of 18 cases from the literature. Head Neck Pathol 2015;9:334–344.

8 Sakuma T, Matsuo K, Koike S, Tagami K: Fine needle aspiration cytology of nodular fasciitis of the breast. Diagn Cytopathol 2015;43:222–229.

9 Wong NL: Fine needle aspiration cytology of pseudosarcomatous reactive proliferative lesions of soft tissue. Acta Cytol 2002;46:1049–1055.

10 Matusik J, Wiberg A, Sloboda J, Andersson O: Fine needle aspiration in nodular fasciitis of the face. Cytopathology 2002;13:128–132.

11 Alkan S, Eltoum IA, Tabbara S, Day E, Karcher DS: Usefulness of molecular detection of human herpesvirus-8 in the diagnosis of Kaposi sarcoma by fine-needle aspiration. Am J Clin Pathol 1999;111:91–96.

12 Raab SS, Silverman JF, McLeod DL, Benning TL, Geisinger KR: Fine needle aspiration biopsy of fibromatoses. Acta Cytol 1993;37:323–328.

13 Berry AB, Jaffee I, Greenberg M, Eisele DW, Ljung BM: Nodular fasciitis: definitive diagnosis by fine needle aspiration. Acta Cytol 2016;60:19–24.

14 Antunes SM, Vieira H, Brito A, Oliveira MH: Cervical nodular fasciitis in a 17-month-old child. BMJ Case Rep 2013;2013:3009794.

15 Wong NL, Di F: Pseudosarcomatous fasciitis and myositis: diagnosis by fine-needle aspiration cytology. Am J Clin Pathol 2009;132:857–865.

16 Dodd LG, Martinez S: Fine-needle aspiration cytology of pseudosarcomatous lesions of soft tissue. Diagn Cytopathol 2001;24:28–35.

17 Erickson-Johnson MR, Chou MM, Evers BR, Roth CW, Seys AR, Jin L, Ye Y, Lau AW, Wang X, Oliveira AM: Nodular fasciitis: a novel model of transient neoplasia induced by MYH9-USP6 gene fusion. Lab Invest 2011;91:1427–1433.

18 Oliveira AM, Chou MM: The TRE17/USP6 oncogene: a riddle wrapped in a mystery inside an enigma. Front Biosci 2012;4:321–334.

19 Domanski HA, Akerman M, Rissler P, Gustafson P: Fine-needle aspiration of soft tissue leiomyosarcoma: an analysis of the most common cytologic findings and the value of ancillary techniques. Diagn Cytopathol 2006;34:597–604.

20 Satish S, Shivalingaiah SC, Ravishankar S, Vimalambika MG: Fine needle aspiration cytology of pseudosarcomatous reactive lesions of soft tissues: a report of two cases. J Cytol 2012;29:264–266.

21 Lundgren L, Kindblom LG, Willems J, Falkmer U, Angervall L: Proliferative myositis and fasciitis: a light and electron microscopic, cytologic, DNA-cytometric and immunohistochemical study. APMIS 1992;100:437–448.

22 Ohjimi Y, Iwasaki H, Ishiguro M, Isayama T, Kaneko Y: Trisomy 2 found in proliferative myositis cultured cell. Cancer Genet Cytogenet 1994;76:157.

23 Vincent J, Maleki Z: Elastofibroma: cytomorphologic, histologic, and radiologic findings in five cases. Diagn Cytopathol 2012;40(suppl 2):E99–E103.

24 Vera-Alvarez J, Garcia-Prats MD, Marigil-Gomez M, Abascal-Agorreta M, Lopez-Lopez JI: Elastofibroma dorsi diagnosed by fine needle aspiration cytology. Acta Cytol 2008;52:264–266.

25 Munoz Arias G, Gonzalez-Campora R, Rios Martin JJ, Otal Salaverri C, Martinez Parra D: Elastofibroma: cytologic findings using fine needle aspiration. Acta Cytol 2007;51:497–499.

26 Domanski HA, Carlen B, Sloth M, Rydholm A: Elastofibroma dorsi has distinct cytomorphologic features, making diagnostic surgical biopsy unnecessary: cytomorphologic study with clinical, radiologic, and electron microscopic correlations. Diagn Cytopathol 2003;29:327–333.

27 Harigopal M, Seshan SV, DeLellis RA, Yankelevitz D, Vazquez M: Aspiration cytology of elastofibroma dorsi: case report with ultrastructural and immunohistochemical findings. Diagn Cytopathol 2002;26:310–313.

28 Mojica WD, Kuntzman T: Elastofibroma dorsi: elaboration of cytologic features and review of its pathogenesis. Diagn Cytopathol 2000;23:393–396.

29 Pisharodi LR, Cary D, Bernacki EG Jr: Elastofibroma dorsi: diagnostic problems and pitfalls. Diagn Cytopathol 1994;10:242–244.

30 Nakamura Y, Ohta Y, Itoh S, Haratake A, Nakano Y, Umeda A, Shima H, Tomoda N: Elastofibroma dorsi: cytologic, histologic, immunohistochemical and ultrastructural studies. Acta Cytol 1992;36: 559–562.

31 Nishio JN, Iwasaki H, Ohjimi Y, Ishiguro M, Koga T, Isayama T, Naito M, Kikuchi M: Gain of Xq detected by comparative genomic hybridization in elastofibroma. Int J Mol Med 2002;10:277–280.

32 Gupta R, Singh S: Cytologic diagnosis of fibrous hamartoma of infancy: a case report of a rare soft tissue lesion. Acta Cytol 2008;52:201–203.

33 Mohanty SK, Dey P: Cytologic diagnosis of fibrous hamartoma of infancy: a case report. Diagn Cytopathol 2003;28:272–273.

34 Jadusingh IH: Fine needle aspiration cytology of fibrous hamartoma of infancy. Acta Cytol 1997; 41:1391–1393.

35 Tassano E, Nozza P, Tavella E, Garaventa A, Panarello C, Morerio C: Cytogenetic characterization of a fibrous hamartoma of infancy with complex translocations. Cancer Genet Cytogenet 2010;201: 66–69.

36 Kurtycz DF, Logrono R, Hoerl HD, Heatley DG: Diagnosis of fibromatosis colli by fine-needle aspiration. Diagn Cytopathol 2000;23:338–342.

37 Owens CL, Sharma R, Ali SZ: Deep fibromatosis (desmoid tumor): cytopathologic characteristics, clinicoradiologic features, and immunohistochemical findings on fine-needle aspiration. Cancer 2007;111:166–172.

38 Dalen BP, Meis-Kindblom JM, Sumathi VP, Ryd W, Kindblom LG: Fine-needle aspiration cytology and core needle biopsy in the preoperative diagnosis of desmoid tumors. Acta Orthop 2006;77: 926–931.

39 Rege TA, Madan R, Qian X: Long fascicular tissue fragments in desmoid fibromatosis by fine needle aspiration: a new cytologic feature. Diagn Cytopathol 2012;40:45–47.

40 Fletcher JA, Naeem R, Xiao S, Corson JM: Chromosome aberrations in desmoid tumors. Trisomy 8 may be a predictor of recurrence. Cancer Genet Cytogenet 1995;79:139–143.

41 Goyal P, Sehgal S, Singh S, Rastogi S: Dermatofibrosarcoma protuberans in a child: a case report. Case Rep Dermatol Med 2012, 2012:796818.

42 Kim L, Park IS, Han JY, Kim JM, Chu YC: Aspiration cytology of fibrosarcomatous variant of dermatofibrosarcoma protuberans with osteoclast-like giant cells in the chest wall: a case report. Acta Cytol 2005;49:644–649.

43 Tsang AK, Wong FC, Ng PW, Loke SL, Tse GM: Fine needle aspiration cytology of dermatofibrosarcoma protuberans in the breast: a case report. Pathology 2005;37:84–86.

44 Domanski HA: FNA diagnosis of dermatofibrosarcoma protuberans. Diagn Cytopathol 2005;32: 299–302.

45 Klijanienko J, Caillaud JM, Lagace R: Fine-needle aspiration of primary and recurrent dermatofibrosarcoma protuberans. Diagn Cytopathol 2004; 30:261–265.

46 Domanski HA, Gustafson P: Cytologic features of primary, recurrent, and metastatic dermatofibrosarcoma protuberans. Cancer 2002;96:351–361.

47 Zee SY, Wang Q, Jones CM, Abadi MA: Fine needle aspiration cytology of dermatofibrosarcoma protuberans presenting as a breast mass: a case report. Acta Cytol 2002;46:741–743.

48 Fukushima H, Suda K, Matsuda M, Tanaka R, Kita H, Hanaoka T, Goya T: A case of dermatofibrosarcoma protuberans in the skin over the breast of a young woman. Breast Cancer 1998;5:407–409.

49 Powers CN, Berardo MD, Frable WJ: Fine-needle aspiration biopsy: pitfalls in the diagnosis of spindle-cell lesions. Diagn Cytopathol 1994;10:232–240; discussion 241.

50 Powers CN, Hurt MA, Frable WJ: Fine-needle aspiration biopsy: dermatofibrosarcoma protuberans. Diagn Cytopathol 1993;9:145–150.

51 Kocjan G, Sams V, Davidson T: Dermatofibrosarcoma protuberans as a diagnostic pitfall in fine-needle aspiration diagnosis of angiosarcoma of the breast. Diagn Cytopathol 1996;14:94–95.

52 Simon MP, Navarro M, Roux D, Pouyssegur J: Structural and functional analysis of a chimeric protein COL1A1-PDGFB generated by the translocation t(17;22)(q22;q13.1) in dermatofibrosarcoma protuberans (DP). Oncogene 2001;20:2965–2975.

53 Patel KU, Szabo SS, Hernandez VS, Prieto VG, Abruzzo LV, Lazar AJ, Lopez-Terrada D: Dermatofibrosarcoma protuberans COL1A1-PDGFB fusion is identified in virtually all dermatofibrosarcoma protuberans cases when investigated by newly developed multiplex reverse transcription polymerase chain reaction and fluorescence in situ hybridization assays. Hum Pathol 2008;39: 184–193.

54 Khairwa A, Dey P, Nada R: Fine needle aspiration cytology of malignant solitary fibrous tumour. Cytopathology 2015;26:391–393.

55 Gupta N, Banik T, Rajwanshi A, Radotra BD, Panda N, Dey P, Srinivasan R, Nijhawan R: Fine-needle aspiration cytology of oral and oropharyngeal lesions with an emphasis on the diagnostic utility and pitfalls. J Cancer Res Ther 2012;8:626–629.

56 Gupta N, Barwad A, Katamuthu K, Rajwanshi A, Radotra BD, Nijhawan R, Dey P: Solitary fibrous tumour: a diagnostic challenge for the cytopathologist. Cytopathology 2012;23:250–255.

57 Bean SM, Baker A, Eloubeidi M, Eltoum I, Jhala N, Crowe R, Jhala D, Chhieng DC: Endoscopic ultrasound-guided fine-needle aspiration of intrathoracic and intra-abdominal spindle cell and mesenchymal lesions. Cancer Cytopathol 2011;119: 37–48.

58 Srinivasan VD, Wayne JD, Rao MS, Zynger DL: Solitary fibrous tumor of the pancreas: case report with cytologic and surgical pathology correlation and review of the literature. JOP 2008;9:526–530.

59 Schmitz S, Weynand B, Lengele B, Hamoir M: Solitary fibrous tumour of the soft tissue of the face: a case report. B-ENT 2006;2:201–204.

60 Wiriosuparto S, Krassilnik N, Bhuta S, Rao J, Firschowitz S: Solitary fibrous tumor: report of a case with an unusual presentation as a spindle cell parotid neoplasm. Acta Cytol 2005;49:309–313.

61 Gerhard R, Fregnani ER, Falzoni R, Siqueira SA, Vargas PA: Cytologic features of solitary fibrous tumor of the parotid gland: a case report. Acta Cytol 2004;48:402–406.

62 Parwani AV, Galindo R, Steinberg DM, Zeiger MA, Westra WH, Ali SZ: Solitary fibrous tumor of the thyroid: cytopathologic findings and differential diagnosis. Diagn Cytopathol 2003;28:213–216.

63 Clayton AC, Salomao DR, Keeney GL, Nascimento AG: Solitary fibrous tumor: a study of cytologic features of six cases diagnosed by fine-needle aspiration. Diagn Cytopathol 2001;25:172–166.

64 Drachenberg CB, Bourquin PM, Cochran LM, Burke KC, Kumar D, White CS, Papadimitriou JC: Fine needle aspiration biopsy of solitary fibrous tumors: report of two cases with histologic, immunohistochemical and ultrastructural correlation. Acta Cytol 1998;42:1003–1010.

65 Ali SZ, Hoon V, Hoda S, Heelan R, Zakowski MF: Solitary fibrous tumor: a cytologic-histologic study with clinical, radiologic, and immunohistochemical correlations. Cancer 1997;81:116–121.

66 Torabi A, Lele SM, DiMaio D, Pinnt JC, Hess MM, Nelson M, Bridge JA: Lack of a common or characteristic cytogenetic anomaly in solitary fibrous tumor. Cancer Genet Cytogenet 2008;181:60–64.

67 Domanski HA: Fine-needle aspiration smears from lipomatous hemangiopericytoma need not be confused with myxoid liposarcoma. Diagn Cytopathol 2003;29:287–291.

68 Bridge JA, Kanamori M, Ma Z, Pickering D, Hill DA, Lydiatt W, Lui MY, Colleoni GW, Antonescu CR, Ladanyi M, Morris SW: Fusion of the ALK gene to the clathrin heavy chain gene, CLTC, in inflammatory myofibroblastic tumor. Am J Pathol 2001;159:411–415.

69 Lawrence B, Perez-Atayde A, Hibbard MK, Rubin BP, Dal Cin P, Pinkus JL, Pinkus GS, Xiao S, Yi ES, Fletcher CD, Fletcher JA: TPM3-ALK and TPM4-ALK oncogenes in inflammatory myofibroblastic tumors. Am J Pathol 2000;157:377–384.

70 Toll AD, Wakely PE Jr, Ali SZ: Acral myxoinflammatory fibroblastic sarcoma: cytopathologic findings on fine-needle aspiration. Acta Cytol 2013;57: 134–138.

71 Alaggio R, Coffin CM, Dall'igna P, Bisogno G, Olivotto A, Di Venosa B, Fassina A: Myxoinflammatory fibroblastic sarcoma: report of a case and review of the literature. Pediatr Dev Pathol 2012; 15:254–258.

72 Wickham MQ, Youens KE, Dodd LG: Acral myxoinflammatory fibroblastic sarcoma fine needle aspiration: a case report. Diagn Cytopathol 2012; 40(suppl 2):E144–E148.

73 Khadilkar NP, Rao PS: Cytological diagnosis of myxoinflammatory fibroblastic sarcoma: a case report and discussion of differential diagnosis. Kathmandu Univ Med J 2006;4:235–237.

74 Gonzalez-Campora R, Rios-Martin JJ, Solorzano-Amoretti A, Vargas de los Monteros MT, Trigo-Sanchez I, Otal-Salaverri C, Galera-Davidson H: Fine needle aspiration cytology of an acral myxoinflammatory fibroblastic sarcoma: case report with cytological and cytogenetic findings. Cytopathology 2008;19:118–123.

75 Garcia-Garcia E, Rodriguez-Gil Y, Suarez-Gauthier A, Martinez-Tello FJ, Lopez-Rios F, Ballestin C: Myxoinflammatory fibroblastic sarcoma: report of a case with fine needle aspiration cytology. Acta Cytol 2007;51:231–234.

76 Pohar-Marinsek Z, Flezar M, Lamovec J: Acral myxoinflammatory fibroblastic sarcoma in FNAB samples: can we distinguish it from other myxoid lesions? Cytopathology 2003;14:73–78.

77 Hallor KH, Sciot R, Staaf J, Heidenblad M, Rydholm A, Bauer HC, Astrom K, Domanski HA, Meis JM, Kindblom LG, Panagopoulos I, Mandahl N, Mertens F: Two genetic pathways, t(1;10) and amplification of 3p11–12, in myxoinflammatory fibroblastic sarcoma, haemosiderotic fibrolipomatous tumour, and morphologically similar lesions. J Pathol 2009;217:716–727.

78 Knezevich SR, McFadden DE, Tao W, Lim JF, Sorensen PH: A novel ETV6-NTRK3 gene fusion in congenital fibrosarcoma. Nat Genet 1998;18:184–187.

79 Dal Cin P, Pauwels P, Sciot R, Van den Berghe H: Multiple chromosome rearrangements in a fibrosarcoma. Cancer Genet Cytogenet 1996;87:176–178.

80 Sheng WQ, Hashimoto H, Okamoto S, Ishida T, Meis-Kindblom JM, Kindblom LG, Hisaoka M: Expression of COL1A1-PDGFB fusion transcripts in superficial adult fibrosarcoma suggests a close relationship to dermatofibrosarcoma protuberans. J Pathol 2001;194:88–94.

81 Olson MT, Ali SZ: Myxofibrosarcoma: cytomorphologic findings and differential diagnosis on fine needle aspiration. Acta Cytol 2012;56:15–24.

82 Colin P, Lagace R, Caillaud JM, Sastre-Garau X, Klijanienko J: Fine-needle aspiration in myxofibrosarcoma: experience of Institut Curie. Diagn Cytopathol 2010;38:343–346.

83 Wong NL, Di F: Fine needle aspiration cytology of myxoid lesions of soft tissues: a study of 24 cases (in Chinese). Zhonghua Bing Li Xue Za Zhi 2007; 36:619–623.

84 Kilpatrick SE, Ward WG, Bos GD: The value of fine-needle aspiration biopsy in the differential diagnosis of adult myxoid sarcoma. Cancer 2000; 90:167–177.

85 Kilpatrick SE, Ward WG: Myxofibrosarcoma of soft tissues: cytomorphologic analysis of a series. Diagn Cytopathol 1999;20:6–9.

86 Merck C, Hagmar B: Myxofibrosarcoma: a correlative cytologic and histologic study of 13 cases examined by fine needle aspiration cytology. Acta Cytol 1980;24:137–144.

87 Willems SM, Debiec-Rychter M, Szuhai K, Hogendoorn PC, Sciot R: Local recurrence of myxofibrosarcoma is associated with increase in tumour grade and cytogenetic aberrations, suggesting a multistep tumour progression model. Mod Pathol 2006;19:407–416.

88 Dawamneh MF, Amra NK, Amr SS: Low grade fibromyxoid sarcoma: report of a case with fine needle aspiration cytology and histologic correlation. Acta Cytol 2006;50:208–212.

89 Lindberg GM, Maitra A, Gokaslan ST, Saboorian MH, Albores-Saavedra J: Low grade fibromyxoid sarcoma: fine-needle aspiration cytology with histologic, cytogenetic, immunohistochemical, and ultrastructural correlation. Cancer 1999;87:75–82.

90 Estrada Villasenor EG, Delgado Cedillo EA, Linares Gonzalez LM, Rico Martinez G: Fine needle aspiration cytology of low grade fibromyxoid sarcoma: report of a case with histologic correlation. Acta Cytol 2004;48:69–72.

91 Domanski HA, Mertens F, Panagopoulos I, Akerman M: Low-grade fibromyxoid sarcoma is difficult to diagnose by fine needle aspiration cytology: a cytomorphological study of eight cases. Cytopathology 2009;20:304–314.

92 Mezzelani A, Sozzi G, Nessling M, Riva C, Della Torre G, Testi MA, Azzarelli A, Pierotti MA, Lichter P, Pilotti S: Low grade fibromyxoid sarcoma. a further low-grade soft tissue malignancy characterized by a ring chromosome. Cancer Genet Cytogenet 2000;122:144–148.

93 Storlazzi CT, Mertens F, Nascimento A, Isaksson M, Wejde J, Brosjo O, Mandahl N, Panagopoulos I: Fusion of the FUS and BBF2H7 genes in low grade fibromyxoid sarcoma. Hum Mol Genet 2003;12:2349–2358.

94 Moller E, Hornick JL, Magnusson L, Veerla S, Domanski HA, Mertens F: FUS-CREB3L2/L1-positive sarcomas show a specific gene expression profile with upregulation of CD24 and FOXL1. Clin Cancer Res 2011;17:2646–2656.

Domanski HA, Walther CS: FNA Cytology of Soft Tissue and Bone Tumors. Monogr Clin Cytol.
Basel, Karger, 2017, vol 22, pp 61–63 (DOI: 10.1159/000475095)

So-Called Fibrohistiocytic Tumors

Tenosynovial Giant Cell Tumor of Localized and Diffuse Type

The localized and diffuse types of tenosynovial giant cell tumor share a common pathogenesis and a similar morphology but differ in their growth patterns, clinical features, and biologic behaviors. Both neoplasms can be intra- or extra-articular. The localized type (giant cell tumor of tendon sheath) is a relatively common neoplasm of the digits with a female predominance. It is a painless, slowly growing, well-circumscribed tumor, usually smaller than 4 cm in size. The diffuse type (pigmented villonodular tenosynovitis) is a locally aggressive neoplasm affecting mainly the knee and hip followed by ankle, elbow, shoulder, and wrist, most commonly in younger patients. It presents as an ill-defined, peri-articular mass, often larger than 5 cm. Both neoplasms are composed of mononuclear cells with round to oval nuclei, admixed with osteoclast-like giant cells, xanthoma cells, and siderophages, embedded in a collagenous, occasionally hyalinized matrix. All these components can be seen in the FNA smears from both subtypes of tenosynovial giant cell tumors [1–5] (Fig. 1).

Cytologic Features
- Variable yield but most often hypercellular smears, limited yield in tumors with hyalinized stroma
- Dissociated and clustered mononuclear histiocytoid cells with round to oval nuclei (sometimes plasma cell-like)
- Mild to moderate cellular and nuclear pleomorphism
- Osteoclast-like giant cells
- Xanthomatous histiocytes and siderophages
- Mitoses may be found

Ancillary Tests
Immunophenotype
Positive for CD68 (histiocytes), CD68, and CD45 (osteoclast-like giant cells); scattered cells are occasionally positive for desmin.

Genetics
These tumors can display simple structural aberrations on cytogenetic examination often involving chromosome 1 and the CSF1 gene. These aberrations are only seen in a few of the tumor cells and frequently involve a translocation with chromosome 2, resulting in the upregulation of the CSF1 expression. This in turn attracts macrophages to the tumor [6]. The genetic change can be detected by cytogenetics, FISH, PCR, and consequently NGS (next-generation sequencing), on fresh and fixated material.

Differential Diagnosis
- Deep benign fibrous histiocytoma
- Reactive synovial hyperplasia
- Giant cell-rich sarcoma

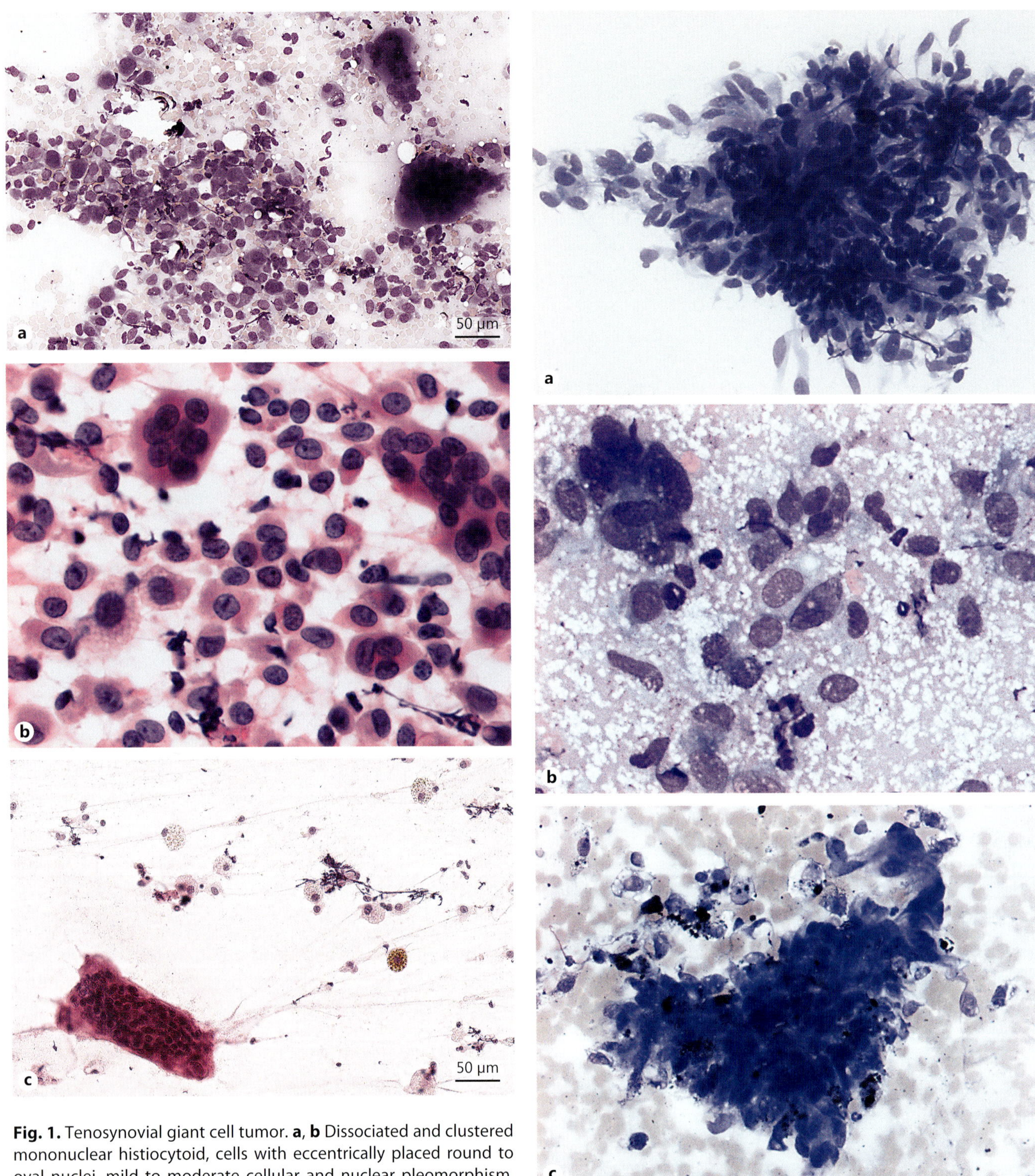

Fig. 1. Tenosynovial giant cell tumor. **a**, **b** Dissociated and clustered mononuclear histiocytoid, cells with eccentrically placed round to oval nuclei, mild to moderate cellular and nuclear pleomorphism, and an admixture of osteoclast-like giant cells. MGG and HE stains. **c** A giant cell, xanthomatous histiocytes, and siderophages. HE stain.

Fig. 2. Benign fibrous histiocytoma. Clustered fibroblasts (**a**) and dispersed cells with a poorly preserved multinucleated histiocytic cell consistent with a Touton giant cell (**b**). MGG stain. **c** Cluster of spindle cells with an admixture of xanthomatous histiocytes containing intracytoplasmic hemosiderin pigment. MGG stain.

Benign Fibrous Histiocytoma

Fibrous histiocytoma commonly arises in the skin of extremities in adults, but may arise in any other location and at any age. A subset of fibrous histiocytomas, most often of a cellular subtype, may be large and deeply penetrating tumors that recur in up to a third of cases. FNA smears show variable cellularity and commonly dispersed and clustered fibroblasts and mononuclear histiocytes with an admixture of fragments of collagenous tissue, hemosiderin-loaded histiocytic cells, and occasional Touton giant cells [7].

Cytologic Features
- Variable yield
- Dispersed and clustered fibroblasts and mononuclear histiocytes
- Fragments of collagenous tissue
- Xanthomatous histiocytes, often with hemosiderin pigment
- Multinucleated histiocytes consistent with Touton giant cells (Fig. 2)

Ancillary Tests
Immunophenotype
Focal SMA and variable focal CD34 positivity. Negative for desmin and epithelial membrane antigen (EMA).

Genetics
No diagnostic recurrent changes are known. A clonal t(16;17)(p13.3;q21.3) has been reported in 1 case [8].

Differential Diagnosis
- Dermatofibrosarcoma protuberans
- Juvenile xanthogranuloma
- Tenosynovial giant cell tumor of localized type

References

1 Abdou AG, Aiad H, Youssef Asaad N: Fine needle aspiration cytology of chondroid tenosynovial giant cell tumor of the hand. Rare Tumors 2015;7: 5814.
2 Gong ZC, Lin ZQ, Moming A, Ling B, Liu H, Hu M, Long X: Extra-articular diffuse tenosynovial giant cell tumour of the infratemporal fossa: report of a case and literature review. Int J Oral Maxillofac Surg 2010;39:820–824.
3 Choudhury M, Jain R, Nangia A, Logani KB: Localized tenosynovial giant cell tumor of tendon sheath: a case report. Acta Cytol 2000;44:463–466.
4 Layfield LJ, Moffatt EJ, Dodd LG, Scully SP, Harrelson JM: Cytologic findings in tenosynovial giant cell tumors investigated by fine-needle aspiration cytology. Diagn Cytopathol 1997;16:317–325.
5 Gonzalez-Campora R, Salas Herrero E, Otal-Salaverri CV-RJL, San Martin Diez V, Hevia Vazquez A, Galera Davidson H: Diffuse tenosynovial giant cell tumor of soft tissues: report of a case with cytologic and cytogenetic findings. Acta Cytol 1995;39:770–776.
6 West RB, Rubin BP, Miller MA, Subramanian S, Kaygusuz G, Montgomery K, Zhu S, Marinelli RJ, De Luca A, Downs-Kelly E, Goldblum JR, Corless CL, Brown PO, Gilks CB, Nielsen TO, Huntsman D, van de Rijn M: A landscape effect in tenosynovial giant-cell tumor from activation of CSF1 expression by a translocation in a minority of tumor cells. Proc Natl Acad Sci USA 2006;103:690–695.
7 Klijanienko J, Caillaud JM, Lagace R: Fine-needle aspiration of primary and recurrent benign fibrous histiocytoma: classic, aneurysmal, and myxoid variants. Diagn Cytopathol 2004;31:387–391.
8 Frau DV, Erdas E, Caria P, Ambu R, Dettori T, Faa G, Fletcher CD, Vanni R: Deep fibrous histiocytoma with a clonal karyotypic alteration: molecular cytogenetic characterization of a t(16;17) (p13.3;q21.3). Cancer Genet Cytogenet 2010;202: 17–21.

Domanski HA, Walther CS: FNA Cytology of Soft Tissue and Bone Tumors. Monogr Clin Cytol.
Basel, Karger, 2017, vol 22, pp 64–67 (DOI: 10.1159/000475096)

Smooth-Muscle Tumors

Leiomyoma of Deep Soft Tissue

Leiomyoma of deep soft tissue is a rare, slowly growing, well-circumscribed benign neoplasm, commonly arising in the deep soft tissue of the extremities or retroperitoneum, and different parts of the abdominal cavity (in this location there is a strong predominance of female patients). Tumor cells in aspirates have morphology reminiscent of normal smooth muscle and myofibroblastic cells. An important diagnostic pitfall is low-grade leiomyosarcoma (LMS), which displays more nuclear pleomorphism and coarser chromatin than leiomyoma.

Cytologic Features
- A mixture of clustered and dispersed, bland-looking spindle cells
- Elongated, blunt-ended, cigar-shaped, occasionally truncated nuclei with insignificant nucleoli
- Collagenous matrix may be seen in the cell clusters
- Occasional mild cellular pleomorphism
- Some cells display a gray or blue-gray cytoplasm with cytoplasmic extensions
- No mitotic figures

Ancillary Tests
Immunophenotype
Positive for smooth muscle actin (SMA), muscle-specific actin (MSA), desmin, rarely focal keratins, and occasionally estrogen receptor in abdominal/pelvic leiomyomas.

Genetics
No known recurrent genetic changes.

Differential Diagnosis
- Extra-abdominal desmoid fibromatosis
- Low-grade LMS
- Gastrointestinal stromal tumor, spindle-cell type
- Schwannoma
- Low-grade malignant peripheral nerve sheath tumor
- Monophasic synovial sarcoma

Leiomyosarcoma

As one of the most common soft tissue sarcomas in adults, LMS accounts for approximately 10% of all primary soft tissue sarcomas. Soft tissue LMS occurs most often in the retroperitoneum and limbs, but also in other locations such as visceral organs and bones. The site of origin is an important prognostic factor, as pure cutaneous LMS most often shows an indolent clinical course, whereas superficial or deep soft tissue or retroperitoneal/intra-abdominal LMS displays aggressive behavior with a high risk of metastasis. LMS smears are usually richly or moderately cellular and show distinctive cytoarchtectural patterns on low-power microscopy – in most cases, a characteristic fascicular/spindle cell/pleomorphic pattern (Fig. 1). Typical tumor cells have elongated, cigar-shaped nuclei, sometimes segmented "in tandem," but an admixture of rounded/polygonal cells is often seen in

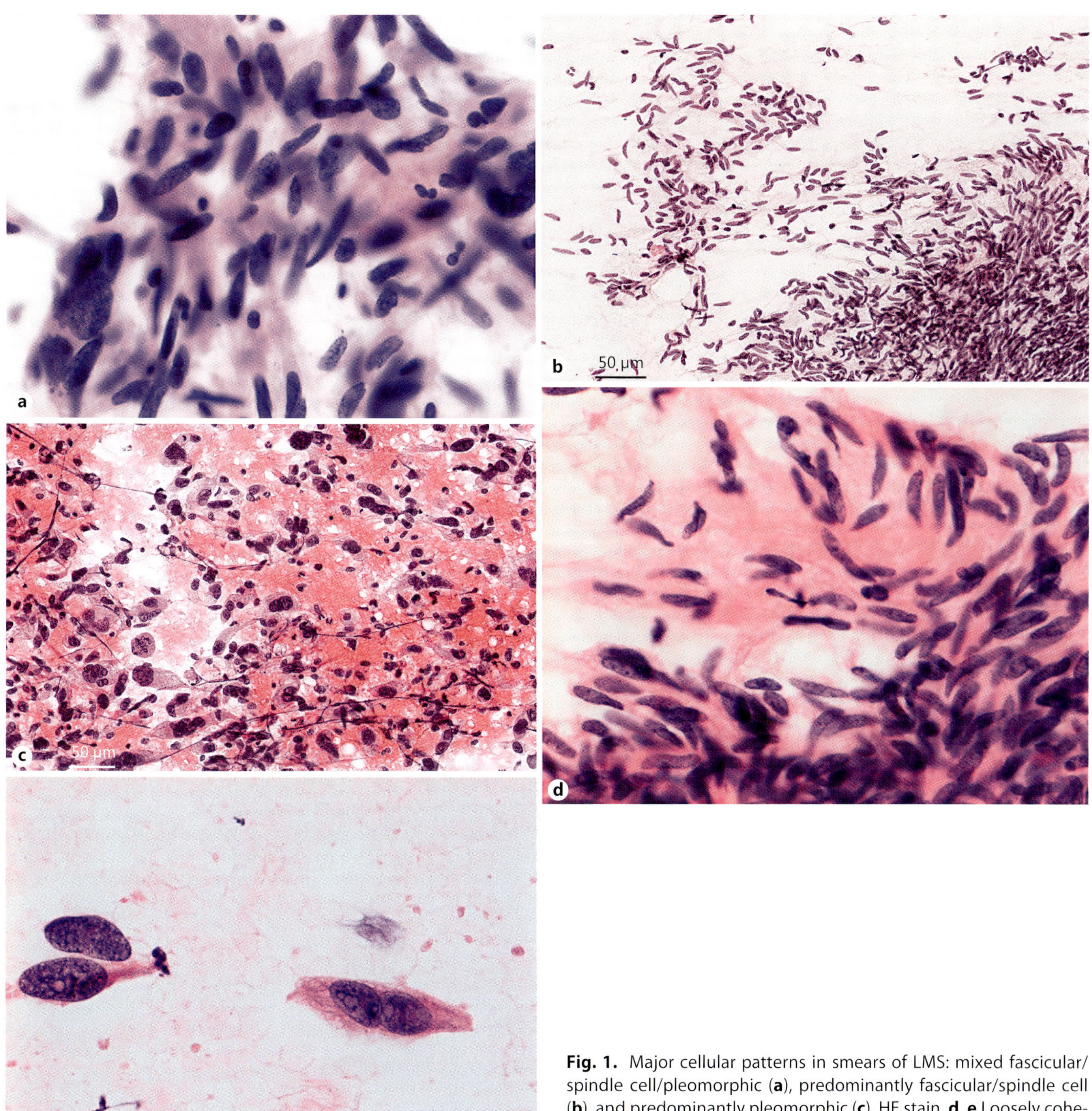

Fig. 1. Major cellular patterns in smears of LMS: mixed fascicular/spindle cell/pleomorphic (**a**), predominantly fascicular/spindle cell (**b**), and predominantly pleomorphic (**c**). HE stain. **d**, **e** Loosely cohesive clusters and dispersed, moderately pleomorphic spindle cells with elongated cigar-shaped, occasionally truncated or "in tandem" position of nuclei, and cytoplasmic extensions. HE stain.

smears. Both spindle cells and rounded/polygonal cells may contain segmented or indented nuclei and occasionally intranuclear vacuoles. In high-grade LMS, the presence of a marked cellular atypia, pleomorphism, necrosis, and multinucleated giant cells, both multinucleated tumor cells and osteoclast-like giant cells, is common [1–4] (Fig. 1, 2). A pure fascicular/spindle cell or epithelioid pattern is less common. The cytomorphology of an uncommon epithelioid variant of LMS can be misinterpreted as carcinoma metastasis.

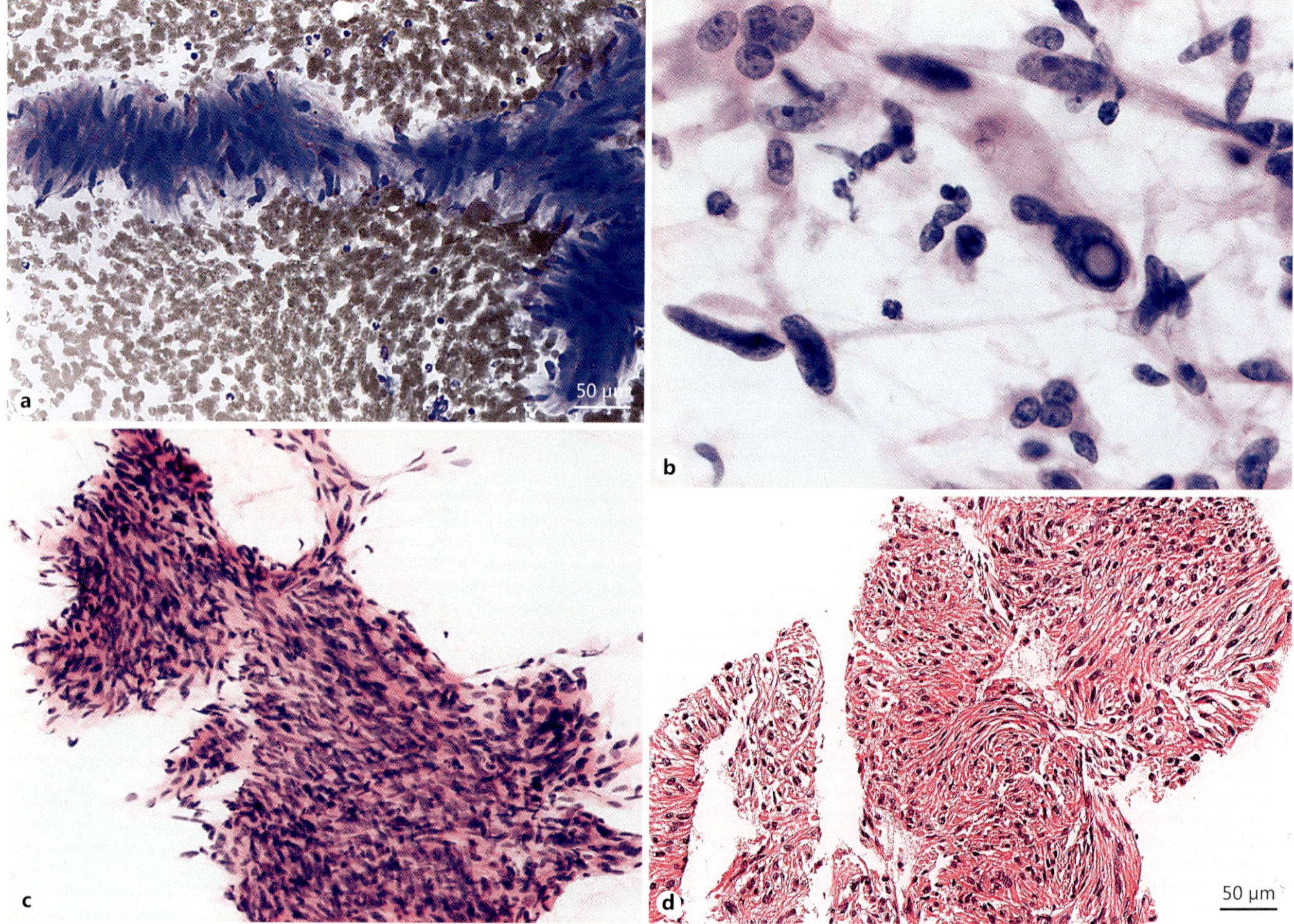

Fig. 2. LMS. **a** Cluster of moderately pleomorphic spindle cells embedded in blue- or magenta-colored collagenous matrix. MGG stain. **b** Mixture of dispersed moderately pleomorphic spindle cells and pleomorphic cells with irregular nuclei – 1 with nuclear "inclusion" and multinucleated cells. HE stain. **c** Cohesive fascicle of moderately pleomorphic spindle cells in the collagenous stroma corresponding to the cell block section (**d**). HE stain.

Cytologic Features
- Hypercellular smears (hypocellular in tumors with hyalinized matrix)
- Major cellular patterns in low power: mixed fascicular/spindle cell/pleomorphic, predominantly fascicular/spindle cell, and predominantly pleomorphic
- Cigar-shaped nuclei with elongated, blunted ends, occasionally segmented "in tandem"
- Stripped atypical, degenerate nuclei, with a blue- or magenta-colored background in fascicles or clusters (May-Grünwald-Giemsa, MGG)
- Minor component of dispersed, well-preserved cells with dense cytoplasm
- Pleomorphic, occasionally bizarre, multinucleated cells

- Epithelioid tumor cells in epithelioid variant
- Occasional intranuclear "inclusions"
- Mitoses and necrosis
- Osteoclast-like giant cells

Ancillary Tests
Immunophenotype
Positive for SMA, MSA, desmin, and h-caldesmon. Focally positive/negative for keratins and epithelial membrane antigen (EMA). Negative for CD117, CD34, ALK1, and S100.

LMS stains for SMA, desmin, and caldesmon, although sometimes only focally. Focal cytokeratin and EMA positivity has been reported in LMS.

Genetics

Often complex karyotypes with numerous structural and numerical changes [5]. Mutations in tumor suppressor TP53 are common and both copies are missing in 50% of cases [6]. Loss at 13q14 affecting the suppressor *RB1* can be seen [7]. The tumor suppressor *PTEN* is frequently lost due to a loss of the 10q region. An amplification of the transcription factor gene *MYOCD* on 17p is seen in the majority of cases [8]. Cytogenetics, FISH, SNP array, PCR, and NGS on both fixed and fresh material can detect these changes.

Differential Diagnosis
- Soft tissue leiomyoma
- Nodular fasciitis
- Schwannoma
- Malignant peripheral nerve sheath tumor
- Myofibroblastic sarcomas
- Undifferentiated pleomorphic/spindle-cell sarcoma
- Dedifferentiated sarcoma
- Metastatic sarcomatoid carcinoma
- Metastatic melanoma

Differentiating LMS from other spindle cell sarcomas is important but it is even more important to differentiate them from benign spindle cell lesions, such as schwannoma and nodular fasciitis. Nodular fasciitis is one of the most important differentials in the cytologic examination of LMS as fine-needle aspiration smears from nodular fasciitis can closely resemble high-grade LMS. The clinical presentation of nodular fasciitis differs from that of LMS as nodular fasciitis often arise in the subcutaneous tissue of the upper extremities and trunk as a rapidly growing and occasionally painful or tender nodule that, in most cases, is regresses spontaneously.

References

1 Domanski HA, Akerman M, Rissler P, Gustafson P: Fine-needle aspiration of soft tissue leiomyosarcoma: an analysis of the most common cytologic findings and the value of ancillary techniques. Diagn Cytopathol 2006;34:597–604.
2 Klijanienko J, Caillaud JM, Lagace R, Vielh P: Fine-needle aspiration of leiomyosarcoma: a correlative cytohistopathological study of 96 tumors in 68 patients. Diagn Cytopathol 2003;28:119–125.
3 Tao LC, Davidson DD: Aspiration biopsy cytology of smooth muscle tumors: a cytologic approach to the differentiation between leiomyosarcoma and leiomyoma. Acta Cytol 1993;37:300–308.
4 Dahl I, Hagmar B, Angervall L: Leiomyosarcoma of the soft tissue: a correlative cytological and histological study of 11 cases. Acta Pathol Microbiol Scand A 1981;89:285–291.
5 Wang R, Lu YJ, Fisher C, Bridge JA, Shipley J: Characterization of chromosome aberrations associated with soft-tissue leiomyosarcomas by twenty-four-color karyotyping and comparative genomic hybridization analysis. Genes Chromosomes Cancer 2001;31:54–64.
6 Perot G, Chibon F, Montero A, Lagarde P, de The H, Terrier P, Guillou L, Ranchere D, Coindre JM, Aurias A: Constant p53 pathway inactivation in a large series of soft tissue sarcomas with complex genetics. Am J Pathol 2010;177:2080–2090.
7 Dei Tos AP, Maestro R, Doglioni C, Piccinin S, Libera DD, Boiocchi M, Fletcher CD: Tumor suppressor genes and related molecules in leiomyosarcoma. Am J Pathol 1996;148:1037–1045.
8 Garraway LA, Sellers WR: Lineage dependency and lineage-survival oncogenes in human cancer. Nat Rev Cancer 2006;6:593–602.

Domanski HA, Walther CS: FNA Cytology of Soft Tissue and Bone Tumors. Monogr Clin Cytol.
Basel, Karger, 2017, vol 22, pp 68–70 (DOI: 10.1159/000475097)

Pericytic (Perivascular) Tumors

Glomus Tumor

Glomus tumor (Fig. 1) is a mesenchymal neoplasm composed of cells resembling smooth muscle of the normal glomus body. The majority of glomus tumors arise under the nails of young women. Glomus tumors arise less frequently in the skin and subcutaneous tissue or in superficial soft tissue elsewhere. Rarely such deep sites as bone, parenchymatous organs, mediastinum, nerves, bladder, and gastrointestinal tract are involved. Morphologic variants of glomus tumor include glomangioma (glomuvenous malformation), which tends to occur in children, glomangiomyoma, and symplastic glomus tumor. The latter tumor displays cytologic atypia but follows a benign clinical course. Glomus tumors are frequently small and painful and are seldom a target for fine-needle aspiration (FNA) cytology examination [1–5]. Radiating paroxysmal pain is common through cold intolerance. Smears from cutaneous and subcutaneous glomus tumors can be easily mistaken for neoplasms of the dermal adnexa, epithelioid vascular neoplasms, and metastatic carcinomas.

Cytologic Features
- Often hemorrhagic aspirates with variable cellularity
- A mixture of clustered and dispersed, medium-sized epithelioid cells with rounded to ovoid bland nuclei containing inconspicuous nucleoli
- Most cells have poorly preserved cytoplasmic borders
- Variable amounts of a myxoid/fibrillary background matrix in cell clusters
- In smears from symplastic glomus tumors, atypical cells with variable anisokaryosis and occasional nuclear inclusions but with fine chromatin pattern

Ancillary Tests
Immunophenotype
Positive for smooth muscle actin (SMA) and caldesmon. Negative for desmin, S100 protein, keratin, and endothelial markers.

Genetics
These exceedingly rare tumors and related genetic information are limited. Inactivation of the tumor suppressor *NF1* on chromosome 17q has been observed in these tumors [6]. Apart from rearrangements involving 17q, *NF1*-associated tumors have displayed both copy number changes and sometimes polyploidy [7]. Fluorescence in situ hybridization (FISH), single nucleotide polymorphism (SNP) array, and next-generation sequencing (NGS) can best visualize this rearrangement on fresh or fixed material.

Differential Diagnosis
- Dermal adnexal neoplasms
- Carcinoma metastasis
- Epithelioid vascular neoplasm
- Angioleiomyoma

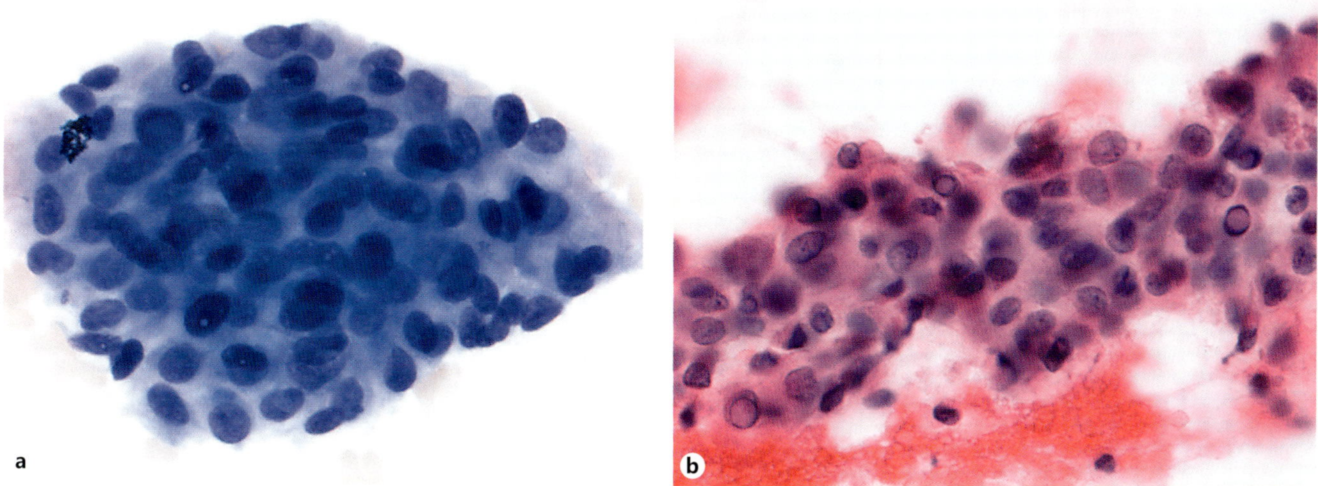

Fig. 1. Glomus tumor. **a** Cluster of middle-sized cells with poorly preserved cytoplasmic borders and bland, round to ovoid nuclei with fine chromatin pattern and occasional inconspicuous nucleoli. MGG stain. **b** Symplastic glomus tumor. A loosely cohesive group of slightly pleomorphic round and ovoid cells showing occasional slight anisonucleosis, inconspicuous nucleoli, and intranuclear "inclusions." HE stain.

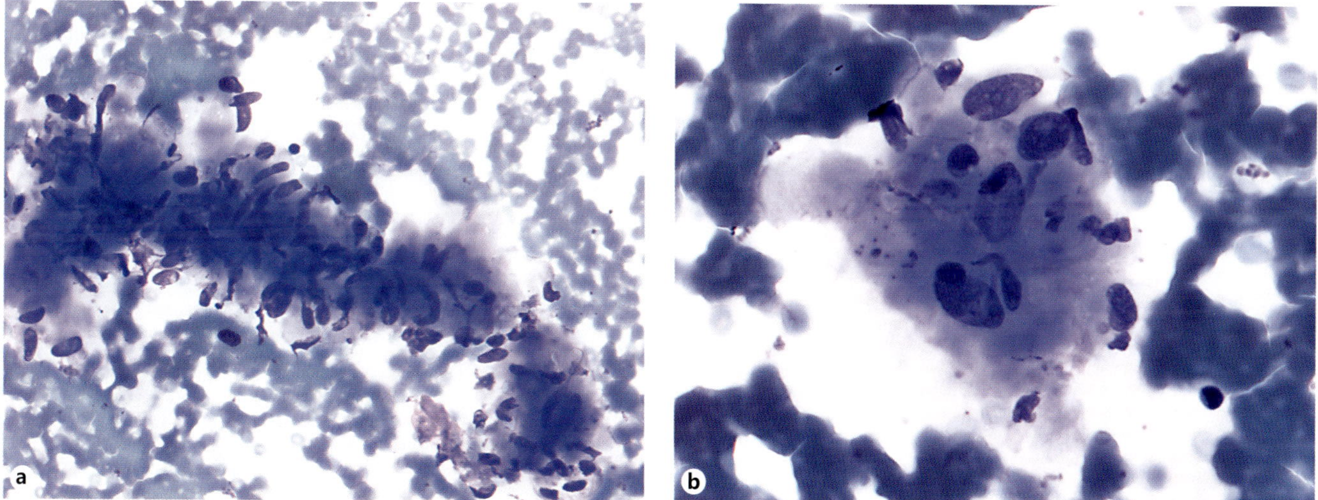

Fig. 2. Angioleiomyoma. **a** A loosely cohesive cluster of slightly pleomorphic smooth muscle cells embedded in blue- or magenta-colored collagenous matrix. MGG stain. **b** Smooth muscle cells with enlarged nuclei showing small nuclei may be occasionally seen in smears of angioleiomyoma. MGG stain.

Glomus tumors are most often painful at aspiration which, together with common sites such as distal extremities, facilitates diagnosis. In other sites it may be difficult to distinguish glomus tumors from epithelial and epithelioid vascular neoplasms. Positive staining for SMA and caldesmon, and negative immunoreactivity for cytokeratins and endothelial cell markers such as CD31 and CD34 helps to exclude epithelial and vascular tumors.

Angioleiomyoma

Angioleiomyoma (Fig. 2) is a benign neoplasm that usually presents as a tender or painful nodule in the skin or subcutaneous tissue in adults. It is commonly located in the lower extremities but can arise almost anywhere. Clinically, angioleiomyoma can be easily confused with glomus tumor, cutaneous cylindroma, and schwannoma. Angioleiomyoma is composed of smooth muscle cells arranged around blood vessels. There is a morphologic overlapping between angioleiomyoma and myopericytoma. One series of FNA of angioleiomyoma has been published to date [8]. The most common findings are variable proportions of benign smooth muscle cells and uniform spindle cells, either dissociated or arranged in small fascicles with small fragments of a collagenous matrix in the background.

Ancillary Tests

Immunophenotype

Positive for SMA and h-caldesmon; variable desmin positivity.

Genetics

The karyotype is often diploid with structural rearrangements including loss of 22q11.2 and gain of Xq [9, 10]. Cytogenetics, FISH, SNP array, and NGS can visualize this on fresh and fixed material.

References

1 Mukherjee S, Bandyopadhyay G, Saha S, Choudhuri M: Cytodiagnosis of glomus tumor. J Cytol 2010;27:104–105.

2 Vidyavathi K, Udayakumar M, Prasad CB, Harendra KM: Glomus tumor mimicking eccrine spiradenoma on fine needle aspiration. J Cytol 2009; 26:46–48.

3 Handa U, Palta A, Mohan H, Punia RP: Aspiration cytology of glomus tumor: a case report. Acta Cytol 2001;45:1073–1076.

4 Daskalopoulou D, Galanopoulou A, Statiropoulou P, Papapetrou S, Pandazis I, Markidou S: Cytologically interesting cases of primary skin tumors and tumor-like conditions identified by fine-needle aspiration biopsy. Diagn Cytopathol 1998;19: 17–28.

5 Daskalopoulou D, Maounis N, Kokalis G, Liodandonaki P, Belezini E, Markidou S: The role of fine needle aspiration cytology in the diagnosis of primary skin tumors. Arch Anat Cytol Pathol 1993; 41:75–81.

6 Brems H, Park C, Maertens O, Pemov A, Messiaen L, Upadhyaya M, Claes K, Beert E, Peeters K, Mautner V, Sloan JL, Yao L, Lee CC, Sciot R, De Smet L, Legius E, Stewart DR: Glomus tumors in neurofibromatosis type 1: genetic, functional, and clinical evidence of a novel association. Cancer Res 2009;69:7393–7401.

7 Stewart DR, Pemov A, Van Loo P, Beert E, Brems H, Sciot R, Claes K, Pak E, Dutra A, Lee CC, Legius E: Mitotic recombination of chromosome arm 17q as a cause of loss of heterozygosity of *NF1* in neurofibromatosis type 1-associated glomus tumors. Genes Chromosomes Cancer 2012;51:429–437.

8 Domanski HA: Cytologic features of angioleiomyoma: cytologic-histologic study of 10 cases. Diagn Cytopathol 2002;27:161–166.

9 Welborn J, Fenner S, Parks R: Angioleiomyoma: a benign tumor with karyotypic aberrations. Cancer Genetics Cytogenetics 2010;199:147–148.

10 Nishio J, Iwasaki H, Ohjimi Y, Ishiguro M, Kobayashi K, Nabeshima K, Naito M, Kikuchi M: Chromosomal imbalances in angioleiomyomas by comparative genomic hybridization. Int J Mol Med 2004;13:13–16.

Domanski HA, Walther CS: FNA Cytology of Soft Tissue and Bone Tumors. Monogr Clin Cytol.
Basel, Karger, 2017, vol 22, pp 71–79 (DOI: 10.1159/000475098)

Skeletal-Muscle Tumors

Rhabdomyosarcoma (RMS) is a malignant tumor with differentiation towards skeletal muscle and is the most common sarcoma of childhood. Four main subtypes are recognized in the current WHO classification: embryonal, alveolar, spindle cell/sclerosing, and pleomorphic. The embryonal subtype of RMS accounts for approximately 60% of cases and the alveolar subtype accounts for 20%. Pediatric RMS belongs to the group of small round blue-cell tumors, neoplasms that are commonly examined by fine-needle aspiration (FNA) cytology [1–10]. The sensitivity and specificity for this group of tumors exceed 90% and with an adequate sampling and the use of ancillary techniques a diagnosis of a specific histologic subtype can be rendered in the majority of cases [4, 11–13]. Benign and malignant striated muscle tumors are uncommon in adults in general, but the rare pleomorphic RMS occurs exclusively in adults.

Adult Rhabdomyoma

Adult rhabdomyoma is a rare benign neoplasm of adults showing mature skeletal muscle differentiation. Most of these neoplasms arise in the head and neck region, often in the soft tissue of the upper aerodigestive tract including the tongue and floor of the mouth [14]. Smears display dispersed cells or syncytial clusters of large, round to polygonal or elongated cells with an abundant eosinophilic finely granular cytoplasm and small, uniform, often eccentric nuclei with large nucleoli [15–21]. Faint cross-striation in the cytoplasm may be seen in careful examination of smears using high-power magnification [22] (Fig. 1).

Cytologic Features
- Large rounded, polygonal or elongated cells, dispersed or arranged in cohesive clusters
- Abundant eosinophilic (hematoxylin and eosin, HE, stained) granular cytoplasm
- Small, peripherally located nuclei with prominent nucleoli
- Occasional cells attached to capillary vessels
- Rare stripped nuclei
- Occasionally visible cross-striation

Ancillary Tests
Immunophenotype
Positive for desmin, myogenin, and MyoD1. Negative for S100 and keratins.

Histochemistry
PAS positive.

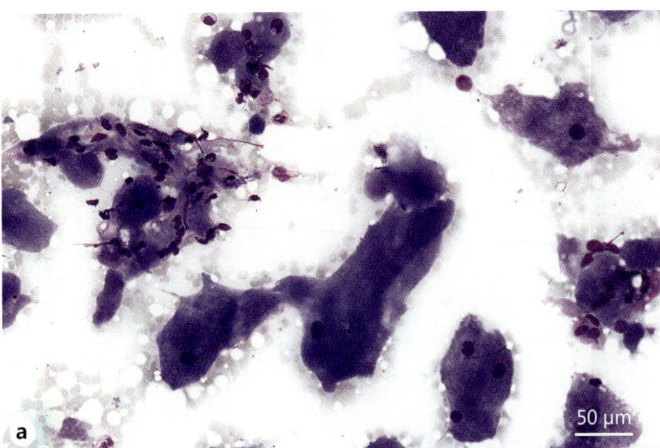

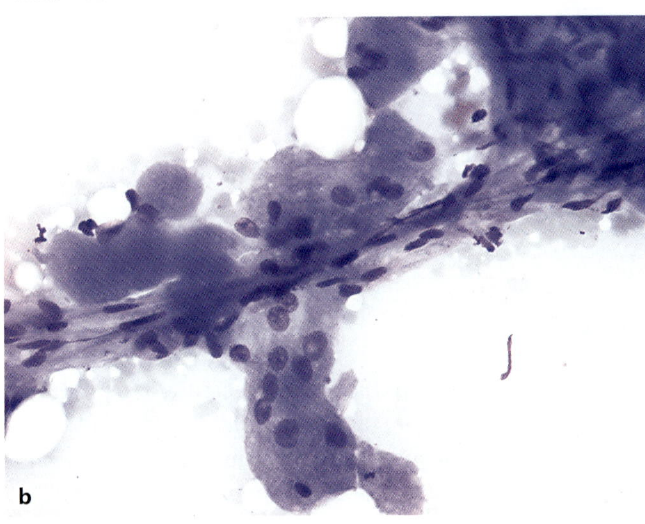

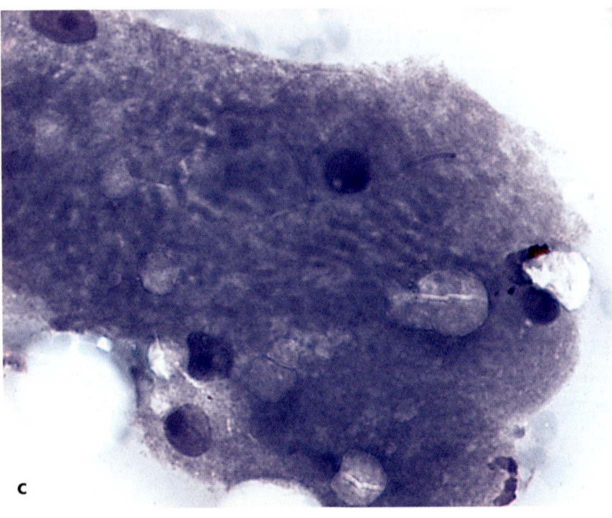

Fig. 1. Adult rhabdomyoma. **a** Large dispersed round to polygonal or elongated tumor cells with an abundant eosinophilic finely granular cytoplasm and small, uniform nuclei. MGG stain. **b** Tumor cells or syncytial clusters of cells with an abundant cytoplasm and eccentric or random situated nuclei attached to capillary vessels. MGG stain. **c** Occasionally visible faint cross-striation in the cytoplasm. MGG stain.

Genetics

The fetal variant of rhabdomyoma is often associated with the basal cell nevus syndrome [23], which is induced by a loss of function of the *PTCH1* tumor suppressor gene [24]. There are no known recurrent genetic changes in adult cases. Single nucleotide polymorphism (SNP) array, fluorescence in situ hybridization (FISH), and next-generation sequencing (NGS) can detect the loss on fresh and fixed material.

Differential Diagnosis

- Granular cell tumor
- Hibernoma

Although the hibernoma cells in FNA are granulated and vacuolated, they are generally smaller than rhabdomyoma cells and display negative immunoreactivity for muscle markers. Cells of granular cell tumors in smears are smaller than those from adult rhabdomyoma and display less distinctive cytoplasmic borders and a fragile cytoplasm. Parts of smears from granular cell tumors show naked nuclei and a granular background of damaged cytoplasm. Diffuse positive S100 protein staining and negative immunoreactivity for muscle markers in granular cell tumors helps to distinguish these neoplasms from adult rhabdomyoma, while desmin and myoglobin are negative.

Embryonal Rhabdomyosarcoma

Embryonal RMS is the most common subtype in children and accounts for approximately 60% of all RMS cases. Most occur in the first decade of life and the majority arise in the head and neck region, genitourinary tract, trunk, and retroperitoneum. Typically, the smears are moderately to highly cellular, with a moderately to marked cellular pleomorphism. Tumor cells vary from small to intermediate-sized and primitive spindle cells and rhabdomyoblast-like cells of various morphology (triangular, rounded, tadpole or strap shaped) are commonly seen. [9, 25–27] (Fig. 2) Embryonal RMS has a better prognosis than alveolar RMS.

Cytologic Features

- Often hypercellular smears
- Mixture of loosely clustered and dispersed tumor cells
- Spindle cells or round cells are the most common cell types
- Cellular and nuclear pleomorphism usually present
- Occasional prominent nucleoli

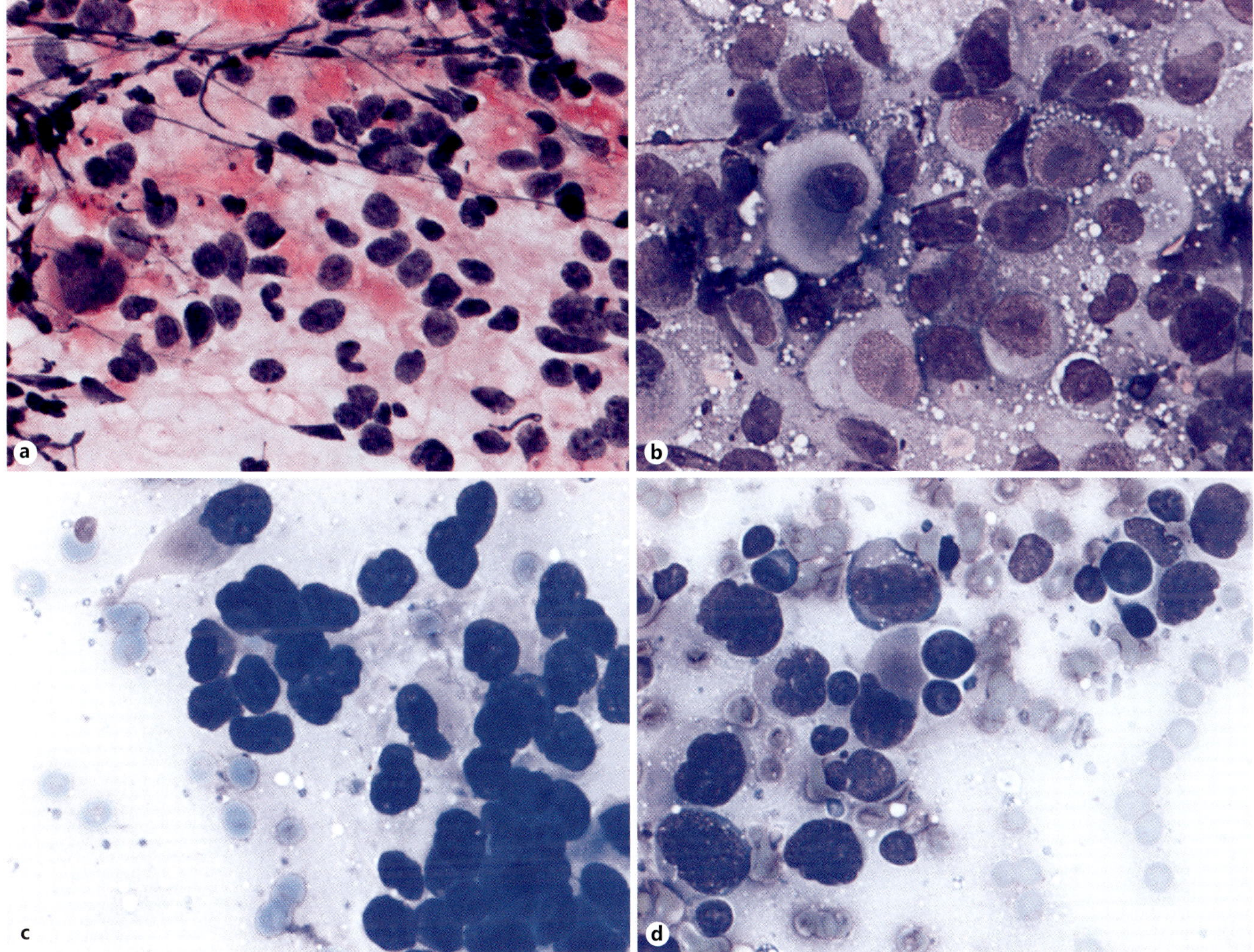

Fig. 2. Embryonal RMS. **a** Cellular smears composed of dispersed round to ovoid, moderately pleomorphic nuclei and poorly preserved cytoplasm. HE stain. **b** Dispersed tumor cells with nuclei of variable shape and size containing large nucleoli; a few binucleated cells and cells with abundant cytoplasm. MGG stain. **c**, **d** Loosely cohesive groups and dispersed single cells and naked nuclei of various morphology: triangular, rounded, tadpole or strap shaped. MGG stain.

- Rhabdomyoblast-like tumor cells (triangular, rounded, tadpole, or strap shaped) variably present
- Occasional rhabdomyoblasts with eosinophilic (HE) or gray-blue (Romanowski stain) dense cytoplasm
- Variably present areas of myxoid matrix

Ancillary Tests
Immunophenotype
Tumor cells express diffuse desmin and nuclear myogenin and MyoD1.

Genetics
Genetical changes with whole chromosome gains involving chromosomes 2, 11, 12, 13, and 20 are common. Loss of chromosomes often involves chromosomes 10 and 15 [28]. Loss of 1 copy of the region 11p15 can be detected and it contains imprinted tumor suppressor genes and growth regulators, indicating that a loss results in the activation of the remaining copy [29]. These changes can bet detected with cytogenetics on fresh material. FISH, SNP array, and NGS can be used on both fresh and fixed material to evaluate the genetic changes.

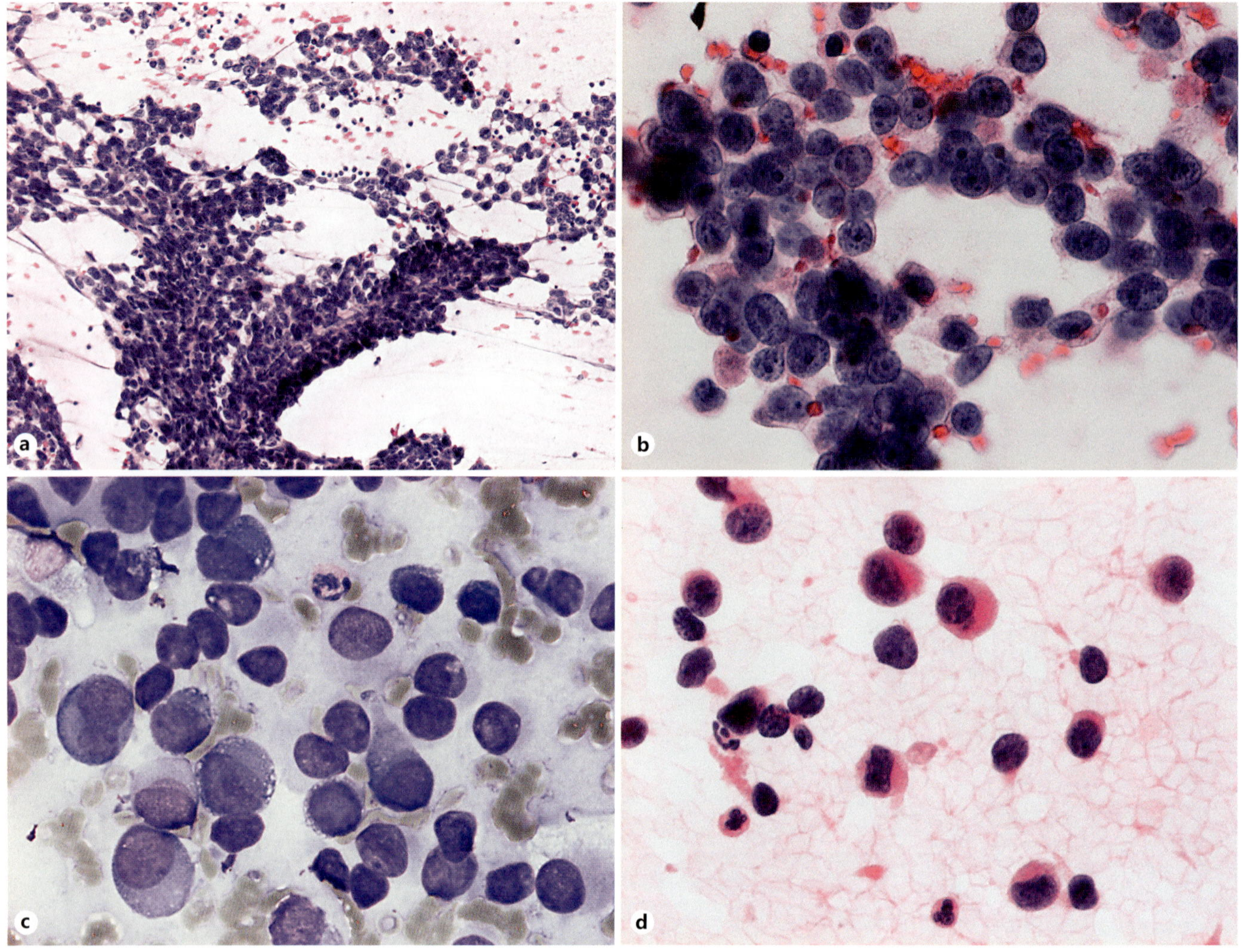

Fig. 3. Alveolar RMS. **a, b** Typically hypercellular smears with loosely cohesive clusters and dispersed more uniformly round to polygonal cells than those seen in smears of embryonal RMS. Most nuclei are hyperchromatic, often with large nucleoli. HE stain. **c** Cells with rhabdomyoblastic morphology showing eccentric nuclei, binucleated cells. MGG stain. **d–f** Cells with cytoplasmic densities (**d, e**; HE stain) and multinucleated tumor cells (**f**; HE stain) are common findings in the FNA smears. **g, h** Diffuse and strong expression of desmin and myogenin support with diagnosis RMS. Cell block; desmin and myogenin.

(Figure continued on next page.)

Differential Diagnosis
- Alveolar RMS
- Leiomyosarcoma (LMS)

Alveolar RMS may be difficult to distinguish from embryonal RMS in smears. Clinical data and molecular genetic examination of tumor cells is important to complement a cytologic examination as most alveolar RMS have either *PAX3-FOXO1* or *PAX7-FOXO1* gene fusion, which can be detected by FISH. LMS is extremely rare in children and, in contrast to RMS, does not express immunoreactivity for either myogenin or MyoD1.

Alveolar Rhabdomyosarcoma

Alveolar RMS belongs to the group of small, round, blue-cell malignant neoplasms and accounts for about 20% of all pediatric RMS. Alveolar RMS occurs most frequently in adolescents and young adults between 10 and 25 years of age. In contrast to embryonal RMS, smears are more uniform with predominantly small- to medium-sized round or ovoid cells with hyperchromatic nuclei, often with large nucleoli. Binucleated and multinucleated tumor giant cells are frequent [30] (Fig. 3). Identification of alveolar RMS is clinically im-

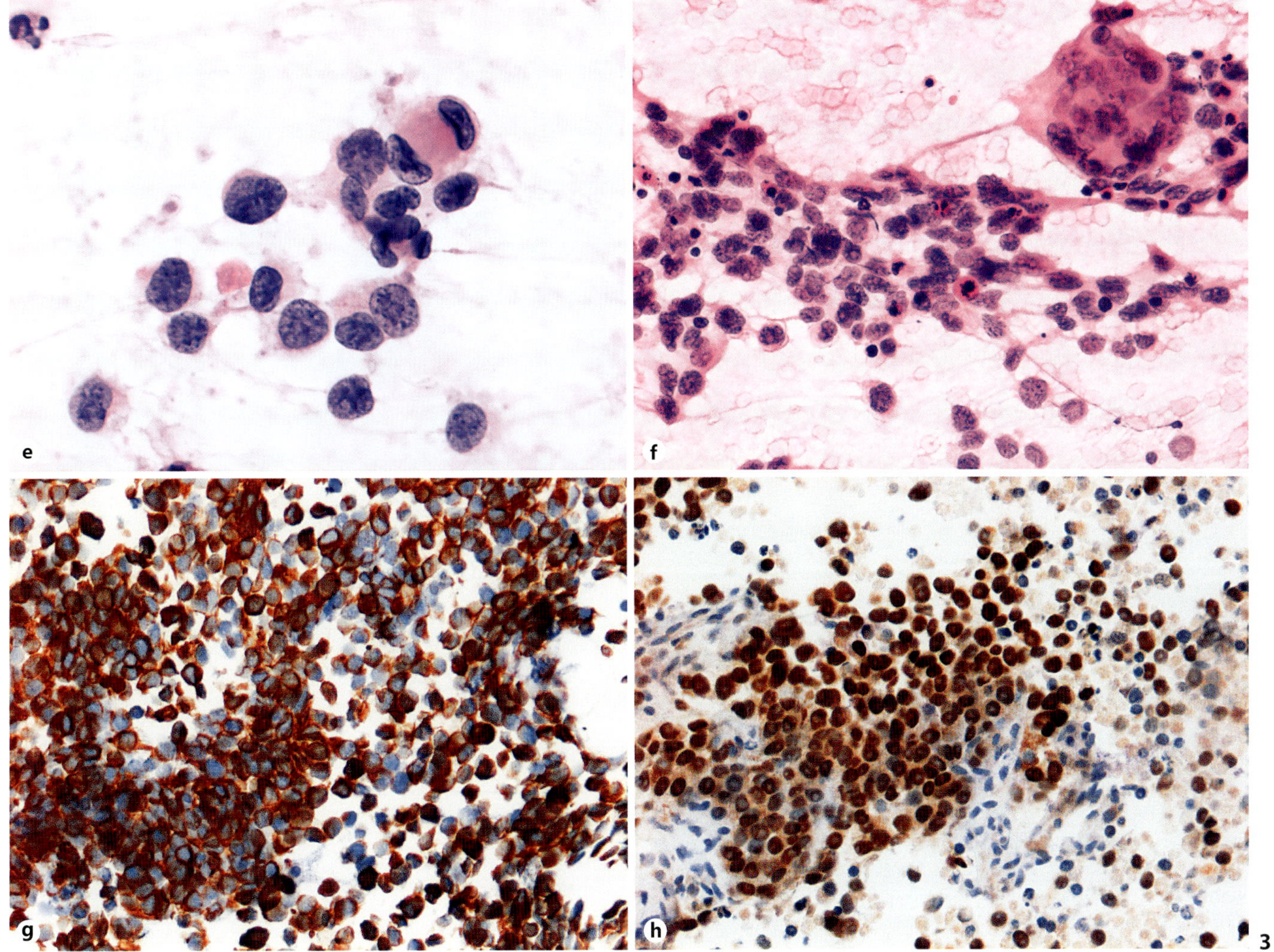

portant as it has an unfavorable prognosis and should be treated more aggressively.

Cytologic Features
- Hypercellular smears
- Cell clusters mixed with dispersed cells
- Stripped nuclei commonly mixed with gray-blue blebs of cytoplasm
- Small- or medium-sized, round to polygonal and ovoid or pear-shaped cells
- Scanty cytoplasm, coarse nuclear chromatin and often large nucleoli
- Cytoplasmic vacuolization
- Mitoses
- Binucleated and multinucleated tumor cells
- Eccentric nuclei, cytoplasmic densities

Ancillary Tests
Immunophenotype
Positive for diffuse desmin, nuclear myogenin, and MyoD1; may show focal expression of keratin, CD99, S100, and neuroendocrine markers.

Genetics
Cytogenetically, alveolar RMS shows recurrent translocations, with t(2;13)(q35;q14) being the most common and t(1;13)(p36;q14) occurring in fewer cases. These translocations result in chimeric genes encoding fusion proteins with strong transcriptional activation and oncogenic effects. The genes involved are *PAX3* located on chromosome 2 and *PAX7* on chromosome 1. They fuse with *FOXO1* on chromosome 13 resulting in the *PAX3/PAX7-FOXO1* fusion genes [31]. The *MYCN* oncogene in 2p24 can also be ampli-

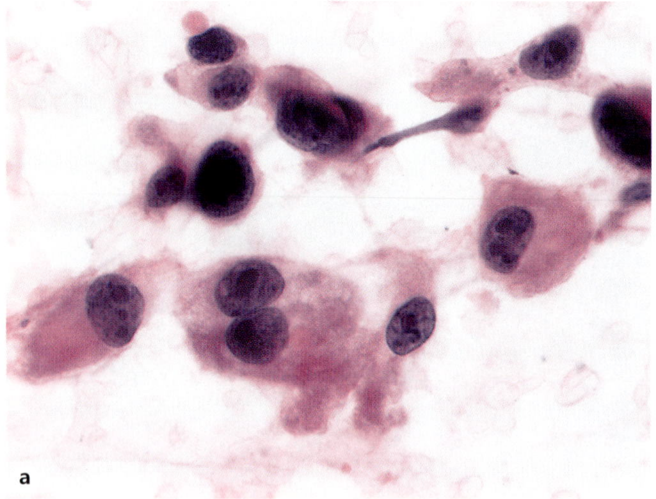

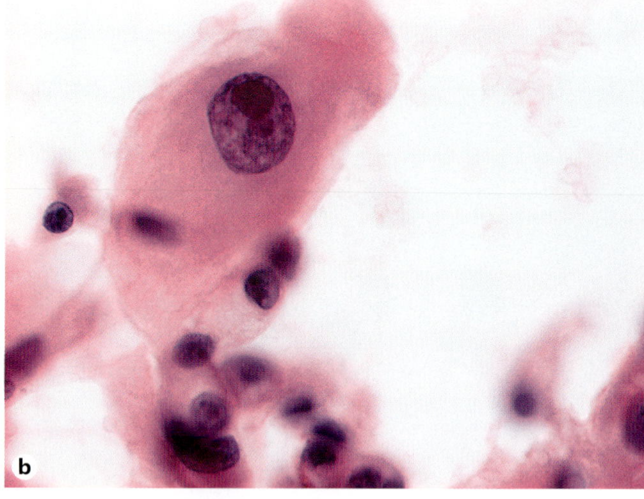

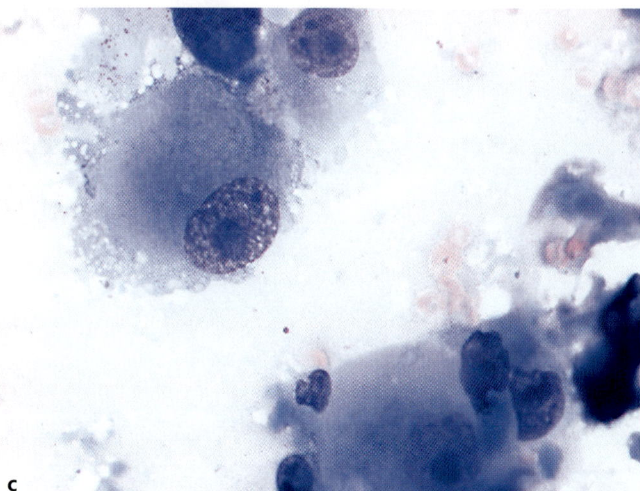

Fig. 4. Pleomorphic RMS. **a**, **b** Highly pleomorphic, spindle or polygonal cells of variable size with round to oval nuclei, prominent nucleoli, and often with an abundant eosinophilic cytoplasm. HE stain. **c** Tumor cells with cytoplasmic densities showing rhabdomyoblastic features may be seen in FNA smears. MGG stain.

fied and overexpressed in fusion-positive cases [32]. These changes can be detected with cytogenetics, FISH, SNP array, PCR, and NGS on fresh and fixed material depending on the material and available method.

Differential Diagnosis
- Embryonal RMS
- Ewing sarcoma
- Neuroblastoma
- Poorly differentiated synovial sarcoma
- Precursor lymphoblastic lymphoma
- Poorly differentiated neuroendocrine carcinoma

Similar to embryonal RMS, tumor cells are immunoreactive with desmin, myogenin, and MyoD1. Aberrant expression of keratins, CD99, S100 protein, neuron-specific enolase, and CD56 may present diagnostic challenges and confusion with other small round blue-cell tumors. Like other small round blue-cell neoplasms, the correct diagnosis of alveolar RMS requires ancillary techniques such as immunocytochemistry and molecular genetics examinations [33, 34].

Pleomorphic Rhabdomyosarcoma

Pleomorphic RMS is an uncommon high-grade sarcoma of adults, usually aged over 50 years, with a median occurrence in the 6th to 7th decades of life, most often arising in the limbs. FNA smears are usually hypercellular and display a marked cellular and nuclear pleomorphism. Highly atypical spindle or polygonal cells, and large cells showing rhabdoid features with abundant eosinophilic cytoplasm (HE) and eccentric nuclei are common findings in FNA smears of this rare neoplasm (Fig. 4).

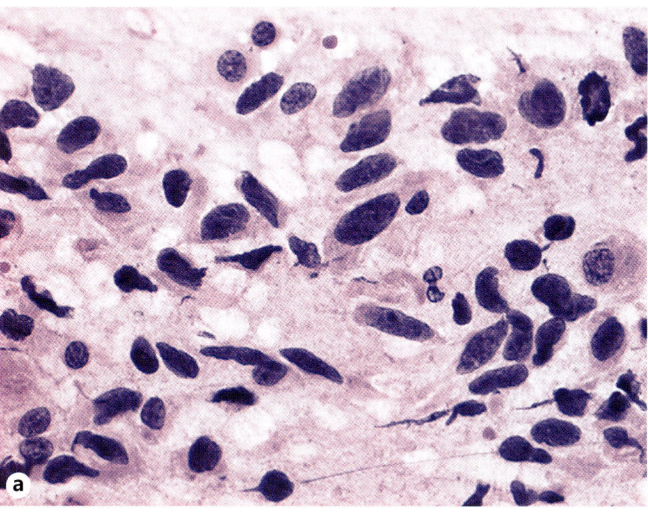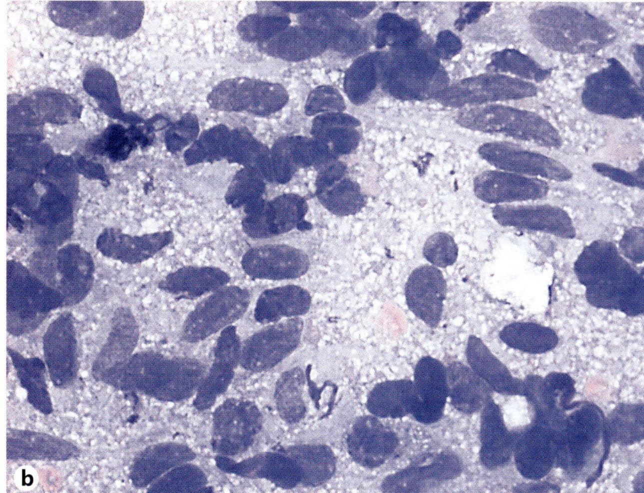

Fig. 5. Spindle cell RMS. **a**, **b** Dispersed cells and bare nuclei with a predominantly spindle cell morphology and variable, usually slight to moderate, nuclear pleomorphism. HE and MGG stains.

Cytologic Features
- Hypercellular smears with both cell clusters and dispersed cells
- Marked cellular and nuclear pleomorphism
- Mixture of atypical spindle cells, epithelioid cells with occasional rhabdoid features, and multinucleated tumor cells

Ancillary Tests
Immunophenotype
Positive for desmin, nuclear myogenin, and MyoD1.

Genetics
Cytogenetics shows complex karyotypes with structural and numerical aberrations but no recurrent changes [35]. Genome-wide analysis has shown multiple losses and gains of varying size spread over several chromosomal regions with a pattern similar to other highly malignant sarcomas, e.g., osteosarcoma [36]. These aberrations can be detected with cytogenetics, FISH, SNP array, and NGS on fresh or fixed material.

Differential Diagnosis
- Pleomorphic variants of other sarcomas
- Malignant peripheral nerve sheath tumor (MPNST) with heterologous rhabdoid differentiation
- Dedifferentiated liposarcoma with heterologous rhabdoid differentiation

The cells with rhabdoid features seen in smears from pleomorphic RMS are similar to those seen as a heterologous component in other high-grade sarcomas, such as MPNST or dedifferentiated liposarcoma. Tumor cells of pleomorphic RMS stain for desmin, myogenin, and MyoD1.

Spindle Cell/Sclerosing Rhabdomyosarcoma

Spindle cell/sclerosing RMS is an uncommon high-grade sarcoma of both children and adults. These neoplasms are closely related to each other but not to embryonal RMS. In the pediatric group, spindle cell RMS usually arises in the paratesticular region, while the majority of cases in adults arise in the deep soft tissue of the head and neck [37]. Sclerosing RMS shows a wide age range, with the median at 30 years, and a strong male predilection. Most cases of sclerotic RMS arise in the extremities, and occasionally in the head and neck area. Smears of spindle cell RMS display predominantly dispersed cells with a spindle cell morphology and variable, usually slight to moderate, nuclear pleomorphism [38, 39] (Fig. 5). Routinely stained smears resemble those from LMS with a predominantly spindle cell or mixed pleomorphic/spindle cell pattern.

Ancillary Tests
Immunophenotype
Spindle cell RMS: positive for desmin, myogenin, and MyoD1; commonly smooth muscle antigen and muscle-specific actin positive. Sclerosing RMS: typically diffuse MyoD1 positivity, variable desmin and myogenin positivity.

Genetics
In this RMS subtype, cytogenetic- and array-based evaluation has shown whole chromosome gains and nonrecurrent structural rearrangements [40, 41]. The material is limited but recent studies have shown *MYOD1* mutations [42], and a study suggests that such mutations are associated with a poor outcome in pediatric sclerosing RMS [43]. These changes can be found by cytogenetics, FISH, SNP array, PCR, and NGS using both fresh and fixed material depending on availability.

Differential Diagnosis
- LMS
- MPNST
- Other spindle cell sarcomas

Cells from most cases of spindle cell RMS strongly express desmin, actins, myogenin, and MyoD1, while cells from the sclerosing subtype stain for MyoD1, but the expression of desmin and myogenin is usually limited. A lack of convincing rhabdoid cells and use of immunostainings along with clinical data can distinguish this subtype of RMS from LMS, MPNST, and other spindle cell sarcomas.

References

1 Cole CD, Wu HH: Fine-needle aspiration in pediatric patients 12 years of age and younger: a 20-year retrospective study from a single tertiary medical center. Diagn Cytopathol 2014;42:600–605.

2 Razack R, Michelow P, Leiman G, Harnekar A, Poole J, Wessels G, Hesseling P, Stefan C, Louw M, Schubert PT, Clarke H, Wright CA: An interinstitutional review of the value of FNAB in pediatric oncology in resource-limited countries. Diagn Cytopathol 2012;40:770–776.

3 Viswanathan S, George S, Ramadwar M, Medhi S, Arora B, Kurkure P: Evaluation of pediatric abdominal masses by fine-needle aspiration cytology: a clinicoradiologic approach. Diagn Cytopathol 2010;38:15–27.

4 Pohar-Marinsek Z: Difficulties in diagnosing small round cell tumours of childhood from fine needle aspiration cytology samples. Cytopathology 2008;19:67–79.

5 Klijanienko J, Caillaud JM, Orbach D, Brisse H, Lagace R, Vielh P, Couturier J, Freneaux P, Theocharis S, Sastre-Garau X: Cyto-histological correlations in primary, recurrent and metastatic rhabdomyosarcoma: the institute Curie's experience. Diagn Cytopathol 2007;35:482–487.

6 Das DK: Fine-needle aspiration (FNA) cytology diagnosis of small round cell tumors: value and limitations. Indian J Pathol Microbiol 2004;47:309–318.

7 Pohar-Marinsek Z, Anzic J, Jereb B: Topical topic: value of fine needle aspiration biopsy in childhood rhabdomyosarcoma: twenty-six years of experience in Slovenia. Med Pediatr Oncol 2002;38:416–420.

8 Kilpatrick SE, Ward WG, Chauvenet AR, Pettenati MJ: The role of fine-needle aspiration biopsy in the initial diagnosis of pediatric bone and soft tissue tumors: an institutional experience. Mod Pathol 1998;11:923–928.

9 Willen H, Akerman M, Carlen B: Fine needle aspiration (FNA) in the diagnosis of soft tissue tumours; a review of 22 years experience. Cytopathology 1995;6:236–247.

10 Akhtar M, Ali MA, Bakry M, Hug M, Sackey K: Fine-needle aspiration biopsy diagnosis of rhabdomyosarcoma: cytologic, histologic, and ultrastructural correlations. Diagn Cytopathol 1992;8:465–474.

11 Gautam U, Srinivasan R, Rajwanshi A, Bansal D, Marwaha RK, Vasishtha RK: Reverse transcriptase-polymerase chain reaction as an ancillary molecular technique in the diagnosis of small blue round cell tumors by fine-needle aspiration cytology. Am J Clin Pathol 2010;133:633–645.

12 Kilpatrick SE, Bergman S, Pettenati MJ, Gulley ML: The usefulness of cytogenetic analysis in fine needle aspirates for the histologic subtyping of sarcomas. Mod Pathol 2006;19:815–819.

13 Udayakumar AM, Sundareshan TS, Appaji L, Biswas S, Mukherjee G: Rhabdomyosarcoma: cytogenetics of five cases using fine-needle aspiration samples and review of the literature. Ann Genet 2002;45:33–37.

14 Gupta N, Banik T, Rajwanshi A, Radotra BD, Panda N, Dey P, Srinivasan R, Nijhawan R: Fine needle aspiration cytology of oral and oropharyngeal lesions with an emphasis on the diagnostic utility and pitfalls. J Cancer Res Ther 2012;8:626–629.

15 Zhang S, Bhalodia A, Swartz B, Abreo F, Fowler M: Fine needle aspiration of parapharyngeal space adult rhabdomyoma: a case report. Acta Cytol 2010;54:775–779.

16 Gupta N, Rajwanshi A, Mohindra S, Vasishta RK, Batra C, Gupta AK: Diagnosis of adult rhabdomyoma by fine needle aspiration cytology: a report of 2 cases. Acta Cytol 2010;54:968–972.

17 Jin B, Saleh H: Pitfalls in the diagnosis of adult rhabdomyoma by fine needle aspiration: report of a case and a brief literature review. Diagn Cytopathol 2009;37:483–486.

18 Bellis D, Torre V, Nunziata R, Demarchi A, Fornaseri V, Coverlizza S, Beatrice F: Submandibular rhabdomyoma: a case report. Acta Cytol 2006;50:557–559.

19 McGregor DK, Krishnan B, Green L: Fine-needle aspiration of adult rhabdomyoma: a case report with review of the literature. Diagn Cytopathol 2003;28:92–95.

20 Cuesta Gil M, Fernandez-Alba Luengo J, Navarro Vila C: Rhabdomyoma of the base of the tongue: a case report. Int J Oral Maxillofac Surg 2000;29:136–137.

21 Tani E, Ersoz C, Silfversward C, Mendel L: Rhabdomyoma: primary diagnosis by fine needle aspiration (FNA) cytology and immunocytochemistry. Cytopathology 1995;6:204–208.

22 Domanski HA, Dawiskiba S: Adult rhabdomyoma in fine needle aspirates: a report of two cases. Acta Cytol 2000;44:223–226.

23 Gorlin RJ: Nevoid basal cell carcinoma syndrome. Dermatol Clin 1995;13:113–125.

24 Gailani MR, Bale SJ, Leffell DJ, DiGiovanna JJ, Peck GL, Poliak S, Drum MA, Pastakia B, McBride OW, Kase R, et al: Developmental defects in Gorlin syndrome related to a putative tumor suppressor gene on chromosome 9. Cell 1992;69:111–117.

25 Valeri RM, Papanikolaou A, Panagiotou A, Michalakis K, Saraboukas T, Chatzichristou D, Destouni C: A rare case of paratesticular embryonal rhabdomyosarcoma diagnosed by fine needle aspiration: a case report. Acta Cytol 2009;53:319–322.

26 Atahan S, Aksu O, Ekinci C: Cytologic diagnosis and subtyping of rhabdomyosarcoma. Cytopathology 1998;9:389–397.

27 Kumar PV, Kazemi H, Khezri A: Testicular embryonal rhabdomyosarcoma diagnosed by fine needle aspiration cytology: a report of two cases. Acta Cytol 1994;38:573–576.

28 Weber-Hall S, Anderson J, McManus A, Abe S, Nojima T, Pinkerton R, Pritchard-Jones K, Shipley J: Gains, losses, and amplification of genomic material in rhabdomyosarcoma analyzed by comparative genomic hybridization. Cancer Res 1996;56:3220–3224.

29 Choufani S, Shuman C, Weksberg R: Beckwith-Wiedemann syndrome. Am J Med Genet C Semin Med Genet 2010;154C:343–354.

30 de Almeida M, Stastny JF, Wakely PE Jr, Frable WJ: Fine-needle aspiration biopsy of childhood rhabdomyosarcoma: reevaluation of the cytologic criteria for diagnosis. Diagn Cytopathol 1994;11:231–236.

31 Barr FG: Gene fusions involving PAX and FOX family members in alveolar rhabdomyosarcoma. Oncogene 2001;20:5736–5746.

32 Barr FG, Duan F, Smith LM, Gustafson D, Pitts M, Hammond S, Gastier-Foster JM: Genomic and clinical analyses of 2p24 and 12q13-q14 amplification in alveolar rhabdomyosarcoma: a report from the Children's Oncology Group. Genes Chromosomes Cancer 2009;48:661–672.

33 Pohar-Marinsek Z, Srebotnik-Kirbis I: Desmin detection in FNAB samples of rhabdomyosarcoma: an immunocytochemical study. Cytopathology 2000;11:171–178.

34 Pohar-Marinsek Z, Bracko M: Rhabdomyosarcoma. Cytomorphology, subtyping and differential diagnostic dilemmas. Acta Cytol 2000;44:524–532.

35 Li G, Ogose A, Kawashima H, Umezu H, Hotta T, Tohyama T, Ariizumi T, Endo N: Cytogenetic and real-time quantitative reverse-transcriptase polymerase chain reaction analyses in pleomorphic rhabdomyosarcoma. Cancer Genet Cytogenet 2009;192:1–9.

36 Gordon A, McManus A, Anderson J, Fisher C, Abe S, Nojima T, Pritchard-Jones K, Shipley J: Chromosomal imbalances in pleomorphic rhabdomyosarcomas and identification of the alveolar rhabdomyosarcoma-associated PAX3-FOXO1A fusion gene in one case. Cancer Genet Cytogenet 2003;140:73–77.

37 Robinson JC, Richardson MS, Neville BW, Day TA, Chi AC: Sclerosing rhabdomyosarcoma: report of a case arising in the head and neck of an adult and review of the literature. Head Neck Pathol 2013;7:193–202.

38 Daneshbod Y, Monabati A, Kumar PV, Rastegar M: Paratesticular spindle cell rhabdomyosarcoma diagnosed by fine needle aspiration cytology: a case report. Acta Cytol 2005;49:331–334.

39 Mahana S, Tomar R, Agarwal A, Sharma D, Khurana N, Gupta R: Spindle-cell rhabdomyosarcoma of the thumb: Rare site, rare tumor in a child. Diagn Cytopathol 2016;44:1094–1097.

40 Chiles MC, Parham DM, Qualman SJ, Teot LA, Bridge JA, Ullrich F, Barr FG, Meyer WH: Sclerosing rhabdomyosarcomas in children and adolescents: a clinicopathologic review of 13 cases from the Intergroup Rhabdomyosarcoma Study Group and Children's Oncology Group. Pediatr Dev Pathol 2004;7:583–594.

41 Bouron-Dal Soglio D, Rougemont AL, Absi R, Barrette S, Montpetit A, Fetni R, Fournet JC: SNP genotyping of a sclerosing rhabdomyosarcoma: reveals highly aneuploid profile and a specific *MDM2/HMGA2* amplification. Hum Pathol 2009;40:1347–1352.

42 Kohsaka S, Shukla N, Ameur N, Ito T, Ng CK, Wang L, Lim D, Marchetti A, Viale A, Pirun M, Socci ND, Qin LX, Sciot R, Bridge J, Singer S, Meyers P, Wexler LH, Barr FG, Dogan S, Fletcher JA, Reis-Filho JS, Ladanyi M: A recurrent neomorphic mutation in MYOD1 defines a clinically aggressive subset of embryonal rhabdomyosarcoma associated with PI3K-AKT pathway mutations. Nat Genet 2014;46:595–600.

43 Agaram NP, Chen CL, Zhang L, LaQuaglia MP, Wexler L, Antonescu CR: Recurrent MYOD1 mutations in pediatric and adult sclerosing and spindle cell rhabdomyosarcomas: evidence for a common pathogenesis. Genes Chromosomes Cancer 2014;53:779–787.

Domanski HA, Walther CS: FNA Cytology of Soft Tissue and Bone Tumors. Monogr Clin Cytol.
Basel, Karger, 2017, vol 22, pp 80–88 (DOI: 10.1159/000475099)

Vascular Tumors

Vascular neoplasms comprise a wide spectrum of entities, including varieties of benign hemangioma, low-grade/intermediate vascular neoplasms, such as pseudomyogenic hemangioendothelioma, and malignant vascular neoplasm, such as epithelioid hemangioendothelioma and angiosarcoma. Cytologic features of benign vascular tumors are usually nonspecific and fine-needle aspiration (FNA) cytology diagnosis must be supplemented by clinical and radiographic findings. Cytologic findings in smears from angiosarcoma and epithelioid hemangioepithelioma are more specific, especially in conjunction with ancillary techniques, and have been reported in some series and case reports.

Hemangioma

Purely cutaneous benign vascular tumors are rarely referred for FNA. The most common targets for FNA are intramuscular and deep subcutaneous hemangiomas, which often present clinically as a soft tissue mass. In many cases of aspiration of hemangioma, the syringe fills with blood without aspiration. Smears from hemangiomas, with the exception of infantile and some capillary hemangiomas [1], show poor cellularity with small sheets and clusters of uniform spindle cells or dispersed spindle cells with thin cytoplasmic processes and fusiform nuclei with pointed ends, corresponding to endothelial cells [2] (Fig. 1). Intramuscular heman-

giomas commonly undergo extensive fatty involution and aspirates from such lesions may be misinterpreted as benign lipomatous tumors.

Cytologic Features
- Often, when a needle reaches the tumor, the syringe is filled with blood before aspiration is even initiated
- Cell-poor, bloody smears
- Small sheets and clusters of uniform spindle cells with thin cytoplasmic processes and fusiform nuclei with pointed ends, corresponding to endothelial cells
- Variable presence of fragments of small capillaries, occasionally with a metachromatic matrix
- Histiocytes in variable numbers, some with hemosiderin pigment
- Small fragments of collagenous matrix and an admixture of adipose tissue may be seen in smears from intramuscular hemangiomas
- Smears of infantile and some capillary hemangiomas contain cohesive sheets and clusters of uniform spindle cells

Ancillary Tests
Immunophenotype
Positive for CD31, CD34, factor VIII, and Fli-1; positive for smooth muscle actin (SMA) in pericytic cells and GLUT1 in infantile hemangioma.

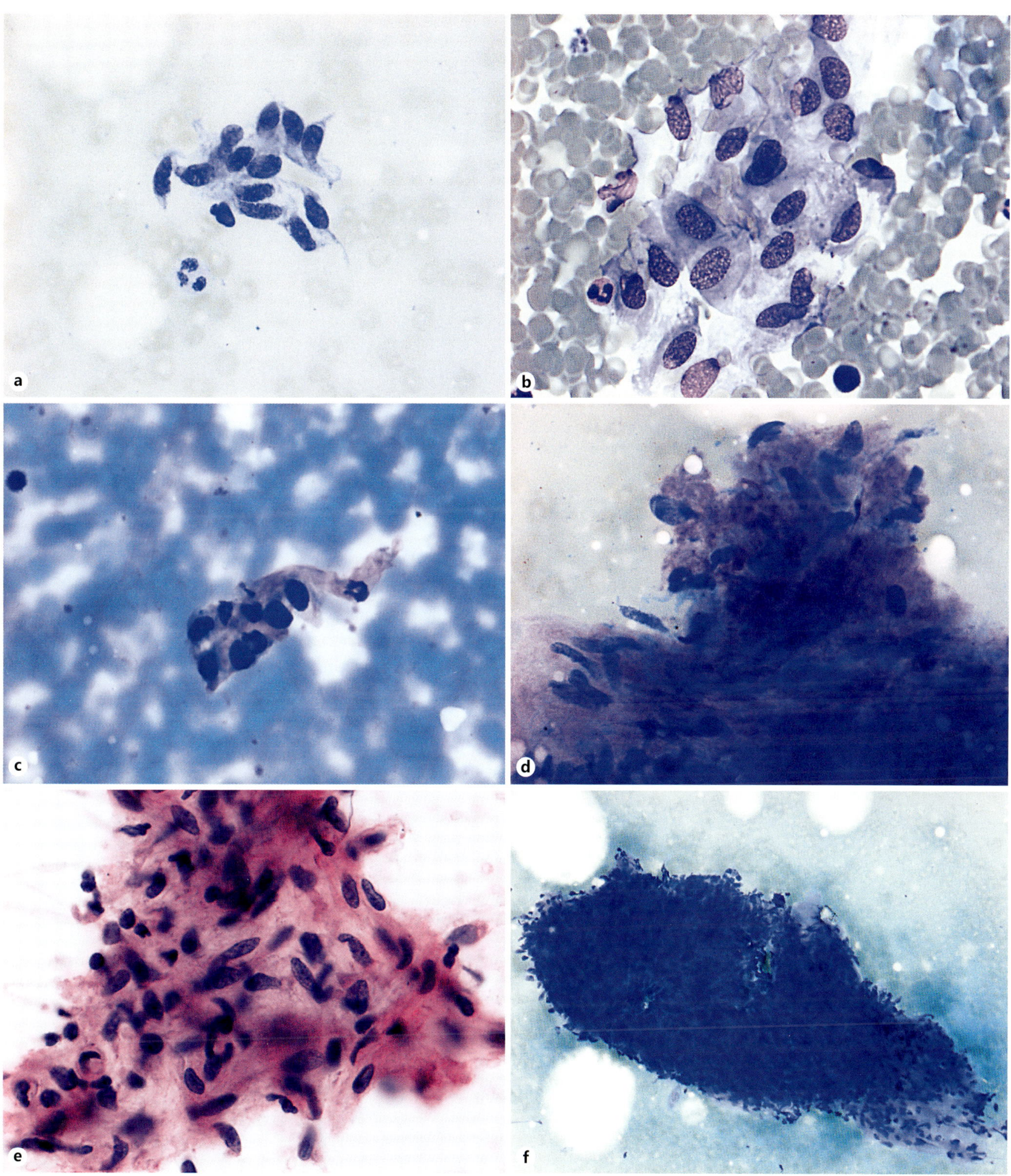

Fig. 1. Hemangioma. **a**, **b** Small sheets of poorly preserved bland spindle cells corresponding to endothelial cells. MGG stain. **c**, **d** Small capillaries and endothelial cells embedded in a collagenous matrix. MGG stain. Larger, loosely cohesive sheets (HE stain; **e**) and a tight cluster of spindle cells (MGG stain; **f**) in smears from juvenile hemangioma.

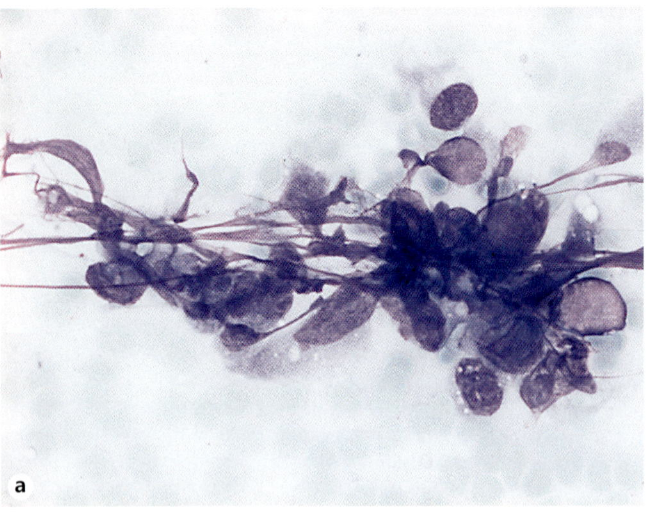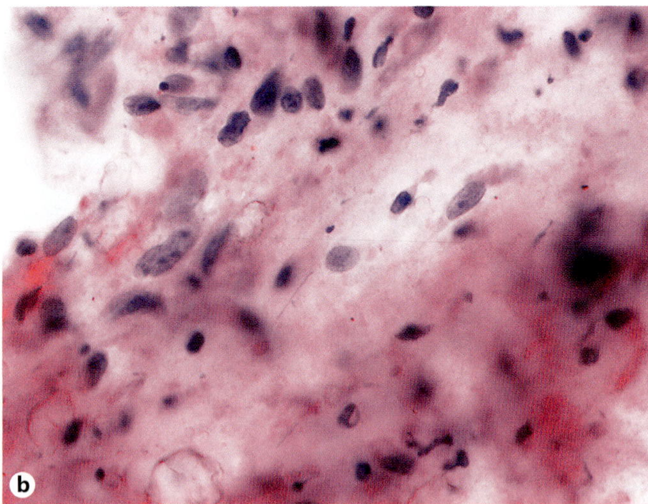

Fig. 2. KS. **a** A sheet of poorly preserved cells (crush artifacts) showing spindled and epithelioid morphology and a bland nuclei. MGG stain. **b** Dispersed and poorly preserved slight to moderately pleomorphic spindle cells and bare spindle-shaped nuclei in a collagenous matrix. HE stain.

Genetics

No known recurrent or specific genetic changes have been described.

Differential Diagnosis
- Benign spindle-cell neoplasms
- Angiomatoid fibrous histiocytoma
- Malignant vascular neoplasms
- Benign lipomatous tumors

A specific diagnosis of hemangioma may be rendered from an FNA specimen when smears contain sheets or clusters of spindle cells that are positive for endothelial markers such as CD31, factor VIII, and Fli-1 (Fig. 1).

Kaposi Sarcoma

Kaposi sarcoma (KS) is a locally aggressive endothelial neoplasm that commonly arises in the skin and is associated with human herpes virus 8 (HHV8) infection. KS may even arise in a wide variety of other locations, including mucosal membranes, visceral organs, and lymph nodes. Four different clinical forms of KS exist. Classic KS arises in the skin of the lower legs in elderly men. An endemic form of KS occurs in children and middle-aged adults in central Africa. This form may be associated with endemic lymphedema but is not associated with HIV infection. An iatrogenic form develops in patients receiving immunosuppressive treatment, and an AIDS-associated form arises in patients with coexisting HIV-1 and HHV8 infections. HIV-associated KS tends to be the most aggressive type and often presents as a disseminated neoplasm. Smears from KS show small sheets and clusters of slightly to moderately atypical spindle cells or dispersed spindle cells with cytoplasmic processes and fusiform nuclei with pointed ends, finely distributed chromatin, and occasional tiny nucleoli, corresponding to atypical endothelial cells [3–10] (Fig. 2).

Cytologic Features
- Mixture of dispersed and small, loosely cohesive sheets of spindle cells
- Spindle cells contain bland-looking, oval, elongated nuclei
- The cytoplasm is often poorly preserved, but in many tumor cells with a preserved cytoplasm small cytoplasmic extensions may be seen

Ancillary Tests

Immunophenotype

Positive for HHV8 in essentially 100% of cases, positive for endothelial markers.

Genetics

The detection of HHV8, also known as KS-associated Herpes virus, can be made with polymerase chain reaction (PCR) on fresh or fixed material [11]. No recurrent clinically relevant genetic changes have been found.

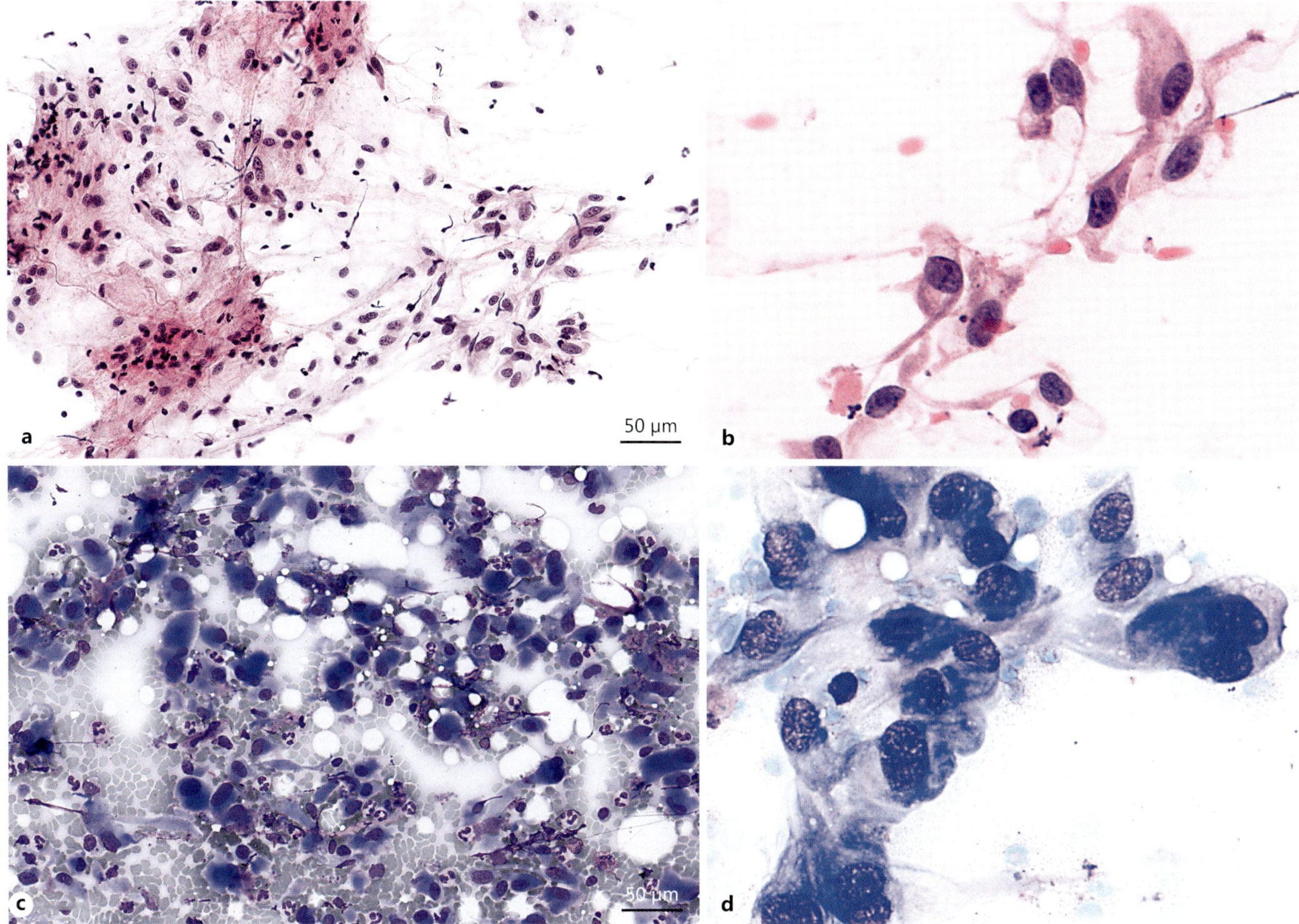

Fig. 3. Pseudomyogenic hemangioendothelioma. **a, b** Loosely cohesive sheets and dispersed atypical spindle cells with fusiform and ovoid nuclei and occasionally abundant cytoplasm with cytoplasmic processes resembling smears of nodular fasciitis. HE stain. **c, d** Dispersed spindle and plump cells with an abundant cytoplasm and fusiform, rounded to oval nuclei with slight anisonucleosis and tiny nucleoli. Some binucleated tumor cells with an abundant cytoplasm resembling "ganglion cells" of nodular/proliferative fasciitis. MGG stain.

Differential Diagnosis

- Angiosarcoma
- Spindle cell sarcomas of various lineages

KS is usually diagnosed by punch biopsy or incisional biopsy and cutaneous/subcutaneous nodules suspected to be manifestations of KS are rare targets for cytologic examination. However, FNA may provide sufficient material for diagnosis, especially when routine cytologic examination is complemented by ancillary studies [12].

Pseudomyogenic Hemangioendothelioma

Pseudomyogenic hemangioendothelioma is a distinctive, intermediate, rarely metastasizing vascular neoplasm, arising often in the superficial and deep soft tissues and bone of the extremities, particularly the lower limbs [13]. Approximately 50% of cases of pseudomyogenic hemangioendothelioma are multicentric, involving different tissue planes in the extremities, trunk, abdomen, and head and neck. Most cases occur in the second and third decades of life with a striking male predominance. No case describing FNA findings has been reported to date, but based on our own experience smears from pseudomyogenic hemangioendothelioma

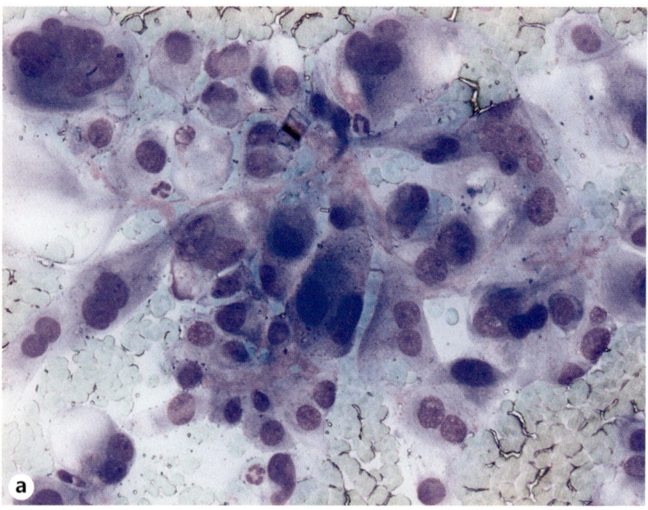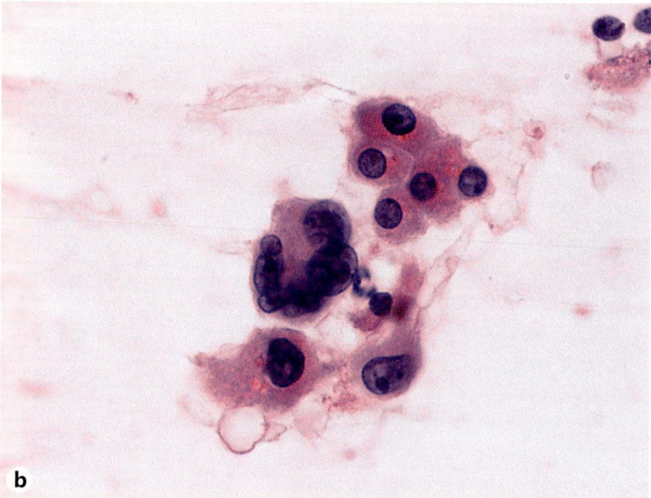

Fig. 4. Epithelioid hemangioendothelioma. **a** A poorly cohesive group of moderately pleomorphic and some binucleated and multinucleated cells, showing round to oval nuclei with tiny nucleoli and an abundant cytoplasm. MGG stain. **b** Epithelioid hemangioendothelioma in the liver. Smears shows a couple of moderately pleomorphic tumor cells with an abundant cytoplasm, 1 multinucleated tumor cell, and a small group of hepatocytes. HE stain.

resemble those from nodular fasciitis, with loosely cohesive fascicles and clusters with an admixture of dispersed variable pleomorphic spindle cells with an abundant cytoplasm with cytoplasmic extensions. Tumor cells contain oval and occasionally rounded, irregular nuclei with relatively finely distributed chromatin and distinct nucleoli. Binuclear ganglion-like cells are easy to find, resembling smears of nodular fasciitis (Fig. 3).

Cytologic Features
- Cellular aspirates
- Occasionally a sparse myxoid background matrix
- Dispersed spindle cells mixed with small- and medium-sized, loosely cohesive clusters and sheets of spindle cells
- Spindle cells often show an abundant cytoplasm and long cytoplasmic extensions
- A collagenous matrix and occasional capillary vessels occur in some cell clusters
- Variable anisocytosis and anisokaryosis and distinct nucleoli
- Mono- and binucleated ganglion-like cells

Ancillary Tests
Immunophenotype
Positive for cytokeratin AE1/AE3, FLI-1, ERG, and CD31 in approximately 50% of cases, retained nuclear INI1.

Genetics
Chromosome banding and fluorescence in situ hybridization (FISH) analyses have shown a balanced t(7;19)(q22;q13) translocation as the sole aberration in several cases [13, 14]. The detected t(7;19)(q22;q13) translocation results in a *SERPINE1-FOSB* fusion gene that acts as a transcription factor. The high frequency of this specific fusion event makes it a useful diagnostic tool to distinguish pseudomyogenic hemangioendothelioma from morphologic mimics [15]. Cytogenetics, FISH, PCR, and next-generation sequencing (NGS) can all provide information regarding the translocation and the resulting gene fusion on both fixed and fresh material.

Differential Diagnosis
- Nodular fasciitis/proliferative fasciitis
- Pleomorphic, spindle-cell, and myxoid sarcomas
  Cytologic features and an occasional clinical presentation of pseudomyogenic hemangioendothelioma resemble those of nodular fasciitis/proliferative fasciitis. A characteristic immunoprofile showing a combination of keratin and endothelial markers helps to distinguish this neoplasm from fasciitis and other neoplasms with an overlapping cytomorphology.

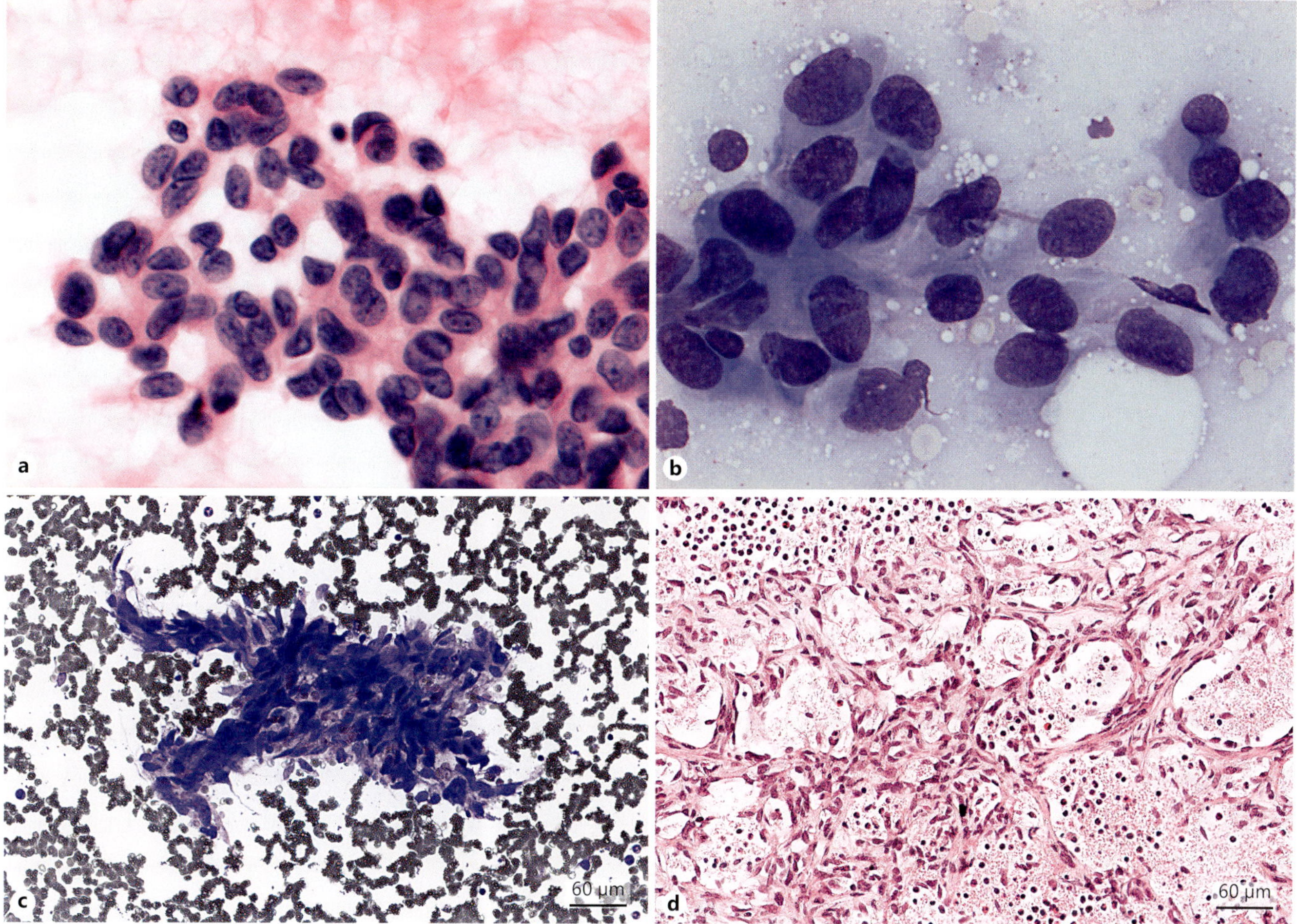

Fig. 5. Angiosarcoma. **a**, **b** Loosely cohesive sheets of moderately pleomorphic cells with variable spindled and epithelioid morphology. It may be difficult to render a specific diagnosis of angiosarcoma without ancillary studies. HE and MGG stains. **c–e** Skeletal metastasis of angiosarcoma: tight cluster of bland or slightly atypical spindle cells embedded in a collagenous matrix (MGG stain; **c**); cell block section and positive immunoreactivity for CD31 confirms the diagnosis of metastatic angiosarcoma (cell block; HE stain and CD31; **d**, **e**). **f**, **g** Epithelioid angiosarcoma in the liver: some pleomorphic tumor cells with epithelioid morphology and molding resembling carcinoma cells adjacent to a group of hepatocytes (HE stain; **f**); positive immunoreactivity for CD31 on a cell block section confirms the diagnosis of angiosarcoma (cell block; CD31; **g**).

(Figure continued on next page.)

Epithelioid Hemangioendothelioma

Epithelioid hemangioendothelioma is a malignant vascular neoplasm arising in middle-aged adults with a wide distribution in both soft tissues of the extremities, trunk, head and neck region, bone, and in visceral organs, particularly the lungs and liver. About 50% of cases show clear angiocentricity involving medium-sized or larger vessels. Histologic features of epithelioid hemangioendothelioma include cords and strands of epithelioid endothelial cells with an eosinophilic cytoplasm and quite often intracytoplasmic vacu-

oles. Tumor cells grow in a characteristic myxohyaline matrix. Smears from epithelioid hemangioendothelioma show small clusters and dispersed epithelioid, polygonal, occasional spindle-shaped cells with a variable nuclear pleomorphism, dense cytoplasm, and distinct cytoplasmic borders. Variable but often slight to moderate anisokaryosis, nuclear grooves, pseudoinclusions, and occasional nucleoli are observed in some tumor cells [16–24] (Fig. 4).

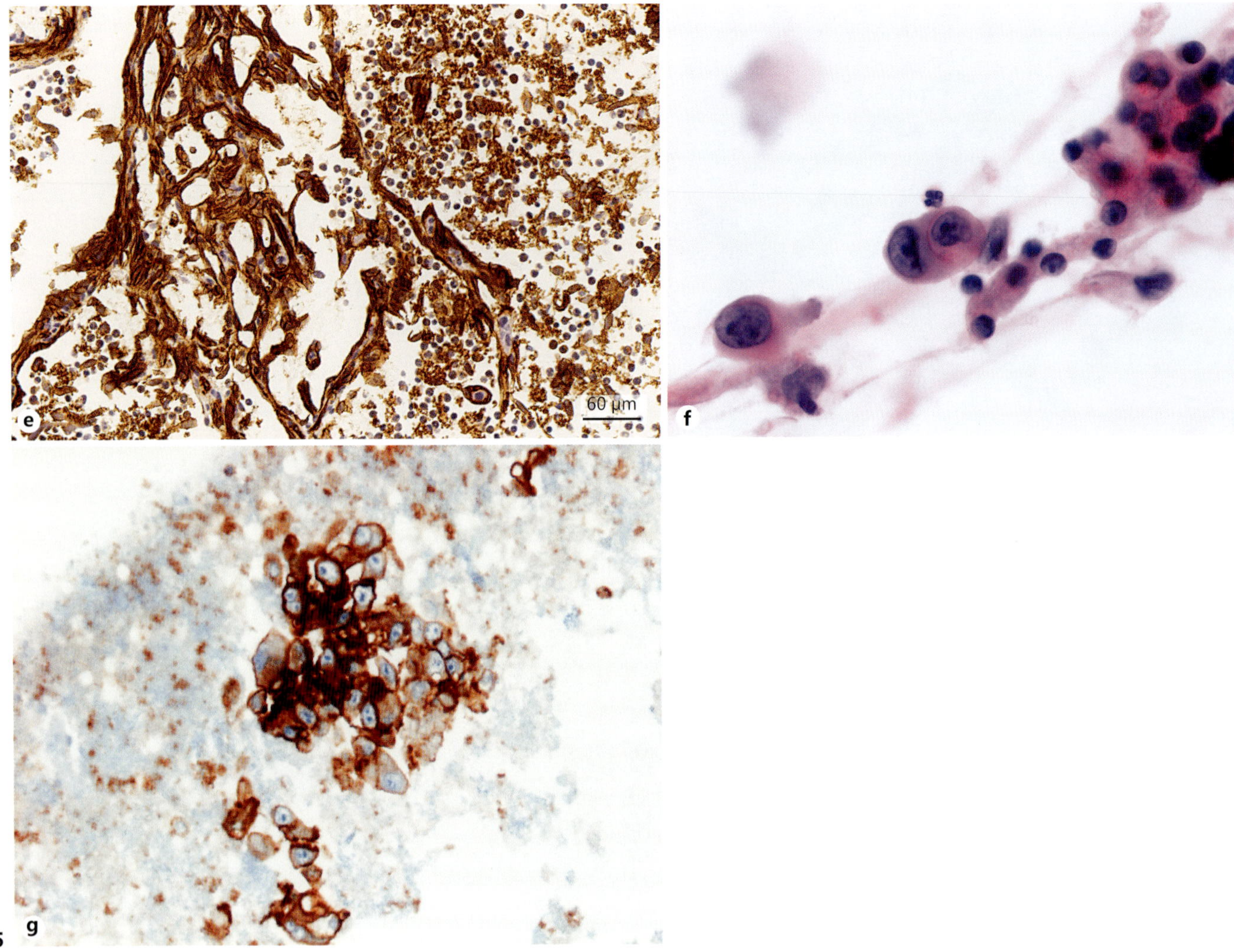

Cytologic Features

- Clustered and dispersed epithelioid, polygonal, occasional spindle-shaped cells with a variable pleomorphism
- Dense cytoplasm with occasional intracytoplasmic lumina
- Binucleated and rare multinucleated cells
- Variable but often slight to moderate anisokaryosis with nuclear grooves, pseudoinclusions, and occasional nucleoli
- Fragments of hyaline and myxohyaline matrix in the background and scant hyaline matrix within the tumor cell clusters

Ancillary Tests

Immunophenotype
Positive for CD31, CD34, ERG, FLI-1, and keratin in a third of cases.

Genetics
No specific or recurrent genetic changes have been detected.

Differential diagnosis
- Epithelioid angiosarcoma [17]
- Epithelioid sarcoma
- Metastatic carcinoma
- Metastatic melanoma
- Mesothelioma

Angiosarcoma

The vast majority of angiosarcomas are cutaneous tumors and only about 20% arise in soft tissue. Smears of angiosarcomas are most often diagnosed as malignant. A specific diagnosis of angiosarcoma is difficult to make in routinely stained smears, however, since aspirates from angiosarcoma show a very variable micromorphology [17, 25–31]. Spindle cell sarcomatoid patterns, a predominance of epithelioid tumor cells with microscopic features resembling metastatic carcinoma, and a variable clustering and pleomorphism of malignant endothelial cells can all be seen (Fig. 5). Immunocytochemical studies to demonstrate endothelial markers are almost always necessary to establish the correct diagnosis (Fig. 5). In the unusual case where vasoformative structures such as small acinar-like formations with central erythrocytes or frequent vacuolated cells containing single erythrocytes are present, a diagnosis of angiosarcoma can be suggested solely on morphologic grounds.

Cytologic Features
- Variable yield
- Often hemorrhagic aspirates
- Mixture of dispersed cells, cells in clusters or groups
- Variable cellular and nuclear pleomorphism
- Variable presence of pleomorphic/polygonal cells and spindle cells
- Occasional acinar structures and signet ring-like cells, often with single erythrocytes within cytoplasmic vacuoles
- Epithelioid cells showing cell molding and nuclei with prominent nucleoli in cases of epithelioid angiosarcoma

Ancillary Tests
Immunophenotype
Positive for CD31, CD34, FLI-1, ERG, and keratin in the majority of epithelioid angiosarcoma cases.

Genetics
These tumors show upregulation of vascular-specific tyrosine kinases, including *TIE1*, *KDR*, *TEK*, and *FLT1*, compared to other tumors. *MYC* amplification in 8q24 is a well-recognized finding in radiation-induced angiosarcoma [32]. These changes can be detected with FISH, single nucleotide polymorphism-array, PCR, and NGS on fresh or fixed material.

Differential Diagnosis
- Spindle cell sarcoma of various lines of differentiation
- Pleomorphic sarcoma of various lines of differentiation
- Epithelioid sarcoma of various lines of differentiation
- Carcinoma metastasis
- Malignant melanoma metastasis

Tumor cells in epithelioid angiosarcoma express cytokeratins in approximately 50% of cases, which can lead to an erroneous diagnosis of metastatic carcinoma [33, 34].

References

1 Sharma S, Mannan R, Bhasin T: Cytological diagnosis of deep-seated cellular hemangioma of the parotid gland by using cell button technique. J Cytol 2016;33:174–176.

2 Layfield LJ, Mooney EE, Dodd LG: Not by blood alone: diagnosis of hemangiomas by fine-needle aspiration. Diagn Cytopathol 1998;19:250–254.

3 Warpe BM: Kaposi sarcoma as initial presentation of HIV infection. N Am J Med Sci 2014;6:650–652.

4 Yergiyev O, Mohanty A, Curran-Melendez S, Latona CR, Bhagavatula R, Greenberg L, Silverman JF: Fine-needle aspiration cytology of disseminated Kaposi sarcoma of the bone in an AIDS patient. Acta Cytol 2015;59:113–117.

5 Michelow P, Dezube BJ, Pantanowitz L: Fine needle aspiration of salivary gland masses in HIV-infected patients. Diagn Cytopathol 2012;40:684–690.

6 Morelli L, Pusiol T, Piscioli I, Del Nonno F, Brenna A, Licci S: Fine needle aspiration cytology determinants of the diagnosis of primary nodal Kaposi's sarcoma as the first sign of unknown HIV infection: a case report. Acta Cytol 2007;51:602–604.

7 Poniecka A, Ghorab Z, Arnold D, Khaled A, Ganjei-Azar P: Kaposi's sarcoma of the thyroid gland in an HIV-negative woman: a case report. Acta Cytol 2007;51:421–423.

8 Gamborino E, Carrilho C, Ferro J, Khan MS, Garcia C, Suarez MC, Yokoyama H, Schmitt FC: Fine-needle aspiration diagnosis of Kaposi's sarcoma in a developing country. Diagn Cytopathol 2000;23:322–325.

9 al-Rikabi AC, Haidar Z, Arif M, al-Ajlan AZ, Ramia S: Fine-needle aspiration cytology of primary Kaposi's sarcoma of lymph nodes in an immunocompetent man. Diagn Cytopathol 1998;19:451–454.

10 Daskalopoulou D, Galanopoulou A, Statiropoulou P, Papapetrou S, Pandazis I, Markidou S: Cytologically interesting cases of primary skin tumors and tumor-like conditions identified by fine-needle aspiration biopsy. Diagn Cytopathol 1998;19:17–28.

11 Folpe AL, Chand EM, Goldblum JR, Weiss SW: Expression of Fli-1, a nuclear transcription factor, distinguishes vascular neoplasms from potential mimics. Am J Surg Pathol 2001;25:1061–1066.

12 Alkan S, Eltoum IA, Tabbara S, Day E, Karcher DS: Usefulness of molecular detection of human herpesvirus-8 in the diagnosis of Kaposi sarcoma by fine-needle aspiration. Am J Clin Pathol 1999;111:91–96.

13 Hornick JL, Fletcher CD: Pseudomyogenic hemangioendothelioma: a distinctive, often multicentric tumor with indolent behavior. Am J Surg Pathol 2011;35:190–201.

14 Trombetta D, Magnusson L, von Steyern FV, Hornick JL, Fletcher CD, Mertens F: Translocation t(7; 19)(q22;q13) – a recurrent chromosome aberration in pseudomyogenic hemangioendothelioma? Cancer Genet 2011;204:211–215.

15 Walther C, Tayebwa J, Lilljebjorn H, Magnusson L, Nilsson J, von Steyern FV, Ora I, Domanski HA, Fioretos T, Nord KH, Fletcher CD, Mertens F: A novel SERPINE1-FOSB fusion gene results in transcriptional up-regulation of FOSB in pseudomyogenic haemangioendothelioma. J Pathol 2014;232:534–540.

16 Campione S, Cozzolino I, Mainenti P, D'Alessandro V, Vetrani A, D'Armiento M: Hepatic epithelioid hemangioendothelioma: pitfalls in the diagnosis on fine needle cytology and "small biopsy" and review of the literature. Pathol Res Pract 2015;211:702–705.

17 VandenBussche CJ, Wakely PE Jr, Siddiqui MT, Maleki Z, Ali SZ: Cytopathologic characteristics of epithelioid vascular malignancies. Acta Cytol 2014;58:356–366.

18 Jurczyk M, Zhu B, Laskin W, Lin X: Pitfalls in the diagnosis of hepatic epithelioid hemangioendothelioma by FNA and needle core biopsy. Diagn Cytopathol 2014;42:516–520.

19 Sehgal S, Agarwal R, Verma S, Kumar Verma A, Singh S: Fine needle aspiration cytology of epithelioid hemangioendothelioma of soft tissue. Diagn Cytopathol 2013;41:179–182.

20 Murali R, Zarka MA, Ocal IT, Tazelaar HD: Cytologic features of epithelioid hemangioendothelioma. Am J Clin Pathol 2011;136:739–746.

21 Kurisu Y, Tsuji M, Kuwabara H, Shibayama Y: Characteristic cytologic findings of epithelioid hemangioendothelioma: a case report and review of literature. Diagn Cytopathol 2011;39:124–127.

22 Tong GX, Hamele-Bena D, Borczuk A, Monaco S, Khosh MM, Greenebaum E: Fine needle aspiration biopsy of epithelioid hemangioendothelioma of the oral cavity: report of one case and review of literature. Diagn Cytopathol 2006;34:218–223.

23 Sharma SG, Aron M, Kapila K, Ray R: Epithelioid hemangioma: morphological presentation on aspiration smears. Diagn Cytopathol 2006;34:830–833.

24 Kilpatrick SE, Koplyay PD, Ward WG, Richards F 2nd: Epithelioid hemangioendothelioma of bone and soft tissue: a fine-needle aspiration biopsy study with histologic and immunohistochemical confirmation. Diagn Cytopathol 1998;19:38–43.

25 Geller RL, Hookim K, Sullivan HC, Stuart LN, Edgar MA, Reid MD: Cytologic features of angiosarcoma: a review of 26 cases diagnosed on FNA. Cancer Cytopathol 2016;124:659–668.

26 Pohar-Marinsek Z, Lamovec J: Angiosarcoma in FNA smears: diagnostic accuracy, morphology, immunocytochemistry and differential diagnoses. Cytopathology 2010;21:311–319.

27 Fleshman R, Mayerson J, Wakely PE Jr: Fine-needle aspiration biopsy of high-grade sarcoma: a report of 107 cases. Cancer 2007;111:491–498.

28 Klijanienko J, Caillaud JM, Lagace R, Vielh P: Cytohistologic correlations in angiosarcoma including classic and epithelioid variants: Institut Curie's experience. Diagn Cytopathol 2003;29:140–145.

29 Boucher LD, Swanson PE, Stanley MW, Silverman JF, Raab SS, Geisinger KR: Cytology of angiosarcoma: findings in fourteen fine-needle aspiration biopsy specimens and one pleural fluid specimen. Am J Clin Pathol 2000;114:210–219.

30 Nguyen GK, Husain M: Fine-needle aspiration biopsy cytology of angiosarcoma. Diagn Cytopathol 2000;23:143–145.

31 Liu K, Layfield LJ: Cytomorphologic features of angiosarcoma on fine needle aspiration biopsy. Acta Cytol 1999;43:407–415.

32 Guo T, Zhang L, Chang NE, Singer S, Maki RG, Antonescu CR: Consistent *MYC* and *FLT4* gene amplification in radiation-induced angiosarcoma but not in other radiation-associated atypical vascular lesions. Genes Chromosomes Cancer 2011;50:25–33.

33 Singh C, Xie L, Schmechel SC, Manivel JC, Pambuccian SE: Epithelioid angiosarcoma of the kidney: a diagnostic dilemma in fine-needle aspiration cytology. Diagn Cytopathol 2012;40(suppl 2):E131–E139.

34 Fulciniti F, Di Mattia D, Bove P, Mastro AA, De Chiara A, Botti G, Petrillo A, Apice G: Fine needle aspiration of metastatic epithelioid angiosarcoma: a report of 2 cases. Acta Cytol 2008;52:612–618.

Domanski HA, Walther CS: FNA Cytology of Soft Tissue and Bone Tumors. Monogr Clin Cytol.
Basel, Karger, 2017, vol 22, pp 89–91 (DOI: 10.1159/000475100)

Gastrointestinal Stromal Tumor

Gastrointestinal stromal tumors (GISTs) are spindle cell or epithelioid neoplasms derived from the interstitial cells of Cajal in the bowel wall and are the most common mesenchymal tumor of the gastrointestinal tract. The majority of GISTs arise in middle-aged or elderly adults and the most common primary site is the stomach, followed by the small intestine, esophagus, colon, and rectum. Rare cases arise in the retroperitoneum, mesentery, and omentum. Clinically, GISTs show a spectrum from benign, through neoplasms having an uncertain malignant potential, to clearly malignant tumors with metastatic potential. The risk of malignant behavior is associated with the anatomic site, tumor size, and mitotic rate.

Cytologic Features [1–10]
- Moderately or richly cellular smears
- Often tight clusters and fascicular tissue fragments of spindle cells showing slight to moderate atypia and a poorly preserved cytoplasm with indistinct cytoplasmic borders
- Bland nuclei with a fine chromatin pattern and indistinct nucleoli
- An admixture of dispersed cells and naked nuclei is common
- A small subset of GISTs display marked cellular and nuclear atypia with occasional nuclei showing an irregular nuclear membrane, coarse chromatin, hyperchromasia, and obvious nucleoli
- Epithelioid, polygonal, and plasmacytoid cells with round to oval nuclei and moderate to abundant, sometimes vacuolated, cytoplasm
- Mitoses rare or absent

Ancillary Tests
Immunophenotype
Positive for c-Kit (CD117), DOG-1, and CD34 in the majority of cases; variable focal immunoreactivity for smooth muscle actin; rare focal immunoreactivity for S100 and desmin.

Genetics
GISTs often display oncogenic mutations in 1 of 2 tyrosine kinases, *C-KIT* or *PDGFRA* [11]. They control cell pathways that stimulate proliferation, downregulate apoptosis, and regulate cell differentiation, adhesion, and motility in normal conditions. Mutations of *C-KIT* and *PDGFRA* lead to activation of these cell pathways, inducing proliferation and tumor growth. Mutations are found in different exons or regions of a single exon as point mutations, deletions, and insertions in the *KIT* (exon 9, 11, 13, and 17) and *PGFRA* (exon 12, 14, and 18) genes. Approximately 80% of GISTs display *C-KIT* mutations and 15% display *PDGFRA* mutations, both situated at chromosome 4q12. The drug imatinib specifically blocks the resulting proteins of both these genes, stopping the tumor cells from dividing and growing. To detect these specific and relatively small mutations, poly-

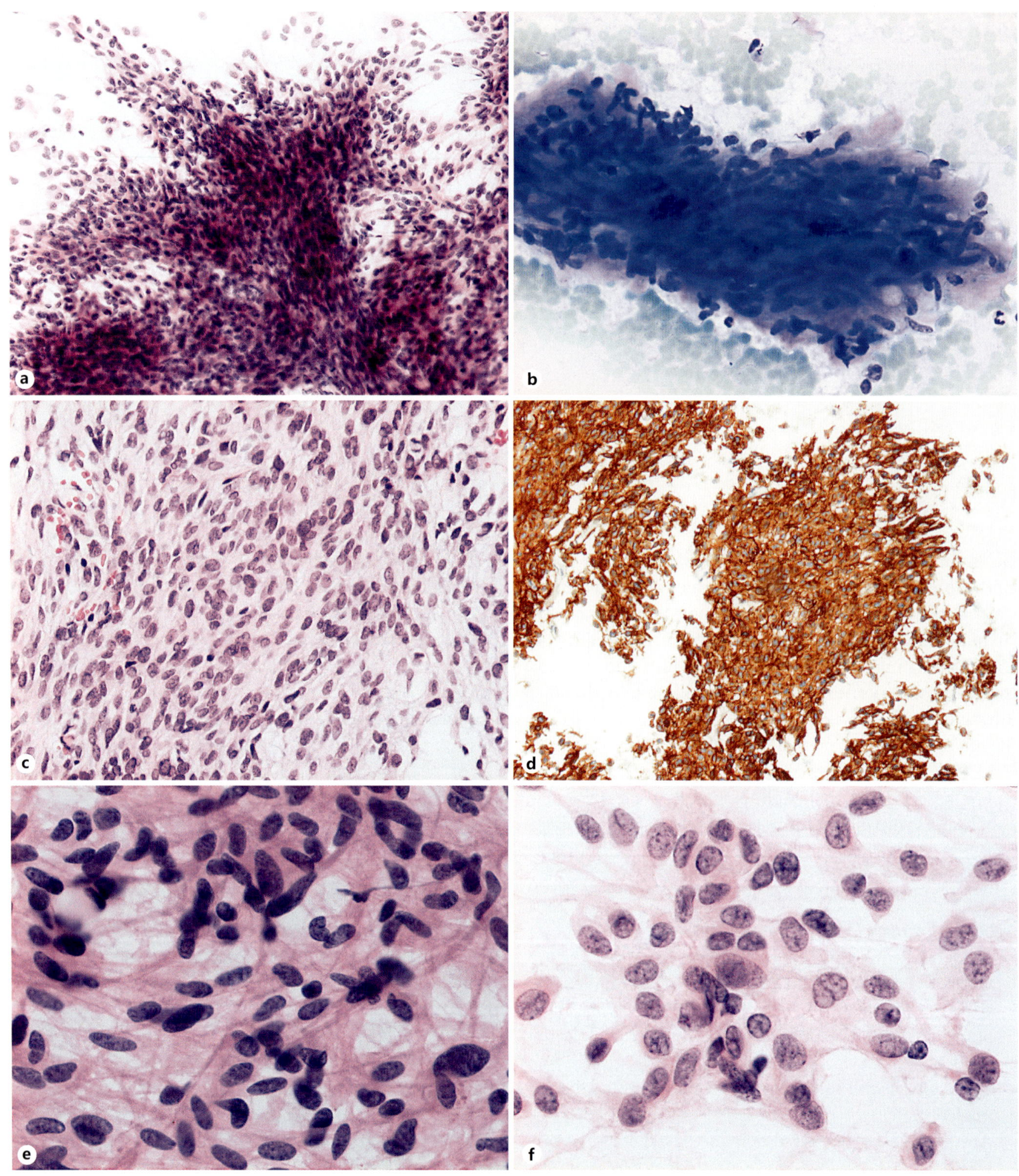

Fig. 1. GIST. **a** Large fascicular tissue fragments of slight to moderately atypical spindle cells with a poorly preserved cytoplasm. HE stain. **b** A cohesive cluster of spindle cells with bland spindled and ovoid nuclei, indistinct cytoplasmic borders, and a collagenous background matrix. MGG stain. **c**, **d** Corresponding cell block section showing fascicular spindle cell neoplasm and CD117 expression. Cell block; HE and CD117 staining. **e** A subset of GISTs including epithelioid variants (**f**) display cells with moderate cellular and nuclear atypia and occasional hyperchromatic nuclei with coarse chromatin and an irregular nuclear membrane. HE stain.

FNA Cytology of Soft Tissue and Bone Tumors

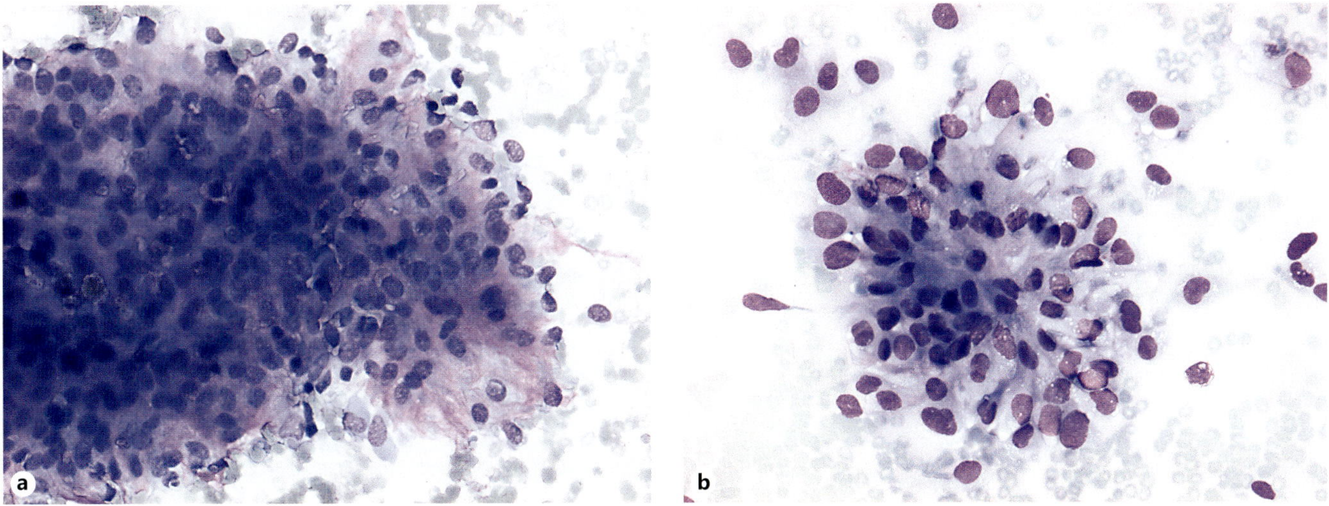

Fig. 2. Epithelioid variants of GIST. Cohesive (**a**) and loosely cohesive (**b**) sheets of uniform or slightly atypical cells and bare nuclei with epithelioid morphology embedded in the collagenous matrix. MGG stain.

merase chain reaction and next-generation sequencing can be used on fresh or fixed material.

Differential Diagnosis
- Spindle cell sarcoma of various lines of differentiation
- Schwannoma
- Solitary fibrous tumor
- Mesenteric desmoid tumor

- Inflammatory myofibroblastic tumor

Although GIST is the most common mesenchymal neoplasm of the gastrointestinal tract, differential diagnoses include spindle cell neoplasms that can resemble GIST in smears, both benign and malignant. Rendering a specific cytologic diagnosis of GIST from fine-needle aspiration smears requires the use of ancillary techniques (Fig. 1) [12, 13]. Rare variants of GIST with epithelioid morphology may be confused with epithelial neoplasm (Fig. 2).

References

1 Vij M, Agrawal V, Kumar A, Pandey R: Cytomorphology of gastrointestinal stromal tumors and extra-gastrointestinal stromal tumors: a comprehensive morphologic study. J Cytol 2013;30:8–12.
2 Kaur G, Manucha V, Verma K: Gastrointestinal stromal tumors: cytomorphologic spectrum in fine needle aspiration smears. Indian J Pathol Microbiol 2010;53:271–275.
3 Yoshida S, Yamashita K, Yokozawa M, Kida M, Takezawa M, Mikami T, Okayasu I: Diagnostic findings of ultrasound-guided fine-needle aspiration cytology for gastrointestinal stromal tumors: proposal of a combined cytology with newly defined features and histology diagnosis. Pathol Int 2009;59:712–719.
4 Chatzipantelis P, Salla C, Karoumpalis I, Apessou D, Sakellariou S, Doumani I, Papaliodi E, Konstantinou P: Endoscopic ultrasound-guided fine needle aspiration biopsy in the diagnosis of gastrointestinal stromal tumors of the stomach: a study of 17 cases. J Gastrointestin Liver Dis 2008; 17:15–20.

5 Akahoshi K, Sumida Y, Matsui N, Oya M, Akinaga R, Kubokawa M, Motomura Y, Honda K, Watanabe M, Nagaie T: Preoperative diagnosis of gastrointestinal stromal tumor by endoscopic ultrasound-guided fine needle aspiration. World J Gastroenterol 2007;13:2077–2082.
6 Elliott DD, Fanning CV, Caraway NP: The utility of fine-needle aspiration in the diagnosis of gastrointestinal stromal tumors: a cytomorphologic and immunohistochemical analysis with emphasis on malignant tumors. Cancer 2006;108:49–55.
7 Vander Noot MR 3rd, Eloubeidi MA, Chen VK, Eltoum I, Jhala D, Jhala N, Syed S, Chhieng DC: Diagnosis of gastrointestinal tract lesions by endoscopic ultrasound-guided fine-needle aspiration biopsy. Cancer 2004;102:157–163.

8 Dong Q, McKee G, Pitman M, Geisinger K, Tambouret R: Epithelioid variant of gastrointestinal stromal tumor: diagnosis by fine-needle aspiration. Diagn Cytopathol 2003;29:55–60.
9 Wieczorek TJ, Faquin WC, Rubin BP, Cibas ES: Cytologic diagnosis of gastrointestinal stromal tumor with emphasis on the differential diagnosis with leiomyosarcoma. Cancer 2001;93:276–287.
10 Seidal T, Edvardsson H: Diagnosis of gastrointestinal stromal tumor by fine-needle aspiration biopsy: a cytological and immunocytochemical study. Diagn Cytopathol 2000;23:397–401.
11 Corless CL, Heinrich MC: Molecular pathobiology of gastrointestinal stromal sarcomas. Annu Rev Pathol 2008;3:557–586.
12 Fatima N, Cohen C, Siddiqui MT: DOG1 utility in diagnosing gastrointestinal stromal tumors on fine-needle aspiration. Cancer Cytopathol 2011; 119:202–208.
13 Hwang DG, Qian X, Hornick JL: DOG1 antibody is a highly sensitive and specific marker for gastrointestinal stromal tumors in cytology cell blocks. Am J Clin Pathol 2011;135:448–453.

Domanski HA, Walther CS: FNA Cytology of Soft Tissue and Bone Tumors. Monogr Clin Cytol.
Basel, Karger, 2017, vol 22, pp 92–102 (DOI: 10.1159/000475101)

Nerve Sheath Tumors

Schwannoma

Schwannoma is a benign nerve sheath tumor composed of Schwann cells. They are typically encapsulated and arise sporadically in the superficial or, less often, the deep soft tissues of the head and neck and the limbs. Schwannomas arise occasionally in the retroperitoneum, posterior mediastinum, or as a pelvic mass (usually larger tumors) [1, 2]. A small subset of these tumors occurs in the gastrointestinal tract and parenchymal organs or involving cranial nerves. Schwannomas occur commonly in adults up to 50 years of age, but may be seen in all age groups. Approximately 10% are associated with syndromes such as neurofibromatosis type 2, schwannomatosis, or multiple meningiomas. Schwannomas are common targets for fine-needle aspiration (FNA) examination. Many patients experience sharp pain when their tumors are punctured, a pain which occasionally radiates along a nerve. This sign can provide a valuable clue to the diagnosis but is not entirely specific, and may be encountered in the aspiration of other soft tissue lesions situated close to a peripheral nerve. Smears from schwannomas vary with respect to cellularity but are often hypercellular, containing irregular tissue fragments of spindle cells embedded in a fibrillary stroma [3–6]. It is often possible to identify both the highly cellular Antoni A and the poorly cellular myxoid Antoni B components corresponding to microscopic patterns of tissue sections. Most of the spindle cells exhibit neurogenic differentiation, including elongated, wavy nuclei that are often pointed or folded and sometimes show a fishhook-like appearance. Many aspirates also contain variable amounts of small- or medium-sized epithelioid cells with round, bland-looking nuclei [7] (Fig. 1).

One of the main reasons that schwannomas may be difficult to diagnose from aspiration smears is that many show cystic changes resulting in poor cellularity or a nondiagnostic yield [7–10]. A subset of schwannoma termed ancient schwannoma may cause problems in the cytologic diagnosis as FNA smears from these contain atypical cells with marked anisonucleosis and hyperchromasia [11, 12]. Nuclei in the majority of these atypical cells, however, show evenly distributed chromatin and some have large intranuclear vacuoles – "Kern-loche" – which are characteristic of ancient schwannoma (Fig. 2). It is also often possible to find other components typical of a usual schwannoma in addition to the scattered atypical cells [7]. Yet another problem in the cytologic diagnosis of schwannoma may be the misinterpreting of smears from a cellular schwannoma as being a low-grade spindle-cell sarcoma. Demonstration of diffuse and strong positivity for S100 protein by immunocytochemistry is very helpful to confirm the benign and specific diagnosis of schwannoma.

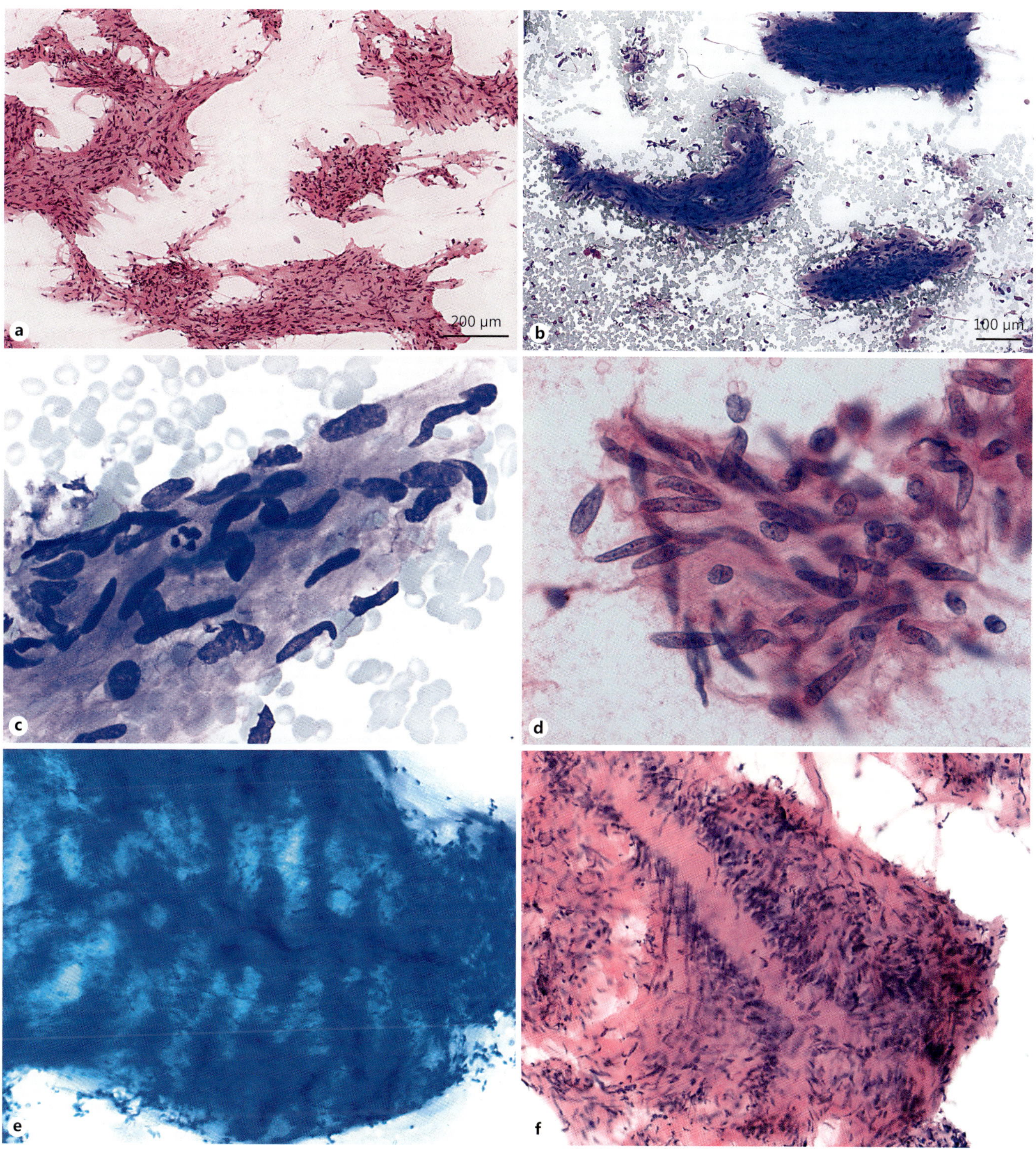

Fig. 1. Schwannoma. **a**, **b** Spindle cells in cohesive fascicles and sheets of variable size and shape with irregular borders – "pieces of a jigsaw puzzle" – and few dispersed cells. HE and MGG stains. **c**, **d** Most of the spindle cells exhibit neurogenic differentiation showing elongated, wavy nuclei that are often pointed or folded and sometimes show a fishhook-like appearance. MGG and HE stains. **e**, **f** Occasional nuclear palisading and Verocay bodies in the tissue fragments corresponding to Antoni A areas. MGG and HE stains. **g**, **h** An admixture of cells with epithelioid morphology showing small round nuclei is occasionally seen in smears of schwannoma. HE and MGG stains.

(Figure continued on next page.)

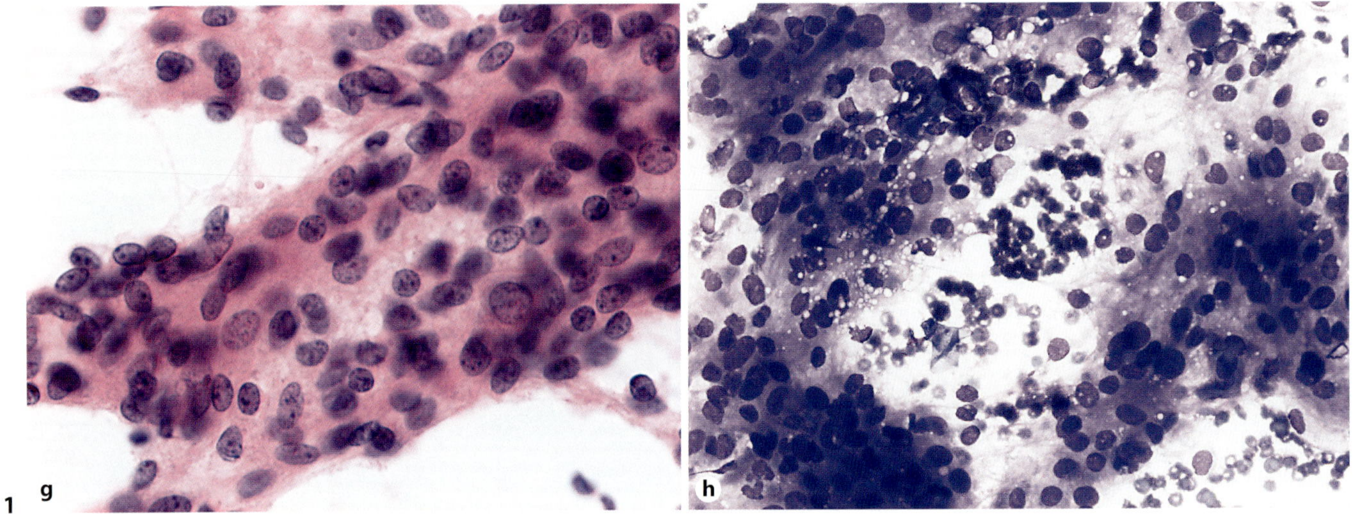

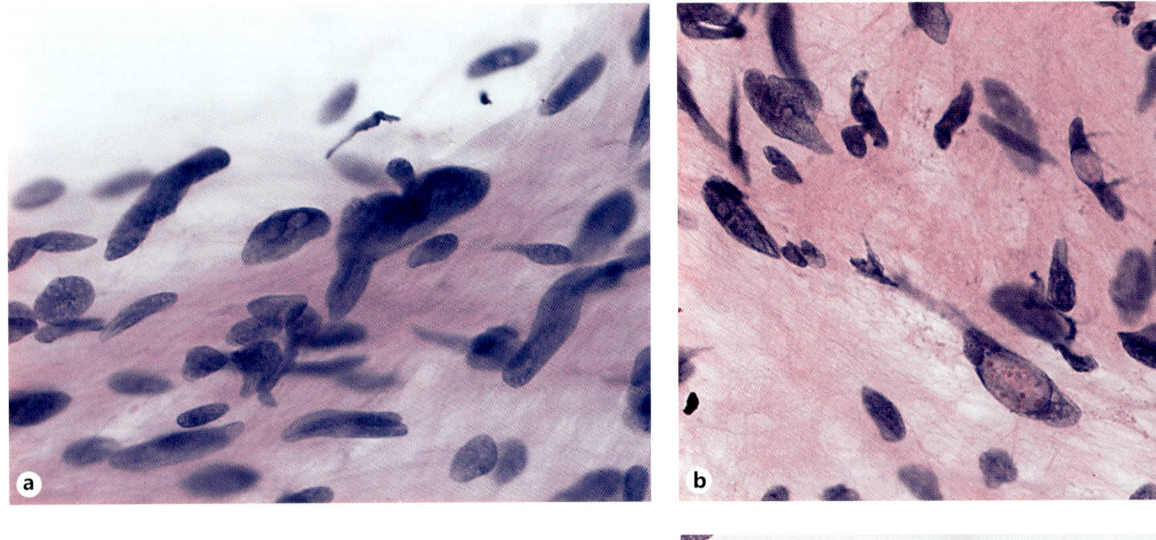

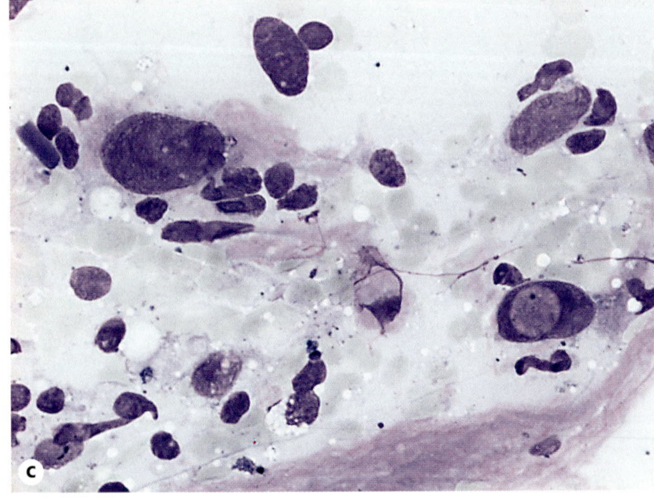

Fig. 2. Ancient schwannoma. **a–c** Cellular smears composed of loosely cohesive sheets and dispersed irregular spindled or epithelioid/polygonal cells with marked anisonucleosis, hyperchromasia, and occasional nuclei containing intranuclear inclusions – "Kern-loche." HE and MGG stains.

Cytologic Features
- Cohesive tissue fragments of different sizes, often with irregular borders ("jigsaw puzzle pieces")
- Occasional nuclear palisading and Verocay bodies in the tissue fragments corresponding to Antoni A areas
- Cell-poor smears with variable areas of myxoid matrix corresponding to Antoni B areas
- Scant dispersed cells
- Dispersed cells more common than in smears from Antoni A areas
- Spindle cells with indistinct cytoplasm and elongated, slender nuclei with pointed ends, boomerang-shaped, or comma-like nuclei ("fishhook" nuclei) embedded in a fibrillary stroma
- Occasionally cells with epithelioid morphology and small round nuclei
- Occasionally slight to moderate nuclear pleomorphism
- Cystic degeneration with the presence of histiocytes and inflammatory cells

Ancillary Tests
Immunophenotype
Strong and diffuse positivity for S100. Occasional focal positivity for glial fibrillary acidic protein (GFAP). Negative for CD34, CD117, and DOG1.

Genetics
Partial or complete loss of chromosome 22 is the most frequent cytogenetic anomaly in schwannomas [13]. Tumorigenesis is linked to inactivating mutations of the *NF2* tumor suppressor gene located at 22q12 and has been detected in 60% of new schwannoma cases [14, 15]. These anomalies and mutations can be detected with cytogenetics, fluorescence in situ hybridization (FISH), single nucleotide polymorphism (SNP) array, and next-generation sequencing (NGS) on both fresh and fixed material.

Differential Diagnosis
- Low-grade malignant peripheral nerve sheath tumor (MPNST)
- Low-grade leiomyosarcoma (LMS)
- Monophasic synovial sarcoma
- Neurofibroma
- Spindle cell lipoma
- Solitary fibrous tumor
- Desmoid-type fibromatosis
- Myxoid soft tissue tumors (Antoni B-type neurilemomas with large foci of myxoid matrix)
- Pleomorphic sarcomas (smears from ancient schwannomas)

The most important differential diagnoses are spindle cell sarcomas such as MPNST, LMS, and monophasic synovial sarcoma, which usually display a distinctive component of dispersed tumor cells in addition to cohesive cell clusters and sheets. A greater degree of nuclear pleomorphism is usually observed in smears from MPNST and LMS compared to smears of benign schwannomas. Ancillary techniques are often necessary to render the correct diagnosis of schwannoma in smears. Positive immunoreactivity for muscle markers helps to distinguish LMS from schwannoma. Focal positivity for epithelial membrane antigen (EMA) and keratin, and diffuse positivity for CD99 as well as 11:22 translocation helps to distinguish monophasic synovial sarcoma from schwannoma.

Neurofibroma

Neurofibroma is a nerve sheath tumor composed of Schwann cells, fibroblasts, and perineurial cells with an admixture of residual axons. Most neurofibromas are sporadic; approximately 10% are associated with neurofibromatosis type 1. The 3 main subtypes of neurofibroma are localized, diffuse, and plexiform neurofibromas. Localized neurofibroma is the most common type arising in the skin of the trunk, head and neck, and limbs in a wide range of ages, but most often in young and middle-aged adults. Diffuse neurofibroma, which is an infiltrative tumor, arises commonly in the head and neck area in children and young adults. Plexiform neurofibroma, which is always associated with neurofibromatosis type 1, arises in superficial or deep soft tissue and occasionally in the large nerve trunks in the head and neck area, trunk, and extremities of children and young adults. Sporadic neurofibromas and neurofibromas in patients with von Recklinghausen disease are occasionally referred for FNA when there is a question of malignant transformation. In the majority of neurofibromas, the tumor matrix is typically fibromyxoid, collagenous, or hyalinized, giving poorly cellular FNA smears [5, 16, 17] (Fig. 3). Neurofibroma cells in smears are often similar to those in smears from schwannoma: cohesive spindle cells with slender and often comma-like, bent, or wavy nuclei (Fig. 3). Different cell types in neurofibroma are indistinguishable in routinely stained smears and a specific diagnosis of neurofibroma based on FNA smears alone can be difficult without immunocytochemical studies [18, 19].

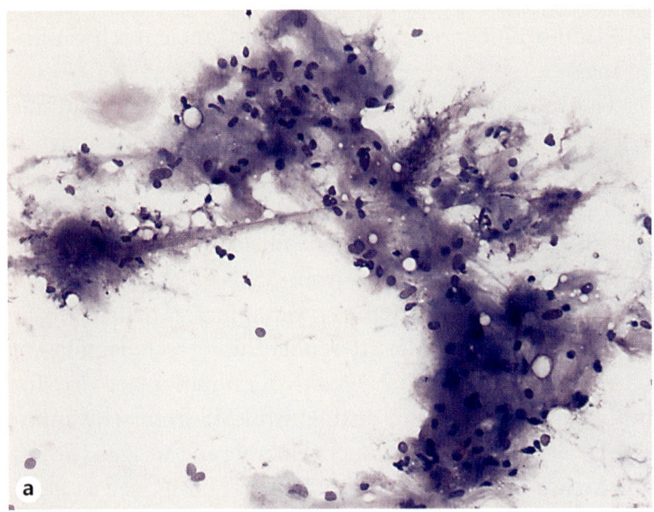

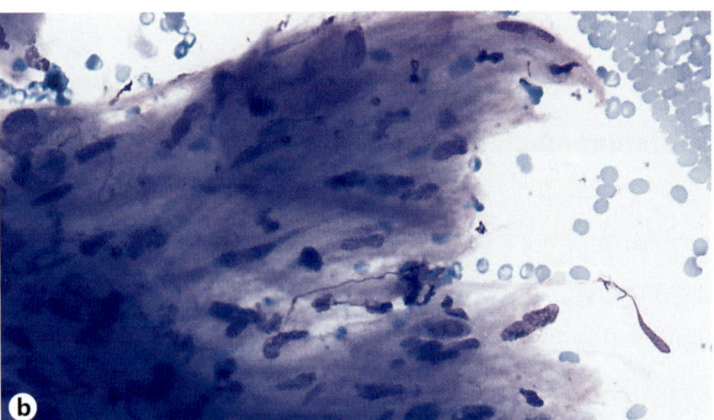

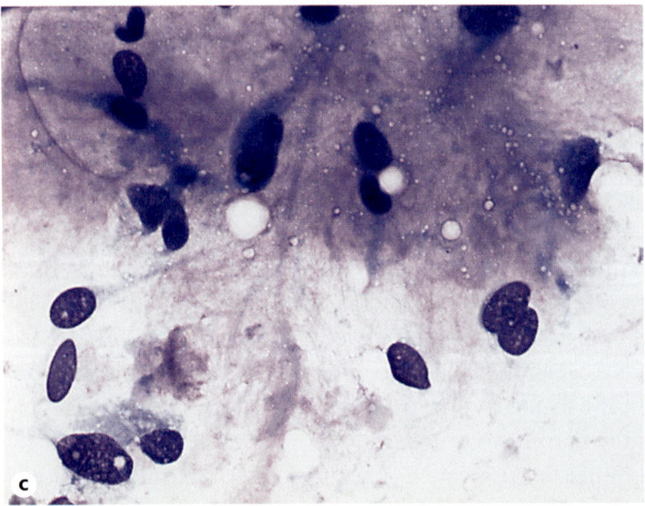

Fig. 3. Neurofibroma. **a** A loosely cohesive cluster of uniform and some slightly atypical cells with bland, round to ovoid nuclei and a fibrillary/myxoid background matrix. MGG stain. **b** A sheet of spindle cells with both Schwannian cells and fibroblast characteristics in a fibrillary/myxoid background matrix. MGG stain. **c** Scattered spindle cells with cytoplasmic extensions and naked nuclei of fibroblast-like cells in a myxoid matrix. MGG stain.

Cytologic Features
- Variable but often poor cellularity
- Occasional myxoid background matrix
- Small, loosely cohesive clusters of spindle cells and dispersed spindle cells with poorly preserved cytoplasm
- Bland, fibroblast-like spindle cells and "nerve" cells with an indistinct cytoplasm and elongated, slender nuclei with pointed ends
- Occasional small round nuclei
- Stripped nuclei

Ancillary Tests
Immunophenotype
Positive for S100 protein and CD34 in stromal cells; scattered perineurial cells show variable positivity for claudin-1, GLUT1, and EMA; scattered axons show positivity for neurofilament.

Genetics
The pathogenesis is loss of or inactivation of both copies of the tumor suppressor gene *NF1* at 17q11 [20]. This can be used for diagnostic purposes and detected by FISH, SNP array, polymerase chain reaction (PCR), and NGS on the available material.

Differential Diagnosis
- Schwannoma
- Low-grade MPNST
- Spindle cell lipoma
- Solitary fibrous tumor
- Intramuscular myxoma

As neurofibromas may be difficult to distinguish from other subtypes of neurogenic and spindle cell/myxoid neoplasms in FNA smears alone, smears from neurofibromas are often diagnosed as mesenchymal neoplasm or suspicious of nerve sheath neoplasm. Clinical data and ancillary studies may help to render the correct cytologic diagnosis.

Perineurioma

Soft tissue perineurioma is a rare benign peripheral nerve sheath neoplasm composed of perineural cells. Perineurioma occurs in superficial soft tissues of the extremities or trunk in patients over a wide age range, but most commonly in adults. FNA smears from perineuriomas share microscopic features with other low-grade and benign spindle cell and myxoid lesions, and a specific diagnosis is most likely

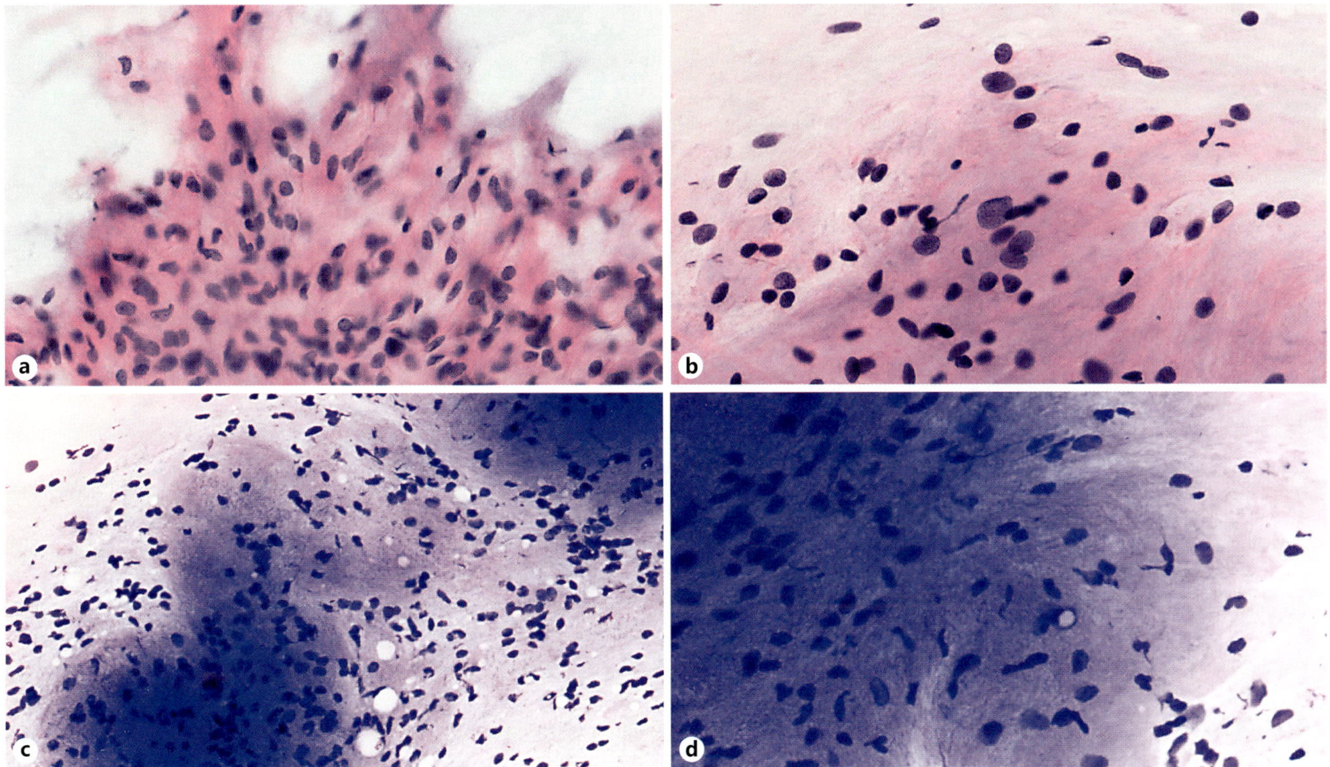

Fig. 4. Perineurioma. **a**, **b** Loosely cohesive clusters of cells with indistinct cytoplasmic borders and naked, bland ovoid, fusiform, or rounded nuclei showing slight to moderate anisonucleosis in a myxoid/collagenous matrix. HE stain. **c**, **d** Dispersed bare nuclei showing a predominant spindle/ovoid cell morphology and variable, usually slight anisonucleosis in the myxoid background matrix, better appreciated in the air-dried smears. MGG stain.

not feasible based on cytology alone. Nevertheless, the presence of elongated spindle cells with bland oval nuclei and characteristic long, thin, bipolar cytoplasmic processes clustered or dispersed in a myxoid matrix is a finding consistent with perineurioma [21, 22] (Fig. 4). Perineurioma cells are positive for CD34, EMA, and claudin-1 (like normal perineural cells), and are negative for S100 protein.

Cytologic Features
- Variable cellularity, but often hypocellular smears
- Often a myxoid or myxoid/collagenous background matrix
- Clusters or dispersed uniform spindle and ovoid cells with bland, slender, elongated, and round to oval nuclei, and a poorly preserved cytoplasm
- Cells with a better preserved cytoplasm show thin bipolar cytoplasmic processes
- Rare fragments of capillaries

Ancillary Tests
Immunophenotype
Most perineuriomas are positive for EMA, claudin-1, and GLUT1, approximately 60% of perineuriomas express CD34. Negative for S100 and GFAP.

Genetics
Chromosome 22 deletions and monosomies can be found in these tumors. However, they are not diagnostically specific and can be found in other soft tissue tumors, like schwannomas. Cytogenetics, FISH, and SNP array can be used on available material.

Differential Diagnosis
- Intramuscular myxoma
- Schwannoma with prominent Antoni B area
- Neurofibroma
- Low-grade fibromyxoid sarcoma
- Low-grade myxofibrosarcoma

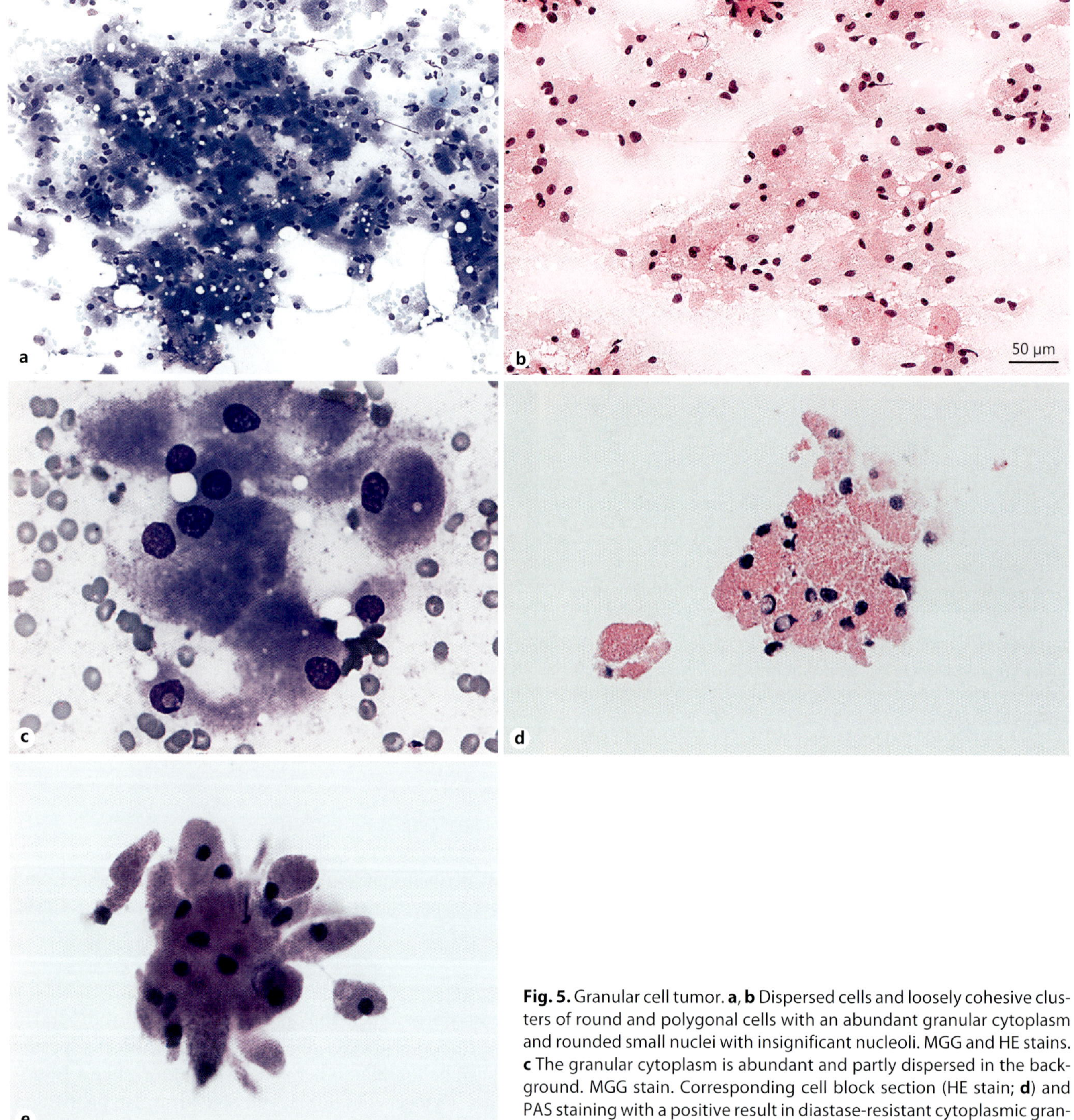

Fig. 5. Granular cell tumor. **a**, **b** Dispersed cells and loosely cohesive clusters of round and polygonal cells with an abundant granular cytoplasm and rounded small nuclei with insignificant nucleoli. MGG and HE stains. **c** The granular cytoplasm is abundant and partly dispersed in the background. MGG stain. Corresponding cell block section (HE stain; **d**) and PAS staining with a positive result in diastase-resistant cytoplasmic granules (**e**).

Fig. 6. MPNST. **a**, **b** Smears of low-grade MPNST: loose fascicles of slightly atypical spindle cells with fusiform, wavy, or comma-like nuclei and occasional bipolar cytoplasmic processes in the fibrillary background matrix may be difficult to distinguish from benign nerve sheath tumors. HE and MGG stains. **c** Smears of high-grade MPNST show a variable morphology: fascicles of moderately to markedly pleomorphic spindle cells with irregular hyperchromatic nuclei. HE stain. **d**, **e** Smears showing cytologic features similar to undifferentiated pleomorphic sarcoma with markedly pleomorphic tumor cells of variable size and shape, irregular hyperchromatic nuclei, and mitoses. HE and MGG stains. **f** The corresponding cell block section with a convincing high-grade morphology. HE stain.

(For figure see next page.)

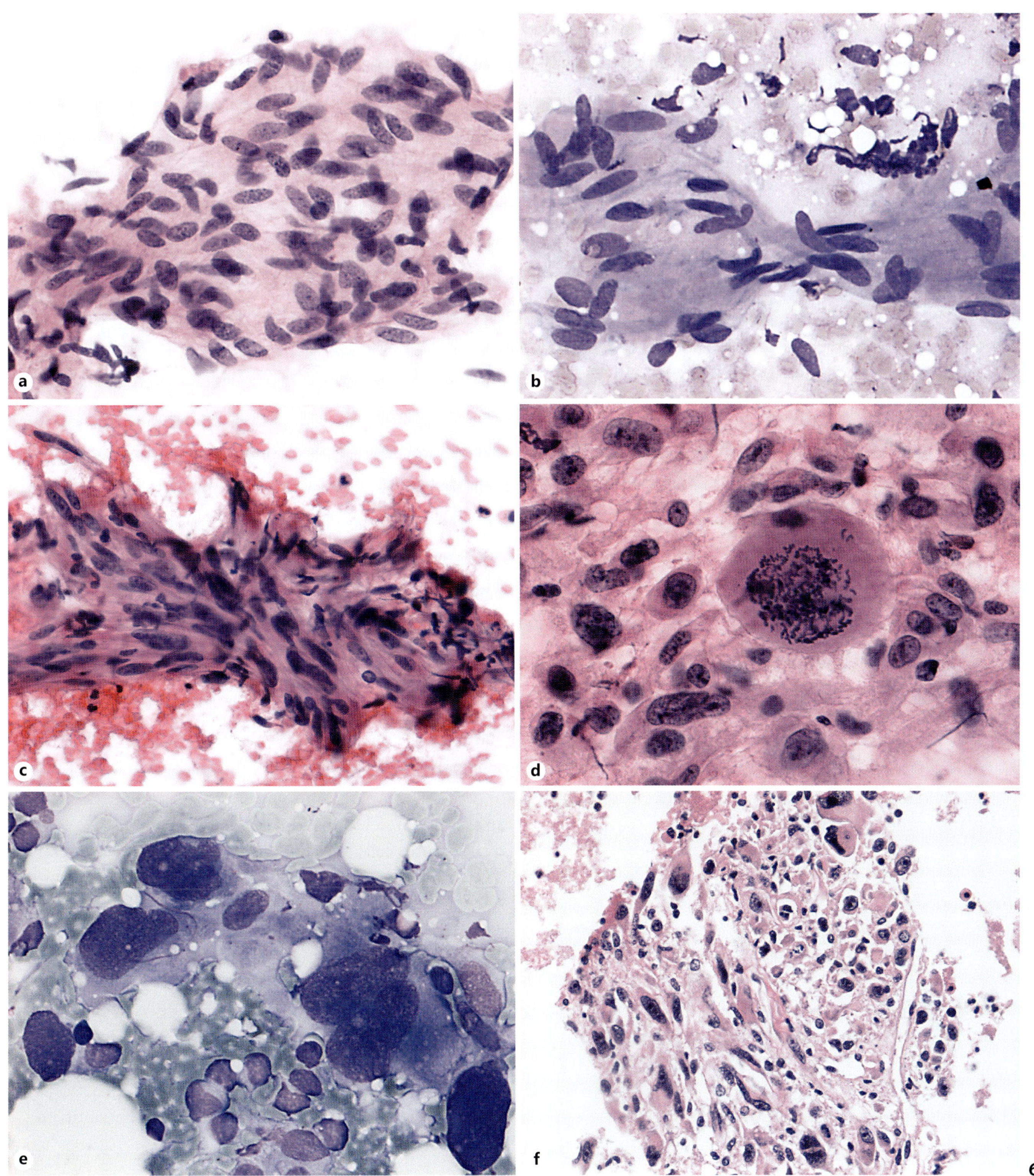

6

Granular Cell Tumor

Granular cell tumor is a benign neoplasm of putative Schwann cell origin with a wide anatomic distribution, but commonly arises in the skin, subcutaneous tissue of the head and neck region, particularly the tongue [23, 24] and oral cavity, aerodigestive tract, genital region, breast, and mediastinum in middle-aged or elderly adults. Granular cell tumors are multicentric in approximately 10% of cases. Because of the fragility of the tumor cells, FNA smears from granular cell tumors are often dominated by naked, bland nuclei in a background of finely granular material [25]. In better-preserved areas there are small clusters and sheets of uniform or slightly atypical tumor cells with round to oval nuclei, inconspicuous nucleoli, and an abundant granular cytoplasm can be seen [26–29] (Fig. 5). Nuclei are small and dark but occasionally with mild to moderate anisokaryosis. Periodic acid-Schiff (PAS)-positive diastase-resistant cytoplasmic granules represent phagolysosomes.

Malignant granular cell tumors are extremely rare, usually arising in adults in deep soft tissues and metastasizing early in up to 50% of cases. Smears from malignant granular cell tumors show a morphologic criteria of malignancy such as a predominance of pleomorphic spindle cells with large nucleoli, mitoses, and necrosis [29, 30].

Cytologic Features
- Dispersed cells and loosely cohesive clusters
- Intact polygonal cells with an abundant granular cytoplasm
- Often naked dissociated nuclei in a granular background
- Rounded, small nuclei with insignificant nucleoli
- Cells with moderate anisokaryosis with coarse chromatin and macronucleoli may be present

Ancillary Tests
Immunophenotype
Strong, diffuse positivity for S100, variable positivity for CD68, CD63, and neuron-specific enolase.

Histochemistry
PAS-positive diastase-resistant cytoplasmic granules.

Genetics
There are no known recurrent genetic changes.

Differential Diagnosis
- Alveolar soft part sarcoma
- Adult rhabdomyoma
- Hibernoma
- Renal cell carcinoma

Access to reliable ancillary tests is of greatest importance in distinguishing granular cell tumor from its main differentials, such as alveolar soft part sarcoma and adult rhabdomyoma. Smears from granular cell tumors display diffuse and strong positivity for S100 in tumor cells, while muscle markers are negative (Fig. 5). Granular cell tumors arising in the breast represent potential pitfalls in breast FNA as many of these lesions overlap clinically and in mammography with breast carcinoma [26, 31–34].

Malignant Peripheral Nerve Sheath Tumor

Malignant peripheral nerve sheath tumor (MPNST) is an uncommon soft tissue sarcoma (comprising about 5% of soft tissue sarcomas) that shows incomplete differentiation toward nerve sheath cells. Approximately 50% of MPNST are associated with neurofibromatosis type 1. Most MPNST arise from peripheral large- and medium-sized nerves in the proximal extremities, buttock, trunk, head and neck region, mediastinum, and retroperitoneum, or from preexisting neurofibromas. Sporadic forms of MPNST occur commonly in young and middle-aged adults between 20 and 50 years of age, while neoplasms associated with NF1 are often present in younger average ages and are more frequent in males.

The cytomorphology of smears is variable and nonspecific [35]. FNA smears are often moderately to highly cellular and the most common cell type is spindle cells in variably sized fascicles mixed with isolated cells and naked nuclei. Tumor cells may be elongated with fusiform, often comma-shaped, wavy, or buckled nuclei, but other forms of neoplastic cells are also present (Fig. 6). Polygonal or rounded cells may predominate in epithelioid MPNST. Pleomorphic cells with a high degree of atypia and multinucleated tumor cells are common findings in high-grade MPNST [36] (Fig. 6). Mitoses are usually easy to find and necrosis and apoptosis can be present. Heterologous components (cartilage, bone, epithelial glands, or rhabdoid cells) present focally in approximately 10–15% of MPNST in tissue sections, but these elements are rarely sampled by FNA.

Cytologic Features
- Hypercellular smears
- Mixture of cell clusters, fascicles, and dispersed cells
- Occasionally a fibrillary background may be found within clusters or fascicles of tumor cells
- Predominantly spindle-shaped cells often with bipolar cytoplasmic processes and fusiform, wavy, or comma-like nuclei
- Rounded or polygonal cells predominate in smears of epithelioid MPNST
- Often hyperchromatic nuclei with large nucleoli
- Variable presence of pleomorphic and/or multinucleated tumor cells
- Infrequent heterologous components
- Mitotic figures

Ancillary Tests

Immunophenotype

Focal positivity for S100 in less than 50% of cases (strong and diffuse positivity in the epithelioid variant) and GFAP in less than 30% of cases.

Genetics

These tumors often display complex karyotypes with both structural and numerical changes [37]. Common aberrations are gains of chromosome arms 7p, 8q, and 17q, and loss of 9p, 11q, 13q, and 17p [38]. Mutations of both copies of the tumor suppressor gene *NF1* at 17q11.2 are found in many MPNSTs [39]. Deletion and inactivation of another known tumor suppressor gene, *CDKN2A*, at 9p21 is also common [40]. These changes at different levels can be can be detected through cytogenetics, FISH, SNP array, PCR, and NGS depending on the available material and sought information.

Differential Diagnosis
- Ancient schwannoma
- Cellular schwannoma
- LMS
- Synovial sarcoma
- Malignant solitary fibrous tumor
- Dedifferentiated liposarcoma
- Sarcomatoid carcinoma
- Spindle cell melanoma
- Metastatic carcinoma (epithelioid MPNS)

A problem that can occur in the cytologic examination of MPNST is an interpretation of morphologically heterologous smears mimicking other subtypes of spindle cell and epithelioid cell sarcomas as well as benign nerve sheaths tumors. Epithelioid features pose a diagnostic challenge because the differential diagnosis involves a variety tumors, such as epithelioid sarcoma, malignant rhabdoid tumor, metastatic carcinomas, and melanoma [41]. Thus, it may be necessary to perform immunochemical stains on cell blocks of FNA aspirates to arrive at a definitive diagnosis. Although focal S100 protein and/or GFAP positivity is helpful in the diagnosis of MPNST, a panel of antibodies (e.g., CD34, cytokeratins, EMA, desmin, MDM2) should be used to exclude morphologic mimics of this tumor.

References

1 Narasimha A, Kumar MH, Kalyani R, Madan M: Retroperitoneal cystic schwannoma: A case report with review of literature. J Cytol 2010;27:136–139.

2 Li Q, Gao C, Juzi JT, Hao X: Analysis of 82 cases of retroperitoneal schwannoma. ANZ J Surg 2007; 77:237–240.

3 Chebib I, Hornicek FJ, Nielsen GP, Deshpande V: Cytomorphologic features that distinguish schwannoma from other low-grade spindle cell lesions. Cancer Cytopathol 2015;123:171–179.

4 Kudo T, Kawakami H, Kuwatani M, Ehira N, Yamato H, Eto K, Kubota K, Asaka M: Three cases of retroperitoneal schwannoma diagnosed by EUS-FNA. World J Gastroenterol 2011;17:3459–3464.

5 Resnick JM, Fanning CV, Caraway NP, Varma DG, Johnson M: Percutaneous needle biopsy diagnosis of benign neurogenic neoplasms. Diagn Cytopathol 1997;16:17–25.

6 Dahl I, Hagmar B, Idvall I: Benign solitary neurilemoma (Schwannoma): a correlative cytological and histological study of 28 cases. Acta Pathol Microbiol Immunol Scand A 1984;92:91–101.

7 Domanski HA, Akerman M, Engellau J, Gustafson P, Mertens F, Rydholm A: Fine-needle aspiration of neurilemoma (schwannoma): a clinicocytopathologic study of 116 patients. Diagn Cytopathol 2006;34:403–412.

8 Bohara S, Dey B, Agarwal S, Gupta R, Khurana N, Gulati A: A case of cystic schwannoma in the neck masquerading as branchial cleft cyst. Rare Tumors 2014;6:5355.

9 Yilmazer R, Yazici ZM, Sayin I, Bakan AA, Kayhan FT: Cervical cystic vagal schwannoma mimicking a type 3 second branchial cleft cyst: a case report. Kulak Burun Bogaz Ihtis Derg 2013;23:192–195.

10 Jadhav CR, Angeline NR, Kumar B, Bhat RV, Balachandran G: Axillary schwannoma with extensive cystic degeneration. J Lab Physicians 2013;5:60–62.

11 Ryd W, Mugal S, Ayyash K: Ancient neurilemmoma: a pitfall in the cytologic diagnosis of soft-tissue tumors. Diagn Cytopathol 1986;2:244–247.

12 Dodd LG, Martinez S: Fine-needle aspiration cytology of pseudosarcomatous lesions of soft tissue. Diagn Cytopathol 2001;24:28–35.

13 Lodding P, Kindblom LG, Angervall L, Stenman G: Cellular schwannoma: a clinicopathologic study of 29 cases. Virchows Arch A Pathol Anat Histopathol 1990;416:237–248.

14 Stemmer-Rachamimov AO, Xu L, Gonzalez-Agosti C, Burwick JA, Pinney D, Beauchamp R, Jacoby LB, Gusella JF, Ramesh V, Louis DN: Universal absence of merlin, but not other ERM family members, in schwannomas. Am J Pathol 1997; 151:1649–1654.

15 Bijlsma EK, Merel P, Bosch DA, Westerveld A, Delattre O, Thomas G, Hulsebos TJ: Analysis of mutations in the *SCH* gene in schwannomas. Genes Chromosomes Cancer 1994;11:7–14.

16 Garg C, Agrawal A, Agrawal R, Kumar P: Neurofibroma at unusual locations: report of two cases in teenage girls. J Clin Diagn Res 2015;9:ED03–ED04.

17 Wakely PE Jr: Myxomatous soft tissue tumors: correlation of cytopathology and histopathology. Ann Diagn Pathol 1999;3:227–242.

18 Mondal P, Basu N, Gupta SS, Bhattacharya N, Mallick MG: Fine needle aspiration cytology of parapharyngeal tumors. J Cytol 2009;26:102–104.

19 Gupta RK, Cheung YK, Al Ansari AG, Naran S, Lallu S, Fauck R: Diagnostic value of image-guided needle aspiration cytology in the assessment of vertebral and intervertebral lesions. Diagn Cytopathol 2002;27:191–196.

20 Serra E, Puig S, Otero D, Gaona A, Kruyer H, Ars E, Estivill X, Lazaro C: Confirmation of a double-hit model for the *NF1* gene in benign neurofibromas. Am J Hum Genet 1997;61:512–519.

21 Yang EJ, Hornick JL, Qian X: Fine-needle aspiration of soft tissue perineurioma: a comparative analysis of cytomorphology and immunohistochemistry with benign and malignant mimics. Cancer Cytopathol 2016;124:651–658.

22 Akerman M, Domanski HA: The cytology of soft tissue tumours. Monogr Clin Cytol 2003;16:1–112.

23 Fitzhugh VA, Maniar KP, Gurudutt VV, Rivera M, Chen H, Wu M: Fine-needle aspiration biopsy of granular cell tumor of the tongue: a technique for the aspiration of oral lesions. Diagn Cytopathol 2009;37:839–842.

24 Domanski HA, Akerman M: Fine-needle aspiration cytology of tongue swellings: a study of 75 cases. Diagn Cytopathol 1998;18:387–392.

25 Koshy J, Schnadig V, Nawgiri R: Is fine needle aspiration cytology a useful diagnostic tool for granular cell tumors? A cytohistological review with emphasis on pitfalls. Cytojournal 2014;11:28.

26 Pieterse AS, Mahar A, Orell S: Granular cell tumour: a pitfall in FNA cytology of breast lesions. Pathology 2004;36:58–62.

27 Mallik MK, Das DK, Francis IM, al-Abdulghani R, Pathan SK, Sheikh ZA, Luthra UK: Fine needle aspiration cytology diagnosis of a cutaneous granular cell tumor in a 7-year-old child: a case report. Acta Cytol 2001;45:263–266.

28 Liu K, Madden JF, Olatidoye BA, Dodd LG: Features of benign granular cell tumor on fine needle aspiration. Acta Cytol 1999;43:552–557.

29 Wieczorek TJ, Krane JF, Domanski HA, Akerman M, Carlen B, Misdraji J, Granter SR: Cytologic findings in granular cell tumors, with emphasis on the diagnosis of malignant granular cell tumor by fine-needle aspiration biopsy. Cancer 2001;93:398–408.

30 Liu Z, Mira JL, Vu H: Diagnosis of malignant granular cell tumor by fine needle aspiration cytology. Acta Cytol 2001;45:1011–1021.

31 Ohnishi H, Nishihara K, Tamae K, Mitsuyama S, Abe R, Toyoshima S, Abe E: Granular cell tumors of the breast: a report of two cases. Surg Today 1996;26:929–932.

32 Hahn HJ, Iglesias J, Flenker H, Kreuzer G: Granular cell tumor in differential diagnosis of tumors of the breast: the role of fine needle aspiration cytology. Pathol Res Pract 1992;188:1091–1097.

33 Rexeena B, Paul A, Nitish RA, Kurian C, Anila RK: Granular cell tumor of breast: a case report and review of literature. Indian J Surg Oncol 2015;6:446–448.

34 McCluggage WG, Sloan S, Kenny BD, Alderdice JM, Kirk SJ, Anderson NH: Fine needle aspiration cytology (FNAC) of mammary granular cell tumour: a report of three cases. Cytopathology 1999;10:383–389.

35 Wakely PE Jr, Ali SZ, Bishop JA: The cytopathology of malignant peripheral nerve sheath tumor: a report of 55 fine-needle aspiration cases. Cancer Cytopathol 2012;120:334–341.

36 Klijanienko J, Caillaud JM, Lagace R, Vielh P: Cytohistologic correlations of 24 malignant peripheral nerve sheath tumor (MPNST) in 17 patients: the Institut Curie experience. Diagn Cytopathol 2002;27:103–108.

37 Lothe RA, Karhu R, Mandahl N, Mertens F, Saeter G, Heim S, Borresen-Dale AL, Kallioniemi OP: Gain of 17q24-qter detected by comparative genomic hybridization in malignant tumors from patients with von Recklinghausen's neurofibromatosis. Cancer Res 1996;56:4778–4781.

38 Brekke HR, Ribeiro FR, Kolberg M, Agesen TH, Lind GE, Eknaes M, Hall KS, Bjerkehagen B, van den Berg E, Teixeira MR, Mandahl N, Smeland S, Mertens F, Skotheim RI, Lothe RA: Genomic changes in chromosomes 10, 16, and X in malignant peripheral nerve sheath tumors identify a high-risk patient group. J Clin Oncol 2010;28:1573–1582.

39 Bottillo I, Ahlquist T, Brekke H, Danielsen SA, van den Berg E, Mertens F, Lothe RA, Dallapiccola B: Germline and somatic *NF1* mutations in sporadic and NF1-associated malignant peripheral nerve sheath tumours. J Pathol 2009;217:693–701.

40 Agesen TH, Florenes VA, Molenaar WM, Lind GE, Berner JM, Plaat BE, Komdeur R, Myklebost O, van den Berg E, Lothe RA: Expression patterns of cell cycle components in sporadic and neurofibromatosis type 1-related malignant peripheral nerve sheath tumors. J Neuropathol Exp Neurol 2005;64:74–81.

41 Jiwani S, Gokden M, Lindberg M, Ali S, Jeffus S: Fine-needle aspiration cytology of epithelioid malignant peripheral nerve sheath tumor: a case report and review of the literature. Diagn Cytopathol 2016;44:226–231.

Domanski HA, Walther CS: FNA Cytology of Soft Tissue and Bone Tumors. Monogr Clin Cytol.
Basel, Karger, 2017, vol 22, pp 103–121 (DOI: 10.1159/000475102)

Tumors of Uncertain Differentiation

Intramuscular Myxoma

Intramuscular myxoma is a benign neoplasm arising within large muscles with a predilection for the thighs, buttocks, and the shoulders and upper arms. Myxomas usually occur in middle-aged or elderly patients and show a female predominance. Most myxomas are sporadic but there is a minor subset of myxomas which are occasionally multiple and associated with fibrous dysplasia (Mazabraud syndrome). A cellular myxoma is a variant of myxoma with increased cellularity and capillary vessels but without the cellular atypia observed in smears from low-grade myxofibrosarcoma. Juxta-articular myxoma is yet another variant of myxoma with similar cytomorphologic features but a different clinical presentation. They are most often seen near the knee. Both cellular myxomas and juxta-articular myxomas carry a risk of local recurrence in contrast to usual intramuscular myxomas that never recur after local excision. Smears from myxomas are hypocellular and contain loosely clustered or isolated spindle cells with small round to oval bland nuclei and long cytoplasmic processes in an abundant myxoid background [1–4] (Fig. 1). Fragments of capillaries are rare or absent. Scattered macrophages with cytoplasmic vacuolization may be seen in smears (Fig. 1).

Cytologic Features

- Droplets of stringy, glue-like, colorless fluid on aspiration
- Abundant myxoid matrix
- Dispersed single cells and small, loose cell clusters
- Slender tumor cells with small, round to oval, bland nuclei and long, thin, uni- or bipolar cytoplasmic processes
- Occasional scattered macrophages with a vacuolated cytoplasm
- Occasional atrophic muscle fibers
- Infrequent small vessel fragments

Ancillary Tests
Immunophenotype
Variable positivity for CD34, desmin, and smooth muscle actin (SMA).

Genetics
Point mutations in a gene called *GNAS* at 20q13 are found in intramuscular myxomas [5]. These mutations are absent in myxofibrosarcomas, which can be used for differential diagnostic purposes [6]. Juxta-articular myxomas do not show any recurrent aberrations and lack *GNAS* mutations

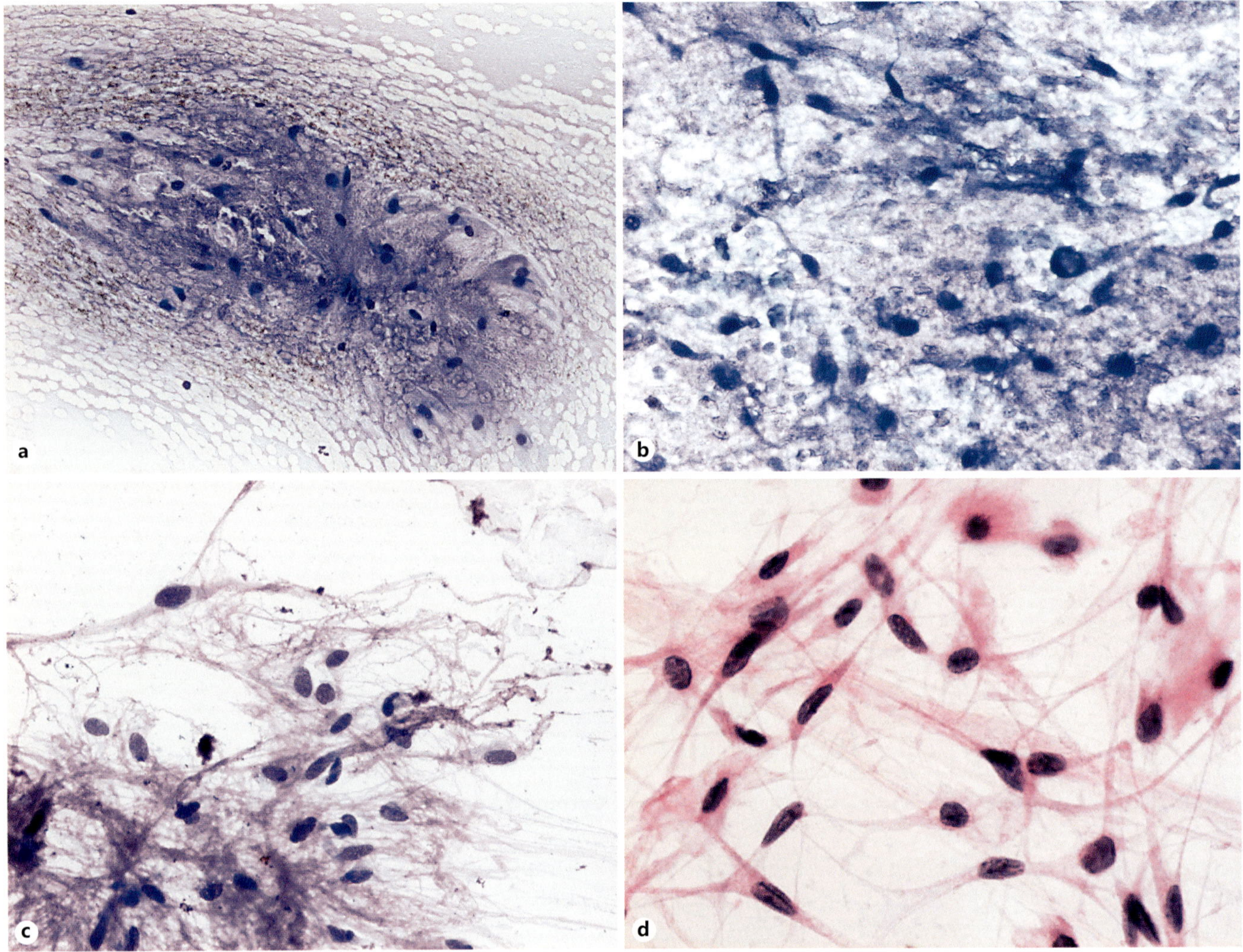

Fig. 1. Intramuscular myxoma. Typically hypocellular smears with an abundant myxoid background and small loosely cohesive clusters (**a**), and dispersed bland spindle cells with long cytoplasmic processes and small uniform round to oval nuclei (**b**, **c**). MGG stain. **d** Spindle cells occasionally exhibit slightly enlarged oval to spindled nuclei with tiny nucleoli but characteristic very long, thin, uni- or bipolar cytoplasmic processes. HE stain.

[7]. These mutations can be found with polymerase chain reaction (PCR) and next-generation sequencing (NGS) on available material.

Differential Diagnosis
- Low-grade myxofibrosarcoma
- Low-grade fibromyxoid sarcoma
- Myxoid loposarcoma
- Schwannoma (Antoni B areas)
- Ganglion cyst
- Soft tissue perineurioma
- Extraskeletal myxoid chondrosarcoma

The main differential diagnoses of myxoma are low-grade myxofibrosarcoma and low-grade fibromyxoid sarcoma. Both show higher cellularity and capillaries or fragments of capillaries are common findings in aspiration smears. In addition, myxomas lack the branching capillary network seen in smears from myxoid liposarcoma and slightly to moderately atypical cells seen in smears from low-grade myxofibrosarcoma and low-grade fibromyxoid sarcoma.

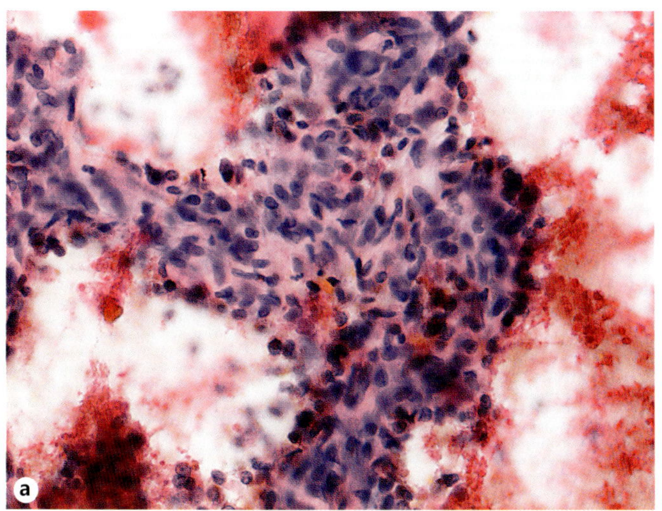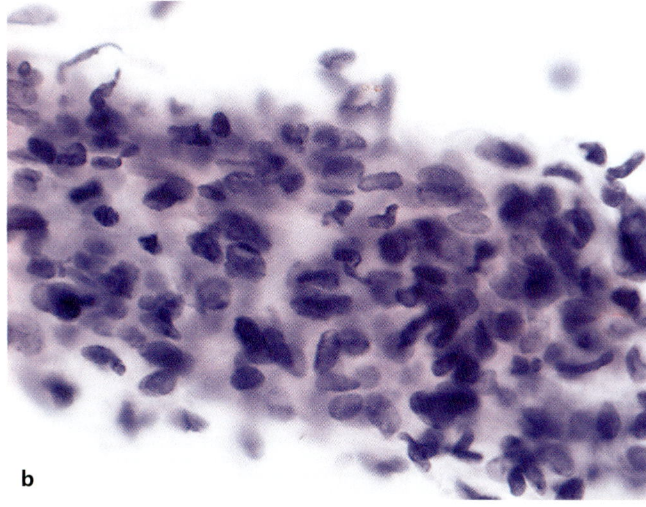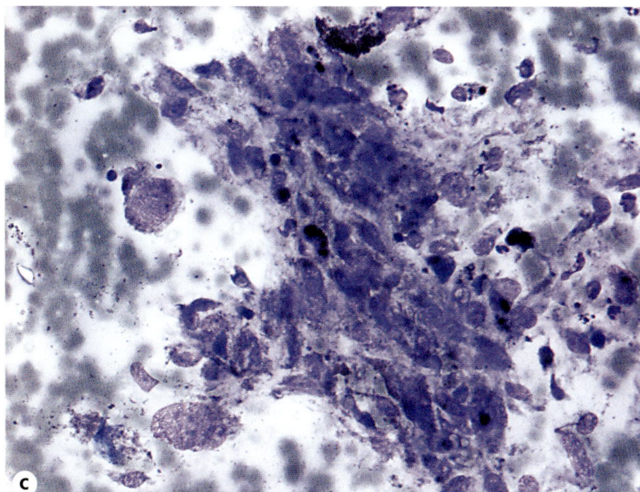

Fig. 2. AFH. **a**, **b** Cellular smears composed of tight or loosely cohesive clusters of oval to spindled or epithelioid histiocytoid cells with poorly preserved cytoplasm and ill-defined cell borders, ovoid to folded nuclei with finely dispersed chromatin and inconspicuous nucleoli. HE stain. **c** Cytologic atypia/anisonucleosis and hemosiderin pigment may be present in some cell clusters. MGG stain.

Angiomatoid Fibrous Histiocytoma

Angiomatoid fibrous histiocytoma (AFH) is an indolent, rarely metastasizing neoplasm of uncertain lineage, commonly arising in the deep dermis and subcutaneous tissue of the extremities in children and young adults. Rarely, AFH may occur in adults and affect other sites such as lung or bone. AFH commonly presents as a partly cystic mass with pseudovascular spaces, hemorrhage, and most often rim of lymphoplasmacytic infiltrate in the periphery of the tumor. Fine-needle aspiration (FNA) smears are usually bloody and show variable cellularity with ovoid to spindled histiocytoid cells that may be isolated or clustered. Some of these cells are slightly atypical and may contain hemosiderin. Large cellular clusters with capillary structures and a whorled arrangement of tumor cells can be appreciated in some cases [8, 9] (Fig. 2).

Cytologic Features
- Often bloody smears with variable cellularity
- Dispersed cells and cell clusters
- Ovoid to spindled histiocytoid cells with poorly defined cell borders
- Often folded nuclei with a finely granular chromatin pattern
- Wispy cytoplasm, intracytoplasmic hemosiderin
- Infrequent lymphoplasmacytic infiltrate
- Occasional whorled arrangement of tumor cells associated with capillaries

Ancillary Tests
Immunophenotype
Positivity, occasionally focal, for desmin, epithelial membrane antigen (EMA), CD99, and CD68 in approximately

50% of cases. Negative for S100 and CD34, and consistent keratin negativity.

Genetics

Over 90% of cases display a t(2;22) translocation resulting in a *EWSR1-CREB1* fusion gene, but the pathogenetic mechanism in not fully understood [10–13]. These aberrations can be found with cytogenetics, fluorescent in situ hybridization (FISH), single nucleotide polymorphism (SNP) array, PCR, and NGS on available material [14].

Differential Diagnosis
- Hemangioma
- Benign fibrous histiocytoma
- Nodular fasciitis
- Inflammatory myofibroblastic tumor
- Follicular dendritic sarcoma

FNA cytologic features are nonspecific and clinical correlation and ancillary studies are necessary to render the correct diagnosis. Tumor cells are positive for desmin and EMA in approximately 50% cases. Most of these tumors show an *EWSR1–CREB1* fusion gene, which can be detected by FISH, SNP array, PCR, and NGS studies [8].

Ossifying Fibromyxoid Tumor

Ossifying fibromyxoid tumor (OFMT) is a rare mesenchymal neoplasm of uncertain lineage commonly arising in the subcutis/superficial soft tissues in adults, with a 2:1 male predominance. The most common primary sites are the extremities (particularly the lower), followed by the trunk and the head and neck region. OFMT is a lobulated, well-circumscribed, and often encapsulated tumor that, in the majority of cases, has an incomplete shell of mature metaplastic bone. Histologically, the tumor is composed of lobules of uniform, round to oval or spindled cells arranged in cords or trabeculae in variable amounts of a fibromyxoid stroma. FNA smears show variable cellularity with mostly dispersed small- and medium-sized round to oval, occasionally spindled cells with a moderate to abundant cytoplasm. Cells have bland, round to oval nuclei with occasional tiny nucleoli [15–19]. Naked nuclei are common findings in smears (Fig. 3).

Cytologic Features
- Variable cellularity (tumors with an extensive shell of bone are difficult to aspirate)

- Dispersed cells, small cell clusters and sheets, and rare acinar-like structures in a variable myxoid matrix
- Often eccentrically situated, rounded (epithelioid) or ovoid nuclei with occasional slight anisonucleosis and small nucleoli
- Naked dispersed nuclei are commonly seen in smears
- Preserved tumor cells contain a moderate to abundant cytoplasm

Ancillary Tests
Immunophenotype
Positive for S100 in the majority of cases and for desmin in less than 50% of cases; occasional focal expression of glial fibrillary acidic protein (GFAP), SMA, and keratins.

Genetics
Rearrangement of the *PHF1* gene at locus 6p21 has been found in most of the typical or atypical classified tumors, but rarely in the malignant lesions that often show loss of chromosome 22 [20]. This rearrangement can be detected by cytogenetics and FISH, or available material.

Differential Diagnosis
- Epithelioid peripheral nerve sheath tumors
- Mixed tumor of soft tissue
- Extraskeletal myxoid chondrosarcoma
- Myxoid liposarcoma
- Thyroid neoplasms (head and neck tumors)

FNA cytology of OFMT has not been sufficiently investigated and only a few case reports have been made. When the FNA material is sufficient, immunocytochemical examinations are of diagnostic value; positivity for S100 protein (>90% cases) and desmin (40–50% cases) would be supportive of a diagnosis of OFMT.

Myoepithelioma/Myoepithelial Carcinoma

Myoepithelial tumor and its morphologic variants – parachordoma and mixed tumor of soft tissue – are neoplasms composed of cells with a myoepithelial phenotype, similar to their counterparts in salivary glands [21, 22]. Parachordoma contains larger epithelioid cells and mixed tumor areas of epithelial differentiation, in addition to a myoepithelial component and most cases contain a chondromyxoid or hyalinized matrix (Fig. 4). Myoepitheliomas arise commonly in the subcutaneous and deep soft tissue of limb, limb girdles, trunk, and head and neck area in adults, but approximately 20% of

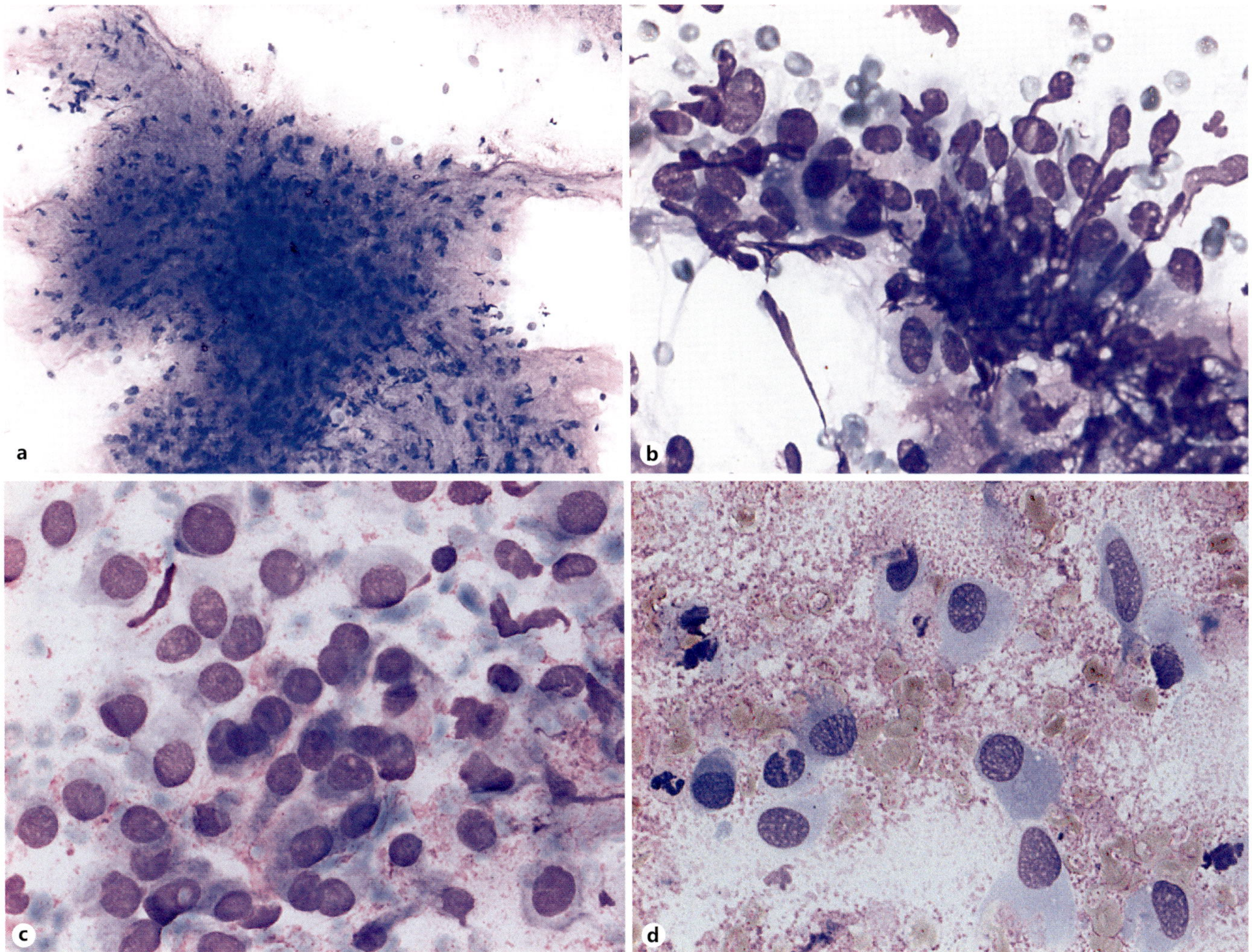

Fig. 3. OFMT. **a** A rare finding in FNA smears: a large loosely cohesive cluster of poorly preserved tumor cells in an abundant myxoid matrix. MGG stain. A loosely cohesive cluster (**b**) and dispersed bland, uniformly round to polygonal cells with a poorly preserved cytoplasm (**c**). MGG stain. **d** Some better-preserved tumor cells with a rather abundant cytoplasm and bland round to oval or spindly shaped nuclei in a variable myxoid background. MGG stain.

cases arise in children. They show a benign clinical course in the majority of cases, and may recur in approximately 20% of cases, but rarely metastasize. Myoepithelial carcinomas show diffuse moderate to severe nuclear atypia and large, epithelioid cell morphology with a high mitotic rate and necrosis, resembling poorly differentiated carcinomas [23].

Ancillary Tests
Immunophenotype
The majority of cases express broad-spectrum keratins, S100, calponin, and EMA; about 50% of cases are positive for GFAP; occasional focal expression of SMA and p63.

Genetics
Myoepithelial tumors from different locations display rearrangement of the *EWSR1* gene in almost 50% of the cases. The tumors negative for *EWSR1* aberrations are more often benign and superficially located [24]. These rearrangements can be detected by FISH, PCR, and NGS on available material.

In FNA smears, cytomorphology of myoepithelioma resembles that of pleomorphic adenoma of the salivary gland and chondroid syringoma. The most important, differential diagnosis is extraskeletal myxoid chondrosarcoma.

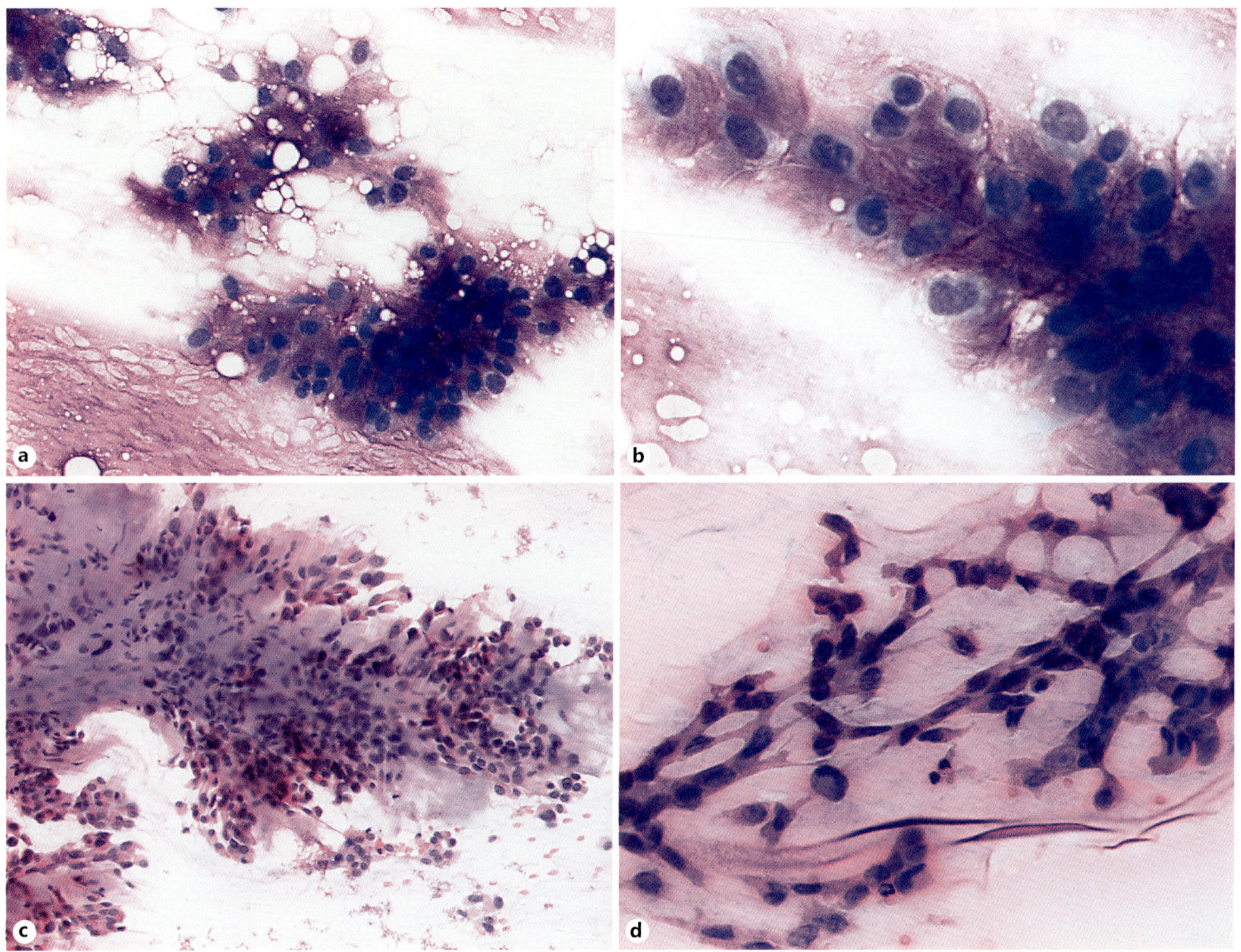

Fig. 4. Mixed tumor of soft tissue. **a, b** Clusters of cells with myoepithelial and epithelial phenotype in a chondromyxoid matrix resembling a pleomorphic adenoma of the salivary gland. MGG stain. **c** Hypercellular smears showing clusters of epithelial/myoepithelial cells with slight nuclear atypia and an abundant chondromyxoid background matrix. HE stain. **d** Branching cords and strands of relatively bland spindle cells with ovoid/fusiform nuclei in the myxoid background matrix resembling extraskeletal myxoid chondrosarcoma. HE stain.

Synovial Sarcoma

Synovial sarcoma (SS) accounts for 5–10% of soft tissue sarcomas. It may occur at any age, but the majority of patients are between the ages of 10 and 40 years. Most SS cases are deep seated and arise in the extremities, trunk, and head and neck region, but they may arise elsewhere in the body, including rare locations in visceral organs, genital tracts, retroperitoneum, and mediastinum. Based on their morphology, SS are divided on monophasic, biphasic, or poorly differentiated subtypes. In addition, 3 morphologic variants of the poorly differentiated SS exist: the small cell variant re-

sembling Ewing sarcoma, the spindle cell variant resembling malignant peripheral nerve sheath tumor (MPNST), and the epithelioid, pleomorphic variant with rhabdoid features [25–28]. SS can be present over a long period, sometimes up to 20 years, and is associated with pain in approximately 50% of cases. SS is a highly aggressive sarcoma with common local recurrences and metastases in approximately 50% of cases.

FNA smears of SS are usually cellular and in low magnification show a distinctive pattern of tight clusters of bland spindle cells alternating with dispersed cells or bare nuclei (Fig. 5). Smears occasionally contain capillaries bordered by

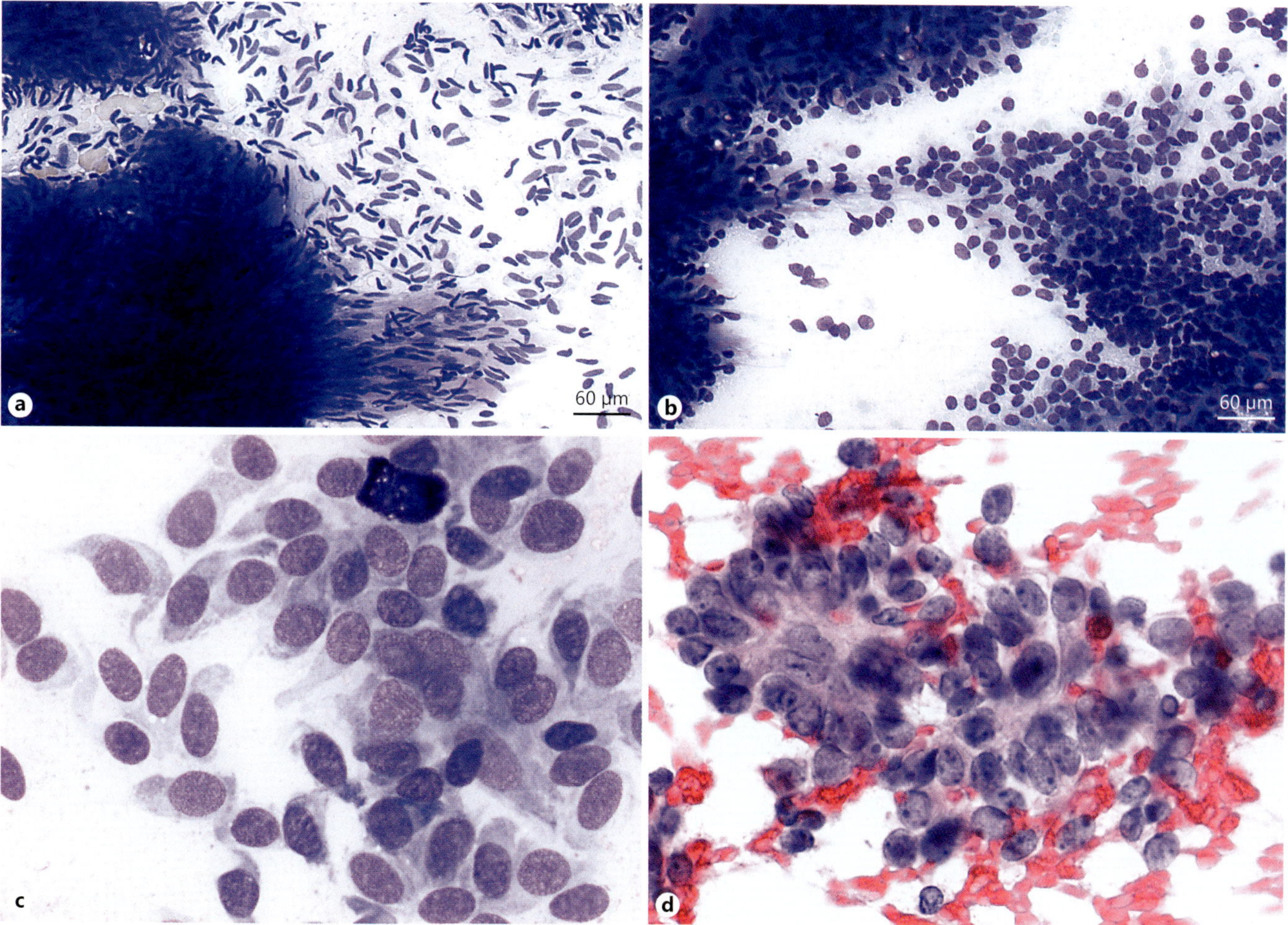

Fig. 5. SS. Typically hypercellular smears with a distinctive pattern of cell clusters alternating with dispersed cells with a poorly preserved cytoplasm and bland spindled (**a**) or ovoid nuclei (**b**). MGG stain. **c** Tumor cells with cytoplasmic processes and bland oval to round and fusiform nuclei that are uniform in size. Mast cells are a characteristic feature (right upper corner). MGG stain. **d** Epithelial elements including glandular structures are a part of smears of biphasic SS. HE stain. **e, f** Poorly differentiated SS of round cell type: the tumor cells have a round cell morphology resembling that of a Ewing sarcoma. MGG and HE stains. **g, h** Cells in smears of monophasic SS may closely resemble those of schwannoma, which is one of the main differential diagnoses of SS. HE and MGG stains.

(Figure continued on next page.)

tumor cells and delicate capillaries within cell clusters. Fragments of fibromyxoid or fibrous matrix and scattered mast cells are other frequent findings in smears (Fig. 5). Aspirates of biphasic SS contain clusters and a dispersed spindle cell mixture with sheets of epithelial cells occasionally arranged in acini glands and tubules resembling well-differentiated adenocarcinomas [26, 29]. A definitive diagnosis of an SS should be supported by ancillary techniques, such as immunocytochemical and molecular genetics examinations [30].

Cytologic Features

- Hypercellular smears
- Tissue fragments and tight clusters of spindle cells mixed with dispersed cells in almost equal proportions
- Occasional capillary strands bordered by tumor cells
- Striking uniformity of cells in the majority of smears
- Spindle cells with bland fusiform or ovoid nuclei end inconspicuous nucleoli
- Scant and delicate cytoplasm in preserved tumor cells
- Many cells with poorly preserved cytoplasm and dispersed naked nuclei
- Mitotic figures usually can be found in smears

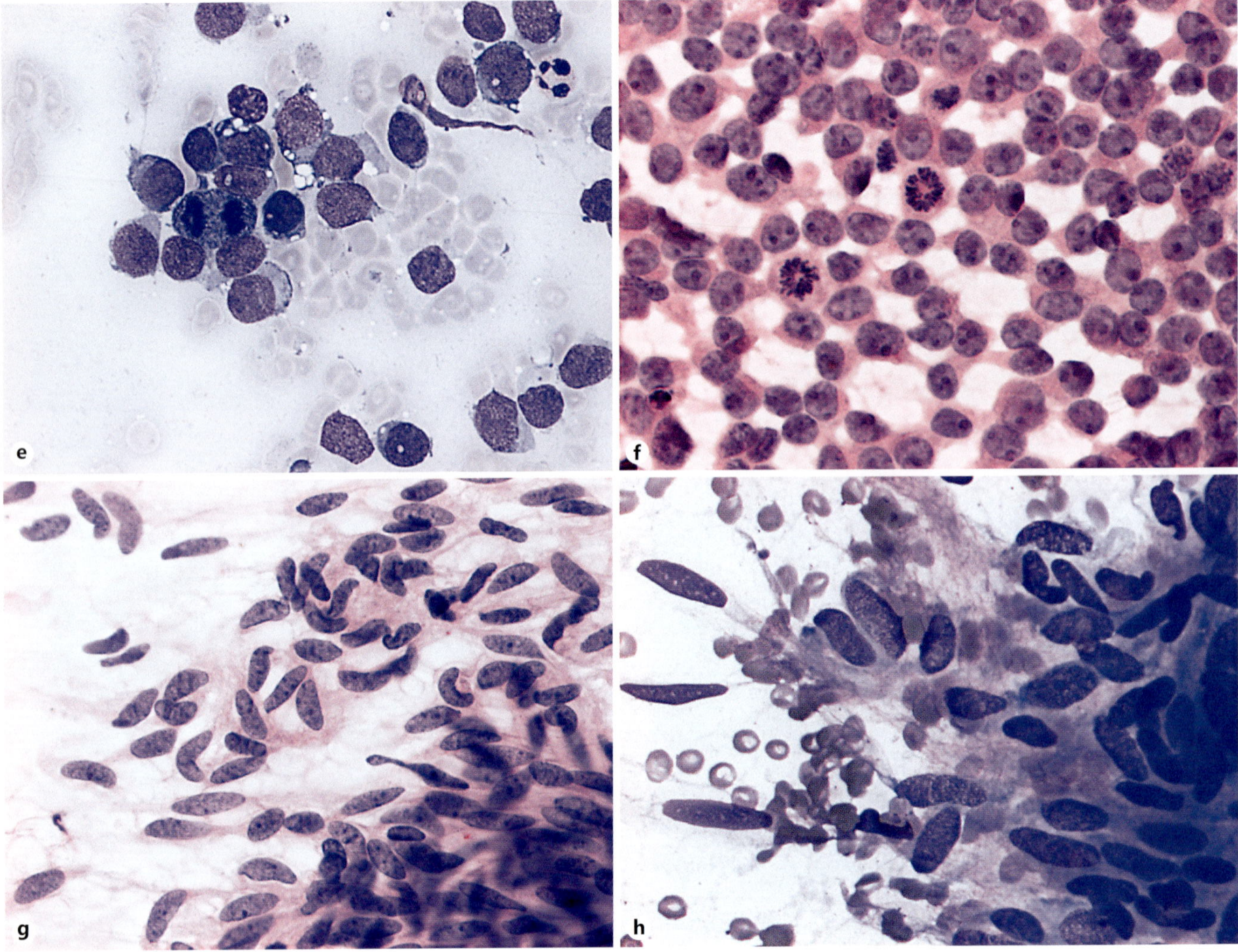

- Often scattered mast cells
- Small sheets, acinar and alveolar structures of epithelioid cells with rounded to oval nuclei in biphasic variants of SS

Ancillary Tests
Immunophenotype
The majority of SS stain positively for EMA and keratins, commonly CK7 and CK19. More than 50% stain positively for CD99 and Bcl-2. These immunostainings may appear focally, especially in poorly differentiated SS.

Genetics
SS has a specific and often sole genetic anomaly of the t(X;18) (p11; q11) translocation which creates a *SS18/SSX* fusion gene that dysregulates gene expression. This can be used for diagnostic purposes using cytogenetics, FISH, PCR, and NGS on available material [31].

Differential Diagnosis
- Schwannoma (monophasic SS)
- Solitary fibrous tumor (monophasic SS)
- MPNST (poorly differentiated or monophasic SS)
- Thymoma (biphasic SS)
- Carcinosarcoma (biphasic SS)
- Ewing sarcoma (poorly differentiated SS)

One of the main differential diagnoses is schwannoma as cells in smears of monophasic SS are remarkably uniform and bland looking, and may closely resemble those of schwannoma. Although SS most often shows a characteristic pattern in smears, with cell clusters alternating with dispersed cells and spindle cells with coarser chromatin and mitoses, some cases of SS are almost indistinguishable from schwannoma in routinely stained smears (Fig. 5). In addition, patients affected by SS may experience pain or tenderness, similarly to patients with schwannoma. In such cases, ancillary techniques are effective tools for a definitive diagnosis.

Epithelioid Sarcoma

Epithelioid sarcoma (ES) is a rare malignant mesenchymal neoplasm showing an epithelioid morphology and phenotype. It arises in the skin and subcutaneous tissue or tendon-aponeurosis of distal extremities, especially the hand and wrist, forearm, and lower leg of adolescents and young adults. They present as a slowly growing superficial mass, often appearing as a nonhealing ulcer or other mimics of infections in the skin and subcutaneous tissues. There are 2 subtypes of ES: the most common classic form, and proximal-type ES, which mainly affects proximal limb girdles, trunk, mediastinum, pelvic regions, and perineum. FNA smears show a mixture of small, loosely cohesive clusters, but predominantly dispersed epithelioid, polygonal, and spindle-shaped cells with eccentrically placed nuclei and eosinophilic to dense cytoplasm [32–35]. Moderate- or large-sized round to oval nuclei are eccentrically placed and contain 1 or more small nucleoli (Fig. 6). It may be difficult to aspirate sufficient material due to necrosis and/or hyalinization commonly occurring in ES. Smears of the proximal type of ES show more prominent cellular and nuclear atypia and cells with rhabdoid morphology.

Cytologic Features
- Variable cellularity
- Small, loosely cohesive clusters, but predominantly dispersed cells
- Dense to eosinophilic cytoplasm
- Epithelioid, polygonal, and spindle-shaped cells with eccentrically placed nuclei
- Large round to oval nuclei with 1 or more small nucleoli
- Necrotic background

Ancillary Tests

Immunophenotype

ES stains positively for EMA and low- and high-molecular keratins, commonly CK8 and CK19; more than 50% stain positively for CD34. Tumor cells are negative for S100, CD31, desmin, and Fli-1; most cases are negative for CK5/6

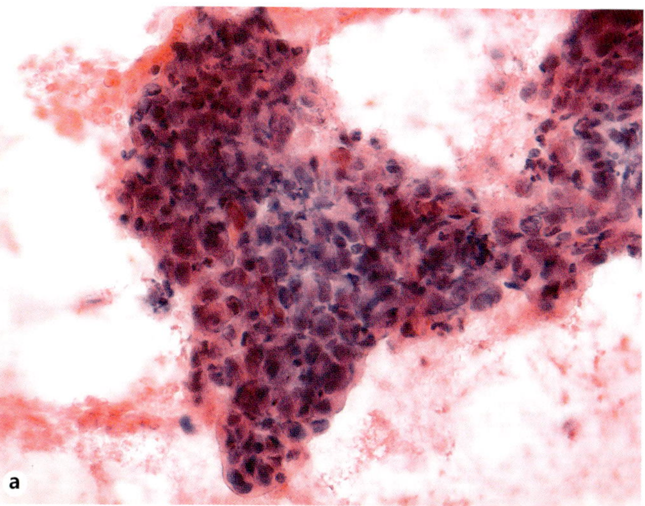

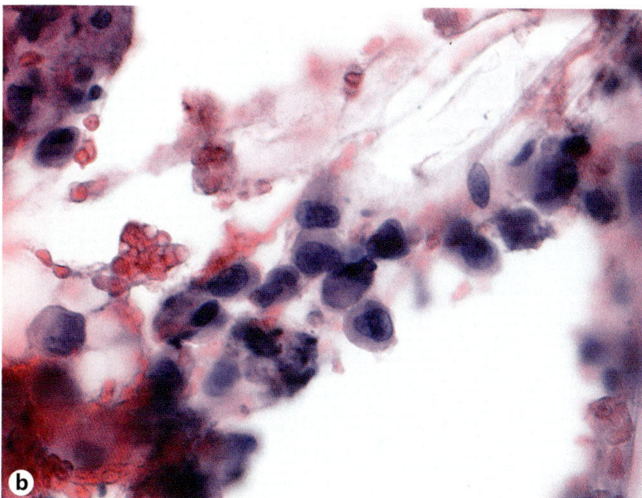

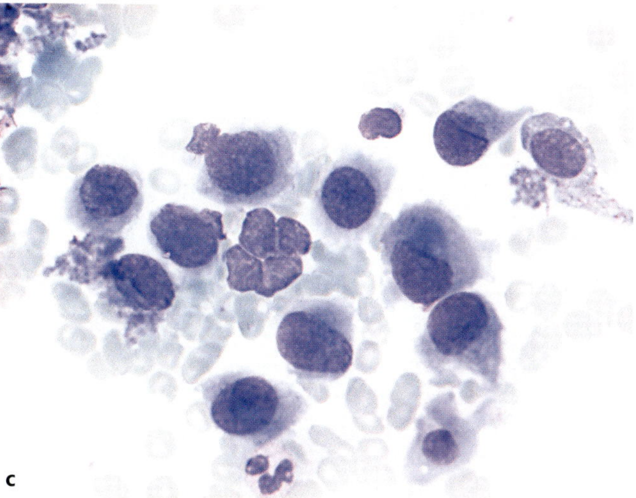

Fig. 6. ES. Loosely cohesive clusters (**a**) but predominantly dispersed epithelioid, polygonal, and spindle-shaped cells with eccentrically placed round to oval or occasionally irregular nuclei (**b**). HE stain. **c** Clear, granular, or dense cytoplasm and large nucleoli. MGG stain.

and P63; loss of nuclear expression of INI1 is characteristic for both types of ES.

Genetics
Genetic alterations of the chromosome region 22q11–12 are thought to be involved in the tumorigenesis of these tumors [36]. Loss of heterozygosity, deletions, and other mutations of this region involve the tumor suppressor gene *SMARCB1* and can be used for diagnostic purposes [37]. These changes can be detected with cytogenetics, FISH, SNP array, PCR, and NGS on available material.

Differential Diagnosis
- Metastatic carcinoma
- Metastatic melanoma
- Epithelioid hemangioendothelioma
- Clear cell sarcoma (CCS)
- Granulomatous inflammation

Alveolar Soft Part Sarcoma

Alveolar soft part sarcoma (ASPS) is a rare, slowly growing soft tissue sarcoma with a variable alveolar growth pattern arising in deep tissue of the lower limbs, limb girdles, buttock, and head and neck region. ASPS accounts for less than 1% of all sarcomas, and commonly occurs in infants, children, and young adults with a slight female predominance. Cytomorphologic features of ASPS include large, dyshesive tumor cells with an abundant granular, fragile cytoplasm and round nuclei with prominent centrally situated nucleoli [38–48]. The presence of stripped nuclei in a cytoplasmic granular background is a useful clue to the diagnosis (Fig. 7). The typical alveolar architecture seen on histology may be found in the cell block section, but is imperceptible on FNA smears. Characteristic rhomboid crystals containing actin filaments may be evident by ultrastructural examination (see Chapter 3, Fig. 5). ASPS is characterized by an *ASPSCR1-TFE3* gene fusion and nuclear overexpression of TFE3 protein.

Cytologic Features
- Variable cellularity
- Large, dyshesive epithelioid and polygonal cells with abundant granular cytoplasm
- Round nuclei with prominent nucleoli
- Bare nuclei and granular cytoplasmic background

Ancillary Tests
Immunophenotype
Approximately 50% of ASPS stain positively for desmin and a small subset of cases for S100. Tumor cells are negative for HBM45, EMA, chromogranin, synaptophysin, and keratins.

Histochemistry
Many cells of ASPS contain rhomboid or rod-shaped intracytoplasmic crystals staining on periodic acid-Schiff (PAS) stains after diastase digestion (Fig. 7).

Genetics
A specific cytogenetic alteration, der(17)t(X;17)(p11;q25), is found in these tumors [49]. The translocation results in a fusion gene between *TFE3* and *ASPSCR1* acting as an aberrant transcription factor [50]. Cytogenetics and FISH are adequate methods for detecting these changes, but PCR and NGS are also able to verify the mutations.

Differential Diagnosis
- Adult rhabdomyoma
- Granular cell tumor
- Paraganglioma
- PEComa
- Metastatic renal cell carcinoma

All those differential diagnoses listed above may resemble ASPS in smears but have different immunoprofiles and lack characteristic PAS-positive intracytoplasmic crystals [51] and ultrastructural findings.

Clear Cell Sarcoma of Soft Tissue

Clear cell sarcoma (CCS), first described by Enzinger in 1965, is a rare, distinct soft tissue neoplasm with melanocytic differentiation. CCS, which is also known as malignant melanoma of soft tissues, arises commonly in the subcutis and deep soft tissue of the extremities, especially the feet in young adults, and is often attached to aponeurotic structures and tendons. Very rare locations are the head and neck area and trunk. FNA smears are moderately to highly cellular, containing small, loosely cohesive clusters, but mostly dispersed, isolated round, polygonal or spindle-shaped cells (Fig. 8). Tumor cells contain a rather abundant, clear or pale cytoplasm, and large round or oval nuclei with prominent nucleoli. Other cytologic features of CCS include intranuclear cytoplasmic pseudoinclusions, melanin, multinucle-

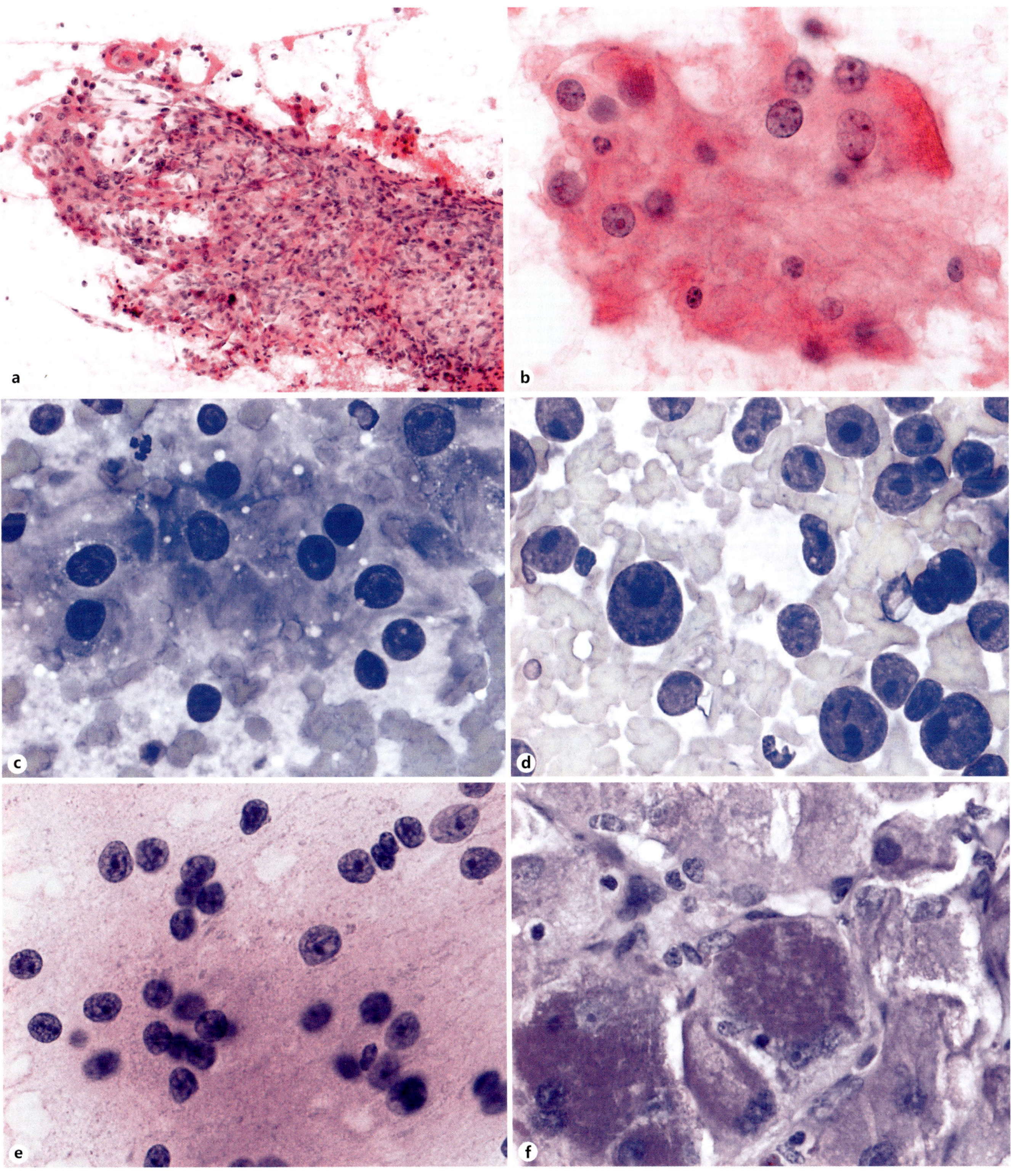

Fig. 7. ASPS. **a**, **b** Loosely cohesive clusters or sheets of tumor cells with abundant finely granular fragile cytoplasm and round nuclei often with prominent nucleoli. HE stain. Dispersed naked nuclei with prominent, centrally situated nucleoli and moderate anisonucleosis (MGG stain; **c**, **d**) in a cytoplasmic granular background (HE stain; **e**) are common findings in smears of ASPS. **f** Characteristic PAS-positive intracytoplasmic crystals appreciated in the cell block sections. Cell block; PAS staining.

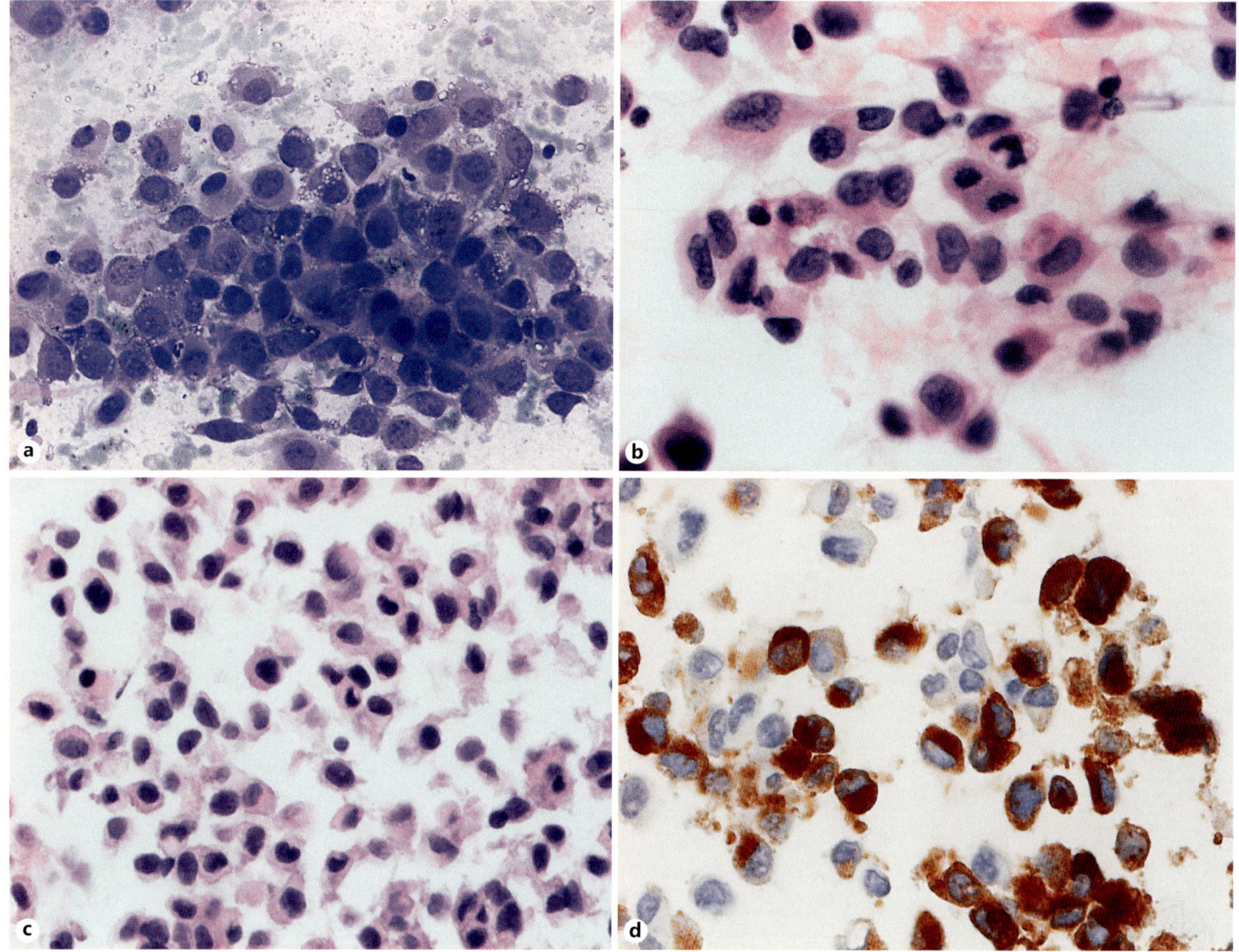

Fig. 8. Clear cell sarcoma. Loosely cohesive sheets (**a**) and mostly dispersed, slightly or moderately atypical round, polygonal, or spindle-shaped cells with a rather abundant clear or pale cytoplasm and large round or oval nuclei (**b**). MGG and HE stains. Corresponding cell block section with cytomorphology similar to FNA smears (HE stain; **c**) and positive immunoreactivity for HMB45 (cell block; HMB45; **d**).

ation, and a tigroid background of the smears. Similarly to malignant melanoma, CCS tumor cells are diffusely and strongly positive for S100 protein, SOX10, and HMB-45, and contain melanosomes as indicated by ultrastructural analysis.

Cytologic Features
- Moderately cellular smears with tigroid background
- Dispersed cells and occasional loose cell clusters
- Round, polygonal, or spindle-shaped cells with an abundant clear to pale cytoplasm
- Round to ovoid nuclei with vesicular chromatin and often prominent nucleoli

Ancillary Tests
Immunophenotype
Tumor cells stain positive for S100, HBM45, SOX10, and typically express the melanoma isoform of microphthalmia transcription factor (MITF-M).

Genetics
The large majority of cases display a specific translocation, t(12;22)(q13;q12), resulting in a fusion gene *EWSR1-ATF1* [52]. This fusion stimulates aberrant cell proliferation resulting in tumor development [53]. These anomalies can be detected by cytogenetics, FISH, PCR, and NGS on available material.

Differential Diagnosis
- Metastatic melanoma
- Metastatic carcinoma with clear cell features

Metastatic malignant melanoma is the most important differential diagnosis. Compared to melanoma, CCS harbors the characteristic translocation t(12;22)(q13;q12) with *EWSR1-ATF1* fusion, which is not present in malignant melanoma.

Extraskeletal Myxoid Chondrosarcoma

Extraskeletal myxoid chondrosarcoma is a malignant mesenchymal tumor of uncertain differentiation in adults with a median age of 50 years. Most extraskeletal myxoid chondrosarcomas arise in the deep soft tissue of the limbs and trunk, with the thigh being the most common site. Other locations include the abdomen, pelvis, head and neck, and pleura. FNA smears show uniform, fusiform to spindle or round epithelioid cells arranged as anastomosing cords, strands, or balls in a fibromyxoid and occasionally fibrillary matrix (Fig. 9) [54–59]. Chondroblast-like lacunar structures mimicking real chondrosarcoma are common findings. The immunophenotype is not specific; up to 20% stain for S100 protein, and about 30% for CD117 (KIT) and occasionally for neuroendocrine markers. A characteristic translocation, t(9;22)(q22/q3;q12), resulting in the *EWSR1-NR4A3* fusion gene, is present in most cases. In about 25% cases, a translocation t(9;17)(q22;q11) is identified, which is probably connected with neuroendocrine differentiation.

Cytologic Features
- Abundant myxoid background matrix
- Dispersed cells, branching cords, strands and cell balls
- Uniform bland spindled, fusiform, or round cells with ovoid or rounded nuclei
- Uniform or slightly variable bland nuclei with small nucleoli
- Chondroblast-like lacunar structures
- Lack of significant vascularity

Ancillary Tests
Immunophenotype
Polyphenotypic differentiation. In about 20–30% of cases tumor cells stain positive for S100 and CD117; in rare cases tumor cells display neuroendocrine differentiation and express chromogranin, synaptophysin, and NSE [60].

Genetics
A t(9;22)(q22;q12) translocation is the cytogenetic hallmark of the tumor. It is often the sole anomaly, but other translocations involving chromosome 9 and trisomies of chromosome 7, 8, 12, and 19 have been detected [61, 62]. The *NR4A3* genes on chromosome 9 fuses with the *EWSR1* gene on chromosome 22, but other fusing partners are present in the different translocations. The gene fusions are thought to be transcriptional activators [63]. Cytogenetics, FISH, SNP array, and NGS can detect the genetic changes on available material.

Differential Diagnosis
- Mixed tumor/myoepithelioma of soft tissue
- Low-grade myxofibrosarcoma
- Low-grade fibromyxoid sarcoma

Desmoplastic Small Round Cell Tumor

Desmoplastic small round cell tumor (DSRCT) is an aggressive malignant mesenchymal tumor of unknown histogenesis. It is predominantly found in the abdominal cavity in adolescents and young adults with a striking male predominance and peak incidence in the third decade of life. Clinical presentation is often dramatic, with a large intra-abdominal/retroperitoneal/pelvic mass with multiple serosal implants. An extra-abdominal location is rare, with the thorax and paratesticular area being the most common sites. The cytomorphology of DSRCT, though similar to other small round cell malignancies, displays some distinct features: relatively low cellularity, some cohesiveness retained, slightly angulated nuclei, and acinar-like structures [64–74] (Fig. 10). Characteristic findings of small nests of tumor cells associated with desmoplastic stroma are better appreciated in cell block sections.

Cytologic Features
- Moderately cellular smears with loosely cohesive, occasionally cohesive cell clusters
- Uniform or slightly pleomorphic undifferentiated cells with round to oval, slightly angulated, irregular nuclei and scant cytoplasm
- Nuclear molding and small acinar-like structures
- Desmoplastic stroma fragments

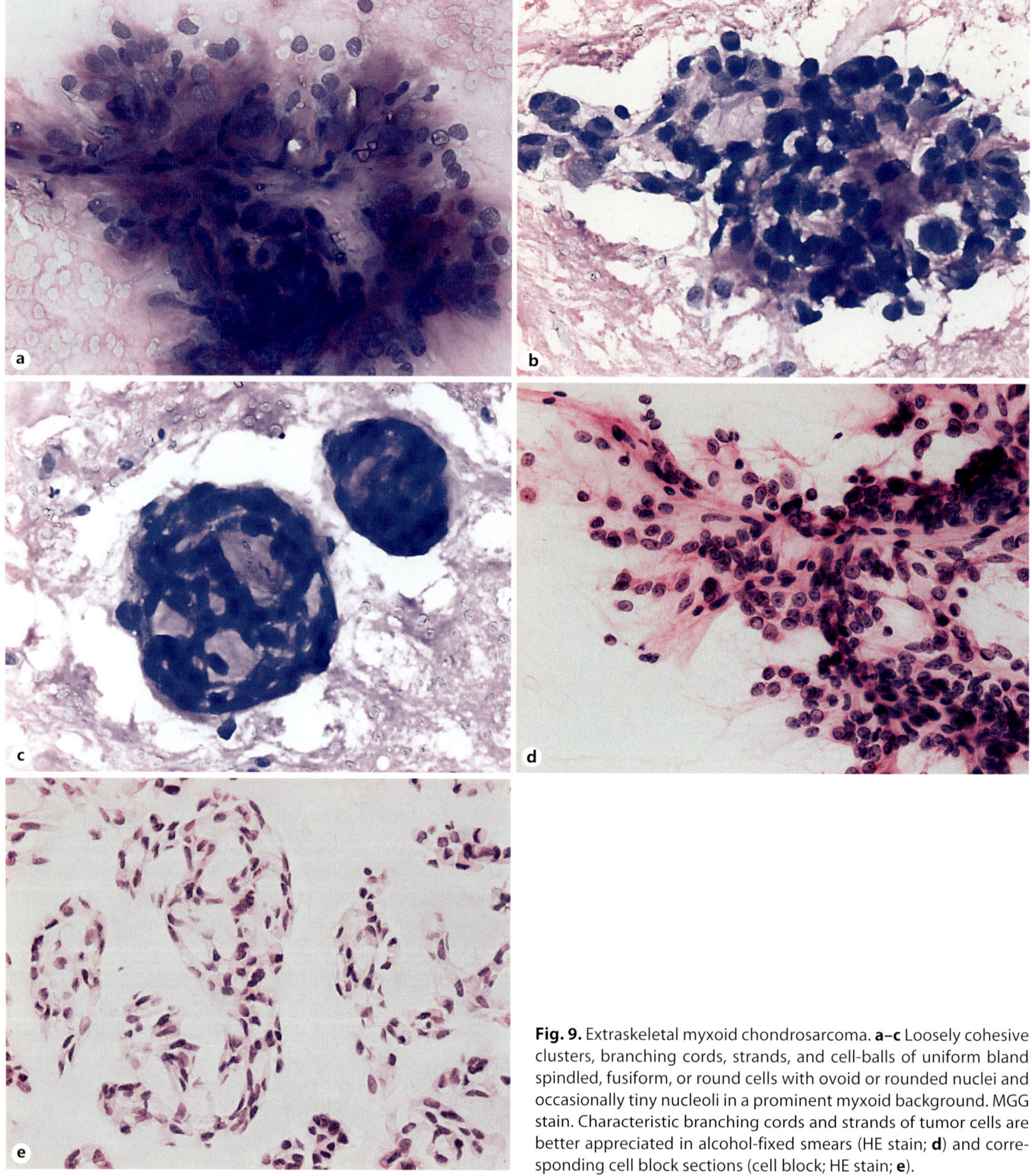

Fig. 9. Extraskeletal myxoid chondrosarcoma. **a–c** Loosely cohesive clusters, branching cords, strands, and cell-balls of uniform bland spindled, fusiform, or round cells with ovoid or rounded nuclei and occasionally tiny nucleoli in a prominent myxoid background. MGG stain. Characteristic branching cords and strands of tumor cells are better appreciated in alcohol-fixed smears (HE stain; **d**) and corresponding cell block sections (cell block; HE stain; **e**).

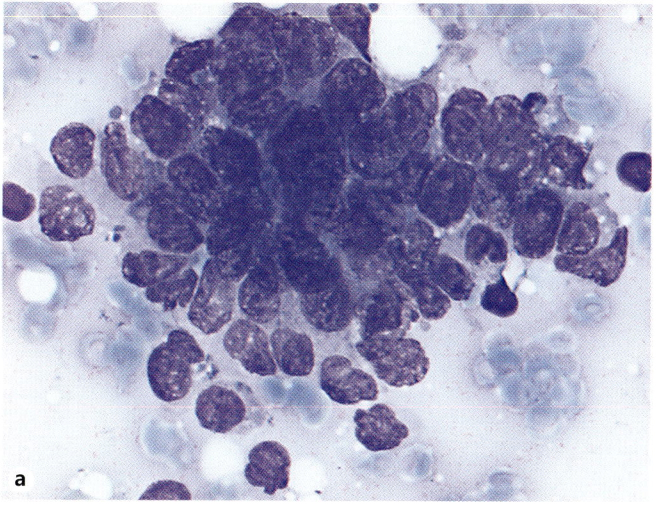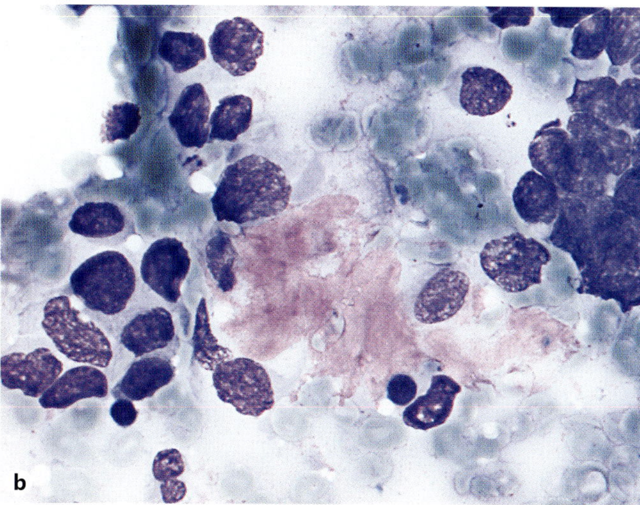

Fig. 10. DSRCT. **a** Cluster of slightly pleomorphic undifferentiated cells with a scant cytoplasm, irregular nuclei and nuclear molding. MGG stain. **b** Dispersed cells with poorly preserved cytoplasm, round to oval, slightly angulated irregular nuclei and desmoplastic stroma fragments. MGG stain.

Ancillary Tests
Immunophenotype
DSRCT exhibits polyphenotypic differentiation: with immunoreactivity for keratins, desmin, EMA, WT1, neuroendocrine markers, and variable positivity for CD99.

Genetics
The tumor displays a characteristic t(11;22)(p13;q12) translocation that fuses *EWSR1* and *WT1* genes on chromosomes 22 and 11, respectively [75]. The fusion results in an aberrant transcription factor [76]. These genetic changes can be detected with cytogenetics, FISH, PCR, and NGS on available material.

Differential Diagnosis
- Ewing sarcoma
- Rhabdomyosarcoma
- Poorly differentiated SS
- Metastatic carcinoma (basaloid squamous cell carcinoma)
- Neuroendocrine tumor

Typical clinical presentation helps to distinguish DSRCT from other small blue round cell tumors and small cell carcinomas in addition to a unique translocation t(11;22)(p13:q12) with *EWSRI-WT1* gene fusion, with can be detected by FISH, PCR, and NGS studies.

Extrarenal Rhabdoid Tumor

Extrarenal rhabdoid tumor is a very rare, highly malignant tumor of infants and young children composed of cells with a rhabdoid morphology. Congenital cases have been reported. Extrarenal rhabdoid tumor arises in deep soft tissue of the neck and paraspinal/retroperitoneal region, but may also affect the skin and visceral organs, such as the liver. The main cytologic feature is a mixture of dispersed cells and cell clusters of large rhabdoid cells and smaller round or polygonal or spindled cells. Cells with a rhabdoid morphology have eccentrically placed large nuclei with macronucleoli and perinuclear cytoplasmic densities (Fig. 11). Although a diagnosis of a malignancy is relatively easy to render from FNA smears, a correct specific diagnosis requires ancillary techniques such as demonstration of *SMARCB1* gene loss by cytogenetic techniques and/or INI1 protein loss by immunohistochemistry.

Cytologic Features
- Variable cellularity with dispersed cells and clusters
- Large rhabdoid cells with eccentric nuclei, prominent nucleoli, and perinuclear density
- Smaller round, polygonal, and spindled cells
- Occasional binucleation and multinucleation
- Brisk mitoses and necrosis

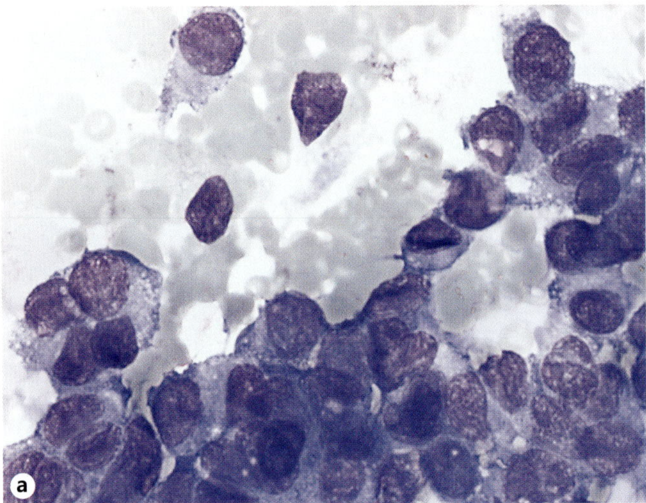

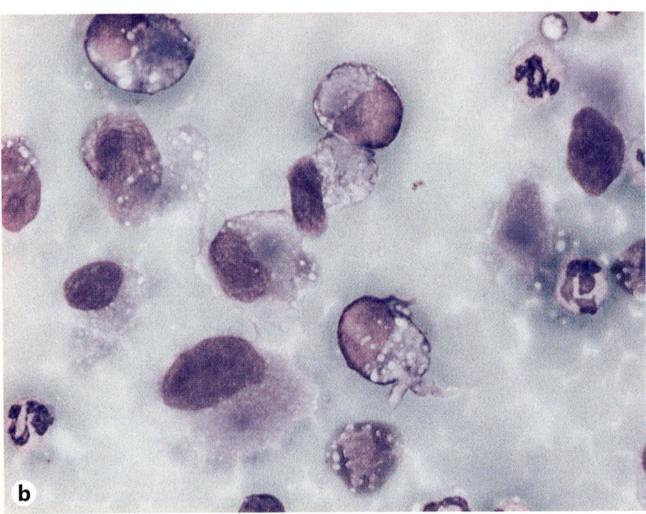

Fig. 11. Extrarenal rhabdoid tumor. **a** Cohesive cluster of medium-sized round, polygonal, and spindled cells with a moderate, somewhat dense cytoplasm. MGG stain. **b** Dispersed single cells showing rhabdoid morphology with eccentrically placed large nuclei and abundant cytoplasm with occasional cytoplasmic densities. MGG stain.

Ancillary Tests

Immunophenotype
Positive for EMA, keratin (most commonly CK8 and CK18), and vimentin; about 50% of cases are positive for CD99 and synaptophysin; occasionally focal expression of S100 and actins; loss of nuclear INI-1 expression.

Histochemistry
PAS diastase resistant positivity.

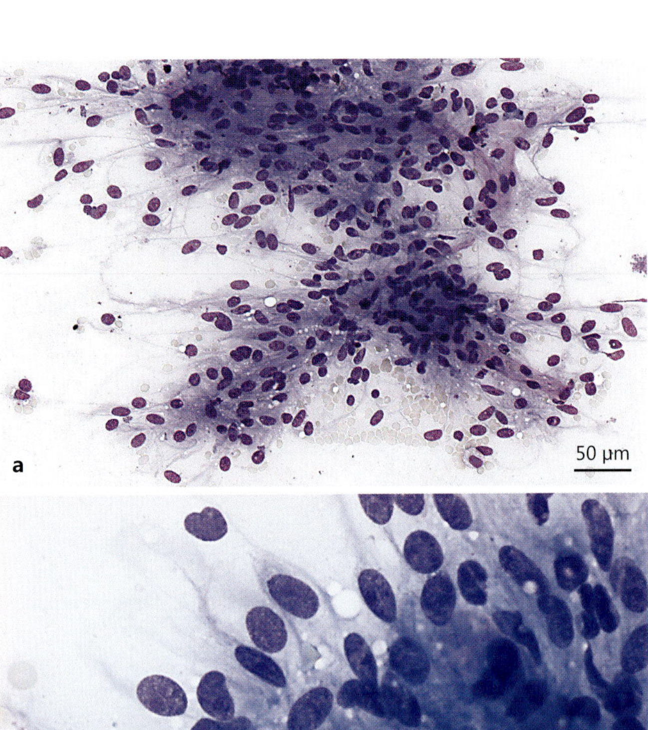

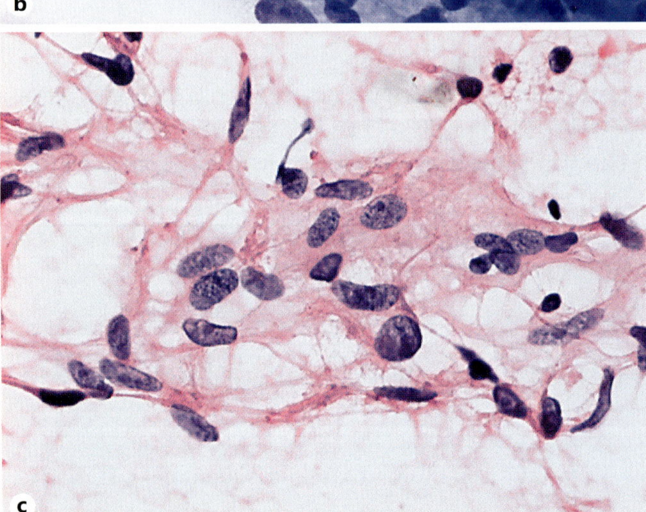

Fig. 12. PEComa. **a**, **b** Loose clusters of uniform or slightly pleomorphic cells containing round to oval and spindled nuclei with small nucleoli and abundant clear or granular cytoplasm with indistinct cytoplasmic borders. MGG stain. **c** Spindle cells with oval and fusiform nuclei, small nucleoli, and occasional spindle cells with cytoplasmic processes. HE stain.

Genetics

These tumors arise due to a complete loss or inactivation of the tumor suppressor gene *SMARCB1* in chromosome band 22q11 [77]. Different mutations, including deletions and translocations, can result in the inactivation and can be investigated with cytogenetics, FISH, SNP array, PCR, and NGS on available material.

Differential Diagnosis
- Rhabdomyosarcoma
- ES
- Other sarcomas with rhabdoid differentiation

Perivascular Epithelioid Cell Tumor

A perivascular epithelioid cell tumor (PEComa) is a distinctive mesenchymal neoplasm arising from perivascular epithelioid cells, usually with a combined melanocytic and smooth muscle phenotype. The PEComa family includes neoplasms that arise in specific organs such as angiomyolipoma (the kidney and liver) [78–80], "sugar" tumor (lung) [81, 82], lymphangioleiomyomatosis (lung), and a variety of histologically and immunophenotypically related neoplasms arising almost in any site, most often in the retroperitoneum, abdomen, pelvis, uterus, and gastrointestinal tract. PEComa occurs over a wide age range, but is most frequent in young and middle-aged adults, with a mean age of 45 and marked female predominance. Histologically, PEComa shows a variable morphology with nests, trabeculae, and sheets of epithelioid to spindled cells with a variable eosinophilic to clear cytoplasm and round to oval nuclei with small nucleoli. In addition, PEComas show unique morphologic features of specific subtypes [83, 84] (Fig. 12).

Cytologic Features
- Variable cellularity with predominantly loosely cohesive clusters
- Uniform or slightly pleomorphic cells with round to oval and spindled nuclei with small nucleoli
- Abundant granular cytoplasm with indistinct cytoplasmic borders
- Smaller round, polygonal, and spindled cells
- Unique morphologic features of specific subtypes

Ancillary Tests
Immunophenotype
Positive for HMB45, melan-A, and MITF; usually positive immunoreactivity for SMA and less common for desmin and h-caldesmon; about 10% of cases express S100 positivity.

Genetics
A variety of genetic gains and losses have been shown in these tumors [85]. Loss of heterozygosity involving the *TSC2* gene has been reported [86].

Differential Diagnosis
- Adult rhabdomyoma
- Granular cell tumor
- ASPS

References

1 Wakely PE Jr, Bos GD, Mayerson J: The cytopathology of soft tissue mxyomas: ganglia, juxta-articular myxoid lesions, and intramuscular myxoma. Am J Clin Pathol 2005;123:858–865.
2 Wakely PE Jr, Geisinger KR, Cappellari JO, Silverman JF, Frable WJ: Fine-needle aspiration cytopathology of soft tissue: chondromyxoid and myxoid lesions. Diagn Cytopathol 1995;12:101–105.
3 Caraway NP, Staerkel GA, Fanning CV, Varma DG, Pollock RE: Diagnosing intramuscular myxoma by fine-needle aspiration: a multidisciplinary approach. Diagn Cytopathol 1994;11:255–261.
4 Akerman M, Rydholm A: Aspiration cytology of intramuscular myxoma: a comparative clinical, cytologic and histologic study of ten cases. Acta Cytol 1983;27:505–510.
5 Delaney D, Diss TC, Presneau N, Hing S, Berisha F, Idowu BD, O'Donnell P, Skinner JA, Tirabosco R, Flanagan AM: *GNAS1* mutations occur more commonly than previously thought in intramuscular myxoma. Mod Pathol 2009;22:718–724.
6 Okamoto S, Hisaoka M, Ushijima M, Nakahara S, Toyoshima S, Hashimoto H: Activating Gs(alpha) mutation in intramuscular myxomas with and without fibrous dysplasia of bone. Virchows Arch 2000;437:133–137.
7 Okamoto S, Hisaoka M, Meis-Kindblom JM, Kindblom LG, Hashimoto H: Juxta-articular myxoma and intramuscular myxoma are two distinct entities. Activating Gs alpha mutation at Arg 201 codon does not occur in juxta-articular myxoma. Virchows Arch 2002;440:12–15.
8 Qian X, Hornick JL, Cibas ES, Dal Cin P, Domanski HA: Angiomatoid fibrous histiocytoma a series of five cytologic cases with literature review and emphasis on diagnostic pitfalls. Diagn Cytopathol 2012;40(suppl 2):E86–E93.
9 Lemos MM, Karlen J, Tani E: Fine-needle aspiration cytology of angiomatoid malignant fibrous histiocytoma. Diagn Cytopathol 2005;33:116–121.
10 Thway K, Fisher C: Angiomatoid fibrous histiocytoma: the current status of pathology and genetics. Arch Pathol Lab Med 2015;139:674–682.
11 Thway K, Stefanaki K, Papadakis V, Fisher C: Metastatic angiomatoid fibrous histiocytoma of the scalp, with *EWSR1-CREB1* gene fusions in primary tumor and nodal metastasis. Hum Pathol 2013;44:289–293.

12 Thway K, Fisher C: Tumors with *EWSR1-CREB1* and *EWSR1-ATF1* fusions: the current status. Am J Surg Pathol 2012;36:e1–e11.

13 Antonescu CR, Dal Cin P, Nafa K, Teot LA, Surti U, Fletcher CD, Ladanyi M: *EWSR1-CREB1* is the predominant gene fusion in angiomatoid fibrous histiocytoma. Genes Chromosomes Cancer 2007;46:1051–1060.

14 Hallor KH, Micci F, Meis-Kindblom JM, Kindblom LG, Bacchini P, Mandahl N, Mertens F, Panagopoulos I: Fusion genes in angiomatoid fibrous histiocytoma. Cancer Lett 2007;251:158–163.

15 Gupta S, Gupta R, Singh S, Pant L: Ossifying fibromyxoid tumour of soft parts: report of a case diagnosed on fine needle aspiration cytology. Cytopathology 2012;23:126–128.

16 Ahmed OI, Qasem SA, Salih ZT: Ossifying fibromyxoid tumor: report of a case with cytomorphologic description. Diagn Cytopathol 2015;43:646–649.

17 Alvarez-Rodriguez F, Jimenez-Heffernan J, Salas C, Pastrana M, Sanz E: Cytological features of ossifying fibromyxoid tumor of soft parts. J Cytol 2012;29:205–207.

18 Mohanty SK, Srinivasan R, Rajwanshi A, Vasishta RK, Vignesh PS: Cytologic diagnosis of ossifying fibromyxoid tumor of soft tissue: a case report. Diagn Cytopathol 2004;30:41–45.

19 Ekfors TO, Kulju T, Aaltonen M, Kallajoki M: Ossifying fibromyxoid tumour of soft parts: report of four cases including one mediastinal and one infantile. APMIS 1998;106:1124–1130.

20 Nishio J, Iwasaki H, Ohjimi Y, Ishiguro M, Isayama T, Naito M, Okabayashi H, Kaneko Y, Kikuchi M: Ossifying fibromyxoid tumor of soft parts: cytogenetic findings. Cancer Genet Cytogenet 2002;133:124–128.

21 Wang G, Tucker T, Ng TL, Villamil CF, Hayes MM: Fine-needle aspiration of soft tissue myoepithelioma. Diagn Cytopathol 2016;44:152–155.

22 Narick C, Velosa C, Pollice P, Silverman J: Fine needle aspiration cytology of a myoepithelioma presenting as a thyroid nodule. Diagn Cytopathol 2015;43:153–157.

23 Machado I, Lopez-Soto MV, Rubio L, Navarro L, Llombart-Bosch A: Soft tissue myoepithelial carcinoma with rhabdoid-like features and *EWSR1* rearrangement: fine needle aspiration cytology with histologic correlation. Diagn Cytopathol 2015;43:421–426.

24 Antonescu CR, Zhang L, Chang NE, Pawel BR, Travis W, Katabi N, Edelman M, Rosenberg AE, Nielsen GP, Dal Cin P, Fletcher CD: *EWSR1-POU5F1* fusion in soft tissue myoepithelial tumors: a molecular analysis of sixty-six cases, including soft tissue, bone, and visceral lesions, showing common involvement of the *EWSR1* gene. Genes Chromosomes Cancer 2010;49:1114–1124.

25 Akerman M, Domanski HA: The complex cytological features of synovial sarcoma in fine needle aspirates, an analysis of four illustrative cases. Cytopathology 2007;18:234–240.

26 Akerman M, Ryd W, Skytting B: Fine-needle aspiration of synovial sarcoma: criteria for diagnosis: retrospective reexamination of 37 cases, including ancillary diagnostics: a Scandinavian Sarcoma Group study. Diagn Cytopathol 2003;28:232–238.

27 Klijanienko J, Caillaud JM, Lagace R, Vielh P: Cytohistologic correlations in 56 synovial sarcomas in 36 patients: the Institut Curie Experience. Diagn Cytopathol 2002;27:96–102.

28 Silverman JF, Landreneau RJ, Sturgis CD, Raab SS, Fox KR, Jasnosz KM, Dabbs DJ: Small-cell variant of synovial sarcoma: fine-needle aspiration with ancillary features and potential diagnostic pitfalls. Diagn Cytopathol 2000;23:118–123.

29 Kottu R, Prayaga AK: Synovial sarcoma with relevant immunocytochemistry and special emphasis on the monophasic fibrous variant. J Cytol 2010;27:47–50.

30 Srinivasan R, Gautam U, Gupta R, Rajwanshi A, Vasistha RK: Synovial sarcoma: diagnosis on fine-needle aspiration by morphology and molecular analysis. Cancer 2009;117:128–136.

31 Ladanyi M, Antonescu CR, Leung DH, Woodruff JM, Kawai A, Healey JH, Brennan MF, Bridge JA, Neff JR, Barr FG, Goldsmith JD, Brooks JS, Goldblum JR, Ali SZ, Shipley J, Cooper CS, Fisher C, Skytting B, Larsson O: Impact of SYT-SSX fusion type on the clinical behavior of synovial sarcoma: a multi-institutional retrospective study of 243 patients. Cancer Res 2002;62:135–140.

32 Kulkarni MM, Deshmukh S, Patil V, Khandeparkar SG: Fine-needle aspiration cytology of recurrent epithelioid sarcoma of the foot: role of immonocytochemistry in definitive diagnosis. J Cytol 2014;31:199–201.

33 Lemos MM, Chaves P, Mendonca ME: Is preoperative cytologic diagnosis of epithelioid sarcoma possible? Diagn Cytopathol 2008;36:780–786.

34 Kitagawa Y, Ito H, Sawaizumi T, Matsubara M, Yokoyama M, Naito Z, Maeda S, Sugisaki Y: Fine needle aspiration cytology of primary epithelioid sarcoma: a report of 2 cases. Acta Cytol 2004;48:391–396.

35 Cardillo M, Zakowski MF, Lin O: Fine-needle aspiration of epithelioid sarcoma: cytology findings in nine cases. Cancer 2001;93:246–251.

36 Lualdi E, Modena P, Debiec-Rychter M, Pedeutour F, Teixeira MR, Facchinetti F, Dagrada GP, Pilotti S, Sozzi G: Molecular cytogenetic characterization of proximal-type epithelioid sarcoma. Genes Chromosomes Cancer 2004;41:283–290.

37 Modena P, Lualdi E, Facchinetti F, Galli L, Teixeira MR, Pilotti S, Sozzi G: *SMARCB1/INI1* tumor suppressor gene is frequently inactivated in epithelioid sarcomas. Cancer Res 2005;65:4012–4019.

38 Agarwal S, Gupta R, Iyer VK, Mathur SR, Ray R: Cytopathological diagnosis of alveolar soft part sarcoma, a rare soft tissue neoplasm. Cytopathology 2011;22:318–322.

39 Wakely PE Jr, McDermott JE, Ali SZ: Cytopathology of alveolar soft part sarcoma: a report of 10 cases. Cancer 2009;117:500–507.

40 Lopez-Ferrer P, Jimenez-Heffernan JA, Vicandi B, Gonzalez-Peramato P, Viguer JM: Cytologic features of alveolar soft part sarcoma: report of three cases. Diagn Cytopathol 2002;27:115–119.

41 Willen H, Akerman M, Carlen B: Fine needle aspiration (FNA) in the diagnosis of soft tissue tumours; a review of 22 years experience. Cytopathology 1995;6:236–247.

42 Drachenberg CB, Papadimitriou JC: Alveolar soft part sarcoma: a case report with correlation of fine needle aspiration and ultrastructural cytologic features. Acta Cytol 1991;35:746–752.

43 Shabb N, Sneige N, Fanning CV, Dekmezian R: Fine-needle aspiration cytology of alveolar soft-part sarcoma. Diagn Cytopathol 1991;7:293–298.

44 Nambirajan A, Jain D, Malik P, Arava S, Mathur SR: Metastatic alveolar soft part sarcoma of the lung: metastatic alveolar soft part sarcoma of the lung – a morphologic pitfall on cytology and aberrant CD10 expression on histology. Diagn Cytopathol 2016;44:250–254.

45 Majumdar K, Saran R, Tyagi I, Jain A, Jagetia A, Sinha S, Singh A: Cytodiagnosis of alveolar soft part sarcoma: report of two cases with special emphasis on the first orbital lesion diagnosed by aspiration cytology. J Cytol 2013;30:58–61.

46 Min KW, Na W, Oh YH, Park YW, Park MH: Fine needle aspiration cytology of alveolar soft part sarcoma of the cheek. Cytopathology 2010;21:205–207.

47 Van Buren R, Stewart J 3rd: Alveolar soft part sarcoma presenting as a breast mass in a 13-year-old female. Diagn Cytopathol 2009;37:122–124.

48 Carter JE, Evans TN, Tucker JA: Cytologic diagnosis of alveolar soft part sarcoma of the lower extremity by fine needle aspiration and correlation with core biopsy: a case report. Acta Cytol 2008;52:459–463.

49 Joyama S, Ueda T, Shimizu K, Kudawara I, Mano M, Funai H, Takemura K, Yoshikawa H: Chromosome rearrangement at 17q25 and xp11.2 in alveolar soft-part sarcoma: a case report and review of the literature. Cancer 1999;86:1246–1250.

50 Tsuda M, Davis IJ, Argani P, Shukla N, McGill GG, Nagai M, Saito T, Lae M, Fisher DE, Ladanyi M: TFE3 fusions activate MET signaling by transcriptional up-regulation, defining another class of tumors as candidates for therapeutic MET inhibition. Cancer Res 2007;67:919–929.

51 Machhi J, Kouzova M, Komorowski DJ, Asma Z, Chivukala M, Basir Z, Shidham VB: Crystals of alveolar soft part sarcoma in a fine needle aspiration biopsy cytology smear: a case report. Acta Cytol 2002;46:904–908.

52 Antonescu CR, Tschernyavsky SJ, Woodruff JM, Jungbluth AA, Brennan MF, Ladanyi M: Molecular diagnosis of clear cell sarcoma: detection of EWS-ATF1 and MITF-M transcripts and histopathological and ultrastructural analysis of 12 cases. J Mol Diagn 2002;4:44–52.

53 Davis IJ, Kim JJ, Ozsolak F, Widlund HR, Rozenblatt-Rosen O, Granter SR, Du J, Fletcher JA, Denny CT, Lessnick SL, Linehan WM, Kung AL, Fisher DE: Oncogenic MITF dysregulation in clear cell sarcoma: defining the MiT family of human cancers. Cancer Cell 2006;9:473–484.

54 Handa U, Singhal N, Punia RS, Garg S, Mohan H: Cytologic features and differential diagnosis in a case of extraskeletal mesenchymal chondrosarcoma: a case report. Acta Cytol 2009;53:704–706.

55 Ananthamurthy A, Nisheena R, Rao B, Correa M: Extraskeletal myxoid chondrosarcoma: diagnosis of a rare soft tissue tumor based on fine needle aspiration cytology. J Cytol 2009;26:36–38.
56 Jakowski JD, Wakely PE Jr: Cytopathology of extraskeletal myxoid chondrosarcoma: report of 8 cases. Cancer 2007;111:298–305.
57 Gonidi M, Athanassiadou P, Petrakakou E, Zerva C, Dimou S: Extraskeletal myxoid chondrosarcoma: a case report with fine needle aspiration (FNA) cytology. Cytopathology 1997;8:130–133.
58 Gordon MD, Vetto J, Meshul CK, Schmidt WA: FNA of extraskeletal myxoid chondrosarcoma: cytomorphologic, EM, and X-ray microanalysis features. Diagn Cytopathol 1994;10:352–356.
59 Gonzalez-Campora R, Otal-Salaverri C, Hevia-Vazquez A, Munoz-Munoz G, Garrido-Cintado A, Galera-Davidson H: Fine needle aspiration in myxoid tumors of the soft tissues. Acta Cytol 1990;34:179–191.
60 Domanski HA, Carlen B, Mertens F, Akerman M: Extraskeletal myxoid chondrosarcoma with neuroendocrine differentiation: a case report with fine-needle aspiration biopsy, histopathology, electron microscopy, and cytogenetics. Ultrastruct Pathol 2003;27:363–368.
61 Attwooll C, Tariq M, Harris M, Coyne JD, Telford N, Varley JM: Identification of a novel fusion gene involving *hTAF$_{II}$68* and *CHN* from a t(9;17)(q22;q11.2) translocation in an extraskeletal myxoid chondrosarcoma. Oncogene 1999;18:7599–7601.
62 Panagopoulos I, Storlazzi CT, Fletcher CD, Fletcher JA, Nascimento A, Domanski HA, Wejde J, Brosjo O, Rydholm A, Isaksson M, Mandahl N, Mertens F: The chimeric *FUS/CREB3l2* gene is specific for low-grade fibromyxoid sarcoma. Genes Chromosomes Cancer 2004;40:218–228.
63 Kim S, Lee HJ, Jun HJ, Kim J: The hTAF$_{II}$68-TEC fusion protein functions as a strong transcriptional activator. Int J Cancer 2008;122:2446–2453.
64 Klijanienko J, Colin P, Couturier J, Lagace R, Freneaux P, Pierron G, Lae M, Klijanienko A, Brisse H, Orbach D, Theocharis S: Fine-needle aspiration in desmoplastic small round cell tumor: a report of 10 new tumors in 8 patients with clinicopathological and molecular correlations with review of the literature. Cancer Cytopathol 2014;122:386–393.
65 Leca LB, Vieira J, Teixeira MR, Monteiro P: Desmoplastic small round cell tumor: diagnosis by fine-needle aspiration cytology. Acta Cytol 2012;56:576–580.
66 Rajwanshi A, Srinivas R, Upasana G: Malignant small round cell tumors. J Cytol 2009;26:1–10.
67 Presley AE, Kong CS, Rowe DM, Atkins KA: Cytology of desmoplastic small round-cell tumor: comparison of pre- and post-chemotherapy fine-needle aspiration biopsies. Cancer 2007;111:41–46.
68 Dave B, Shet T, Chinoy R: Desmoplastic round cell tumor of childhood: can cytology with immunocytochemistry serve as an alternative for tissue diagnosis? Diagn Cytopathol 2005;32:330–335.
69 Granja NM, Begnami MD, Bortolan J, Filho AL, Schmitt FC: Desmoplastic small round cell tumour: cytological and immunocytochemical features. Cytojournal 2005;2:6.
70 Crapanzano JP, Cardillo M, Lin O, Zakowski MF: Cytology of desmoplastic small round cell tumor. Cancer 2002;96:21–31.
71 Ferlicot S, Coue O, Gilbert E, Beuzeboc P, Servois V, Klijanienko J, Delattre O, Vielh P: Intraabdominal desmoplastic small round cell tumor: report of a case with fine needle aspiration, cytologic diagnosis and molecular confirmation. Acta Cytol 2001;45:617–621.
72 Insabato L, Di Vizio D, Lambertini M, Bucci L, Pettinato G: Fine needle aspiration cytology of desmoplastic small round cell tumor: a case report. Acta Cytol 1999;43:641–646.
73 Ali SZ, Nicol TL, Port J, Ford G: Intraabdominal desmoplastic small round cell tumor: cytopathologic findings in two cases. Diagn Cytopathol 1998;18:449–452.
74 el-Kattan I, Redline RW, el-Naggar AK, Grimes MC, Abdul-Karim FW: Cytologic features of intraabdominal desmoplastic small round cell tumor: a case report. Acta Cytol 1995;39:514–520.
75 Biegel JA, Conard K, Brooks JJ: Translocation (11;22)(p13;q12): primary change in intra-abdominal desmoplastic small round cell tumor. Genes Chromosomes Cancer 1993;7:119–121.
76 Gerald WL, Haber DA: The *EWS-WT1* gene fusion in desmoplastic small round cell tumor. Semin Cancer Biol 2005;15:197–205.
77 Biegel JA, Zhou JY, Rorke LB, Stenstrom C, Wainwright LM, Fogelgren B: Germ-line and acquired mutations of INI1 in atypical teratoid and rhabdoid tumors. Cancer Res 1999;59:74–79.
78 Xie L, Jessurun J, Manivel JC, Pambuccian SE: Hepatic epithelioid angiomyolipoma with trabecular growth pattern: a mimic of hepatocellular carcinoma on fine needle aspiration cytology. Diagn Cytopathol 2012;40:639–650.
79 Alatassi H, Sahoo S: Epithelioid angiomyolipoma of the liver with striking giant cell component: fine-needle aspiration biopsy findings of a rare neoplasm. Diagn Cytopathol 2009;37:192–194.
80 Handa U, Nanda A, Mohan H: Fine-needle aspiration of renal angiomyolipoma: a report of four cases. Cytopathology 2007;18:250–254.
81 Policarpio-Nicolas ML, Covell J, Bregman S, Atkins K: Fine needle aspiration cytology of clear cell "sugar" tumor (PEComa) of the lung: report of a case. Diagn Cytopathol 2008;36:89–93.
82 Edelweiss M, Gupta N, Resetkova E: Preoperative diagnosis of clear cell "sugar" tumor of the lung by computed tomography-guided fine-needle biopsy and core-needle biopsy. Ann Diagn Pathol 2007;11:421–426.
83 Collins K, Buckley T, Anderson K, Karasik M, Ligato S: Perivascular epithelioid cell tumor (PEComa) of pancreas diagnosed preoperatively by endoscopic ultrasound-guided fine-needle aspiration: a case report and review of literature. Diagn Cytopathol 2017;45:59–65.
84 Okuwaki K, Kida M, Masutani H, Yamauchi H, Katagiri H, Mikami T, Miyazawa S, Iwai T, Takezawa M, Imaizumi H, Koizumi W: A resected perivascular epithelioid cell tumor (PEComa) of the pancreas diagnosed using endoscopic ultrasound-guided fine-needle aspiration. Intern Med 2013;52:2061–2066.
85 Pan CC, Jong YJ, Chai CY, Huang SH, Chen YJ: Comparative genomic hybridization study of perivascular epithelioid cell tumor: molecular genetic evidence of perivascular epithelioid cell tumor as a distinctive neoplasm. Hum Pathol 2006;37:606–612.
86 Pan CC, Chung MY, Ng KF, Liu CY, Wang JS, Chai CY, Huang SH, Chen PC, Ho DM: Constant allelic alteration on chromosome 16p (*TSC2* gene) in perivascular epithelioid cell tumour (PEComa): genetic evidence for the relationship of PEComa with angiomyolipoma. J Pathol 2008;214:387–393.

Domanski HA, Walther CS: FNA Cytology of Soft Tissue and Bone Tumors. Monogr Clin Cytol.
Basel, Karger, 2017, vol 22, pp 122–124 (DOI: 10.1159/000475103)

Undifferentiated/Unclassified Sarcomas

Undifferentiated/unclassified sarcomas are defined in the 2013 World Health Organization (WHO) monograph as a heterogeneous group of sarcomas without evidence of a particular line of differentiation. Most undifferentiated sarcomas with round cell morphology arise in young patients, while those of pleomorphic morphology (previously pleomorphic malignant fibrous histiocytoma; MFH) usually occur in elderly adults. Morphologically, they can be either spindle cell, epithelioid, round cell, or pleomorphic (Fig. 1) (previous MFH). MFH was considered to be a distinct entity for many years [1]. Retrospective examinations of a series of cases diagnosed as pleomorphic MFH have identified lipogenic, myogenic, and Schwann cell differentiation, as well as nonmesenchymal histogenesis in the majority of re-examined cases [2]. A diagnosis of undifferentiated/unclassified sarcoma diagnosis should only be rendered from fine-needle aspiration smears if there is access to immunocytochemical and molecular studies that exclude any specific subtype of sarcoma.

Cytologic Features [3, 4]
- Hypercellular smears
- Mixture of dispersed cells, cell clusters, and small tissue fragments in variable proportions
- Variable cellular morphology, commonly spindle-, polygonal-, and epithelioid cells with marked cellular and nuclear pleomorphism, coarse chromatin, and large nucleoli
- Uni- and multinucleated giant cells
- Necrosis and hemorrhage
- Atypical mitoses

Ancillary Tests
Immunophenotype
Immunocytochemical examinations exclude specific histologic subtypes of sarcoma and other diagnoses.

Genetics
In undifferentiated round cell and spindle cell sarcomas the *EWSR1* gene is involved in fusions with genes such as *POU5F1* [5]. Another recurrent mutation is the *CIC-DUX4* fusion gene [6]. However, it is not yet fully understood if

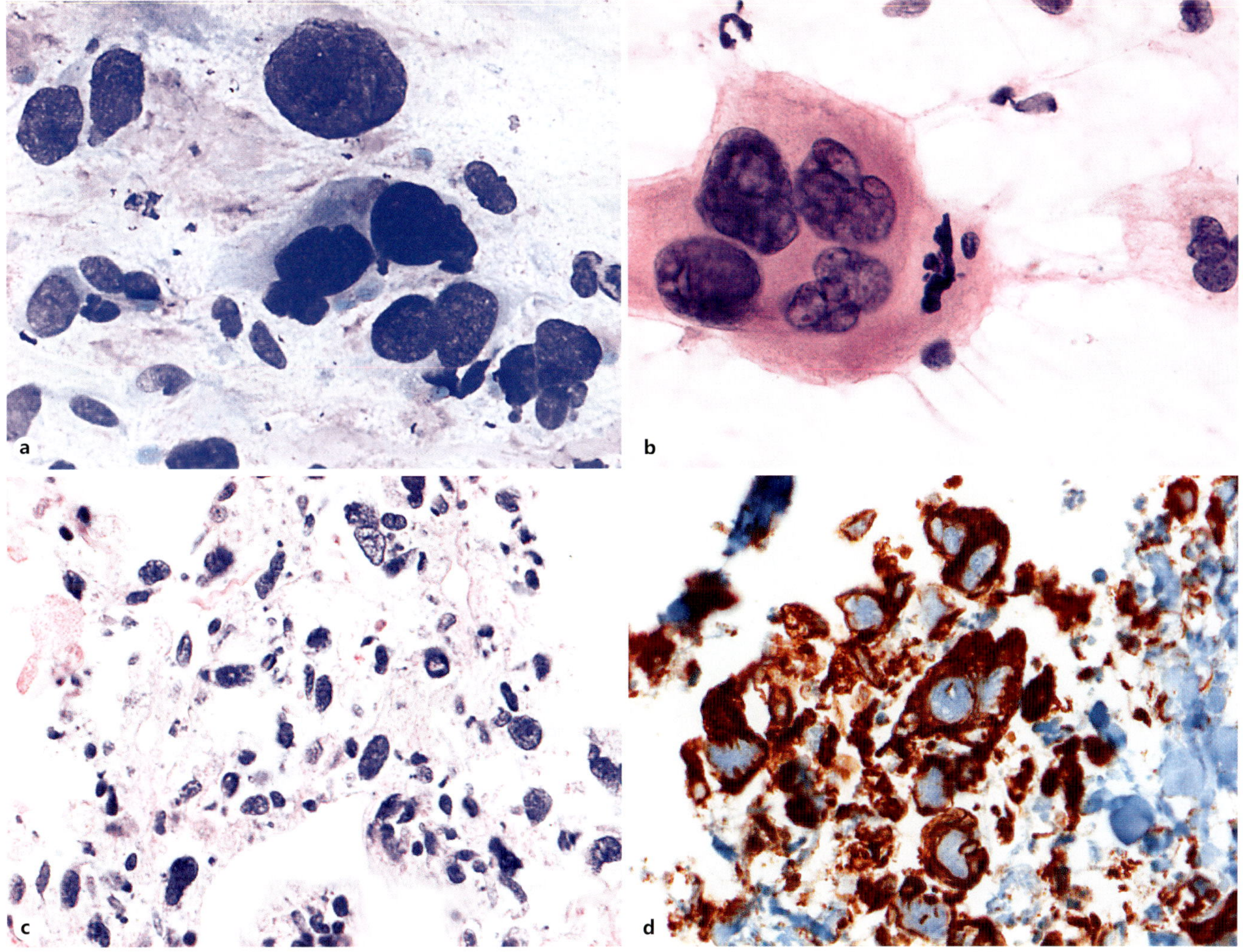

Fig. 1. Undifferentiated sarcoma. **a** Small cell groups and single spindle-, polygonal-, and epithelioid cells with a marked cellular and nuclear pleomorphism and coarse chromatin. MGG stain. **b** Occasional bizarre multinucleate tumor cells. HE stain. The corresponding cell block section shows features of high-grade undifferentiated sarcoma (HE stain; **c**) and positive immunoreactivity for vimentin only (**d**).

these changes represent specific entities, and therefore the diagnostic usefulness is still limited.

Undifferentiated pleomorphic sarcoma was previously termed MFH. These tumors tend to have highly complex karyotypes with a wide variety of molecular changes. The intercellular variation in each tumor can also vary considerably. [7] Therefore, the genetic information in these tumors is difficult to use for specific diagnostic purposes, but can be indicative.

Differential Diagnosis

- Other pleomorphic sarcomas with a specific line of differentiation (pleomorphic liposarcoma, pleomorphic leiomyosarcoma, pleomorphic malignant peripheral nerve sheath tumor, and pleomorphic rhabdomyosarcoma)
- Dedifferentiated sarcomas
- Radiation-associated pleomorphic sarcoma
- Nonmesenchymal tumors (anaplastic large cell lymphoma, soft tissue metastases of anaplastic carcinoma, and sarcoma-like malignant melanoma)
- Sarcomatoid mesothelioma

References

1 Walaas L, Angervall L, Hagmar B, Save-Soder-bergh J: A correlative cytologic and histologic study of malignant fibrous histiocytoma: an analysis of 40 cases examined by fine-needle aspiration cytology. Diagn Cytopathol 1986;2:46–54.

2 Meis-Kindblom JM, Bjerkehage B, Bohling T, Domanski H, Halvorsen TB, Larsson O, Lilleng P, Myhre-Jensen O, Stenwig E, Virolainen M, Willen H, Akerman M, Kindblom LG: Morphologic review of 1,000 soft tissue sarcomas from the Scandinavian Sarcoma Group (SSG) Register: the peer-review committee experience. Acta Orthop Scand Suppl 1999;285:18–26.

3 Klijanienko J, Caillaud JM, Lagace R, Vielh P: Comparative fine-needle aspiration and pathologic study of malignant fibrous histiocytoma: cyto-diagnostic features of 95 tumors in 71 patients. Diagn Cytopathol 2003;29:320–326.

4 Berardo MD, Powers CN, Wakely PE Jr, Almeida MO, Frable WJ: Fine-needle aspiration cytopathology of malignant fibrous histiocytoma. Cancer 1997;81:228–237.

5 Deng FM, Galvan K, de la Roza G, Zhang S, Souid AK, Stein CK: Molecular characterization of an *EWSR1-POU5F1* fusion associated with a t(6;22) in an undifferentiated soft tissue sarcoma. Cancer Genet 2011;204:423–429.

6 Italiano A, Sung YS, Zhang L, Singer S, Maki RG, Coindre JM, Antonescu CR: High prevalence of *CIC* fusion with double-homeobox (DUX4) transcription factors in *EWSR1*-negative undifferentiated small blue round cell sarcomas. Genes Chromosomes Cancer 2012;51:207–218.

7 Fletcher CD, Dal Cin P, de Wever I, Mandahl N, Mertens F, Mitelman F, Rosai J, Rydholm A, Sciot R, Tallini G, van den Berghe H, Vanni R, Willen H: Correlation between clinicopathological features and karyotype in spindle cell sarcomas: a report of 130 cases from the CHAMP study group. Am J Pathol 1999;154:1841–1847.

Domanski HA, Walther CS: FNA Cytology of Soft Tissue and Bone Tumors. Monogr Clin Cytol.
Basel, Karger, 2017, vol 22, pp 125–131 (DOI: 10.1159/000475104)

Neuroectodermal Tumors

Neuroblastoma

Neuroblastoma, a small blue round cell tumor derived from pluripotent sympathetic cells, is the most common extracranial solid malignant tumor in infants. Ninety percent are diagnosed before the age of 5 years. As neuroblastoma and ganglioneuroblastoma originate in sympathetic ganglia, they are commonly found in a paramidline position, with the retroperitoneum being the most frequent site followed by the mediastinum and the sacral region. About two-thirds of all cases present clinically as metastatic deposition in the skeleton, lymph nodes, liver, and skin.

A risk assessment aiding the choice of treatment as well as the assessment of prognosis of neuroblastoma requires a histopathologic examination of tumor tissue. Fine-needle aspiration (FNA) cytology is most frequently used as a primary tool in the examination of metastatic deposits of neuroblastoma. In addition, FNA cytology allows an initial rapid verification of the clinical-radiologic diagnosis of primary tumors, usually followed by biopsy. The utility of FNA cytology in the diagnosis and evaluation of biologic prognostic parameters has been widely reported [1–4]. Smears of neuroblastoma are usually hypercellular with predominantly isolated cells, but also small clusters of tumor cells often have eccentric, rounded, or irregular, kidney-shaped nuclei with a finely granular, clumped chromatin. Nucleoli are inconspicuous. Between the cells and in the background of the smears there is a variable amount of a delicate fibrillary background (neuropil) of neurotic cell processes. Cell clusters are composed of neuroblasts or differentiating cells with nuclear molding and rosette-like structures with a central core of fibrillary neuropil (Homer-Wright rosettes) (Fig. 1). In smears of undifferentiated neuroblastoma, the fibrillary matrix may be missing while large ganglion-like cells are present in more mature tumors. Positive immunostaining for neuron-specific enolase (NSE), chromogranin, and synaptophysin is a common finding, although staining for chromogranin and synaptophysin may be negative in undifferentiated tumors. At electron microscopic examination, neuritic processes with neurotubules and uniform dense-core granules are characteristic features.

Cytologic Features
- Most commonly a rich yield with predominantly dispersed cells
- Cells with irregular, hyperchromatic nuclei
- Nuclear molding and neuroblasts often in small molded clusters
- Variable presence of rosette-like structures with a central neuropil

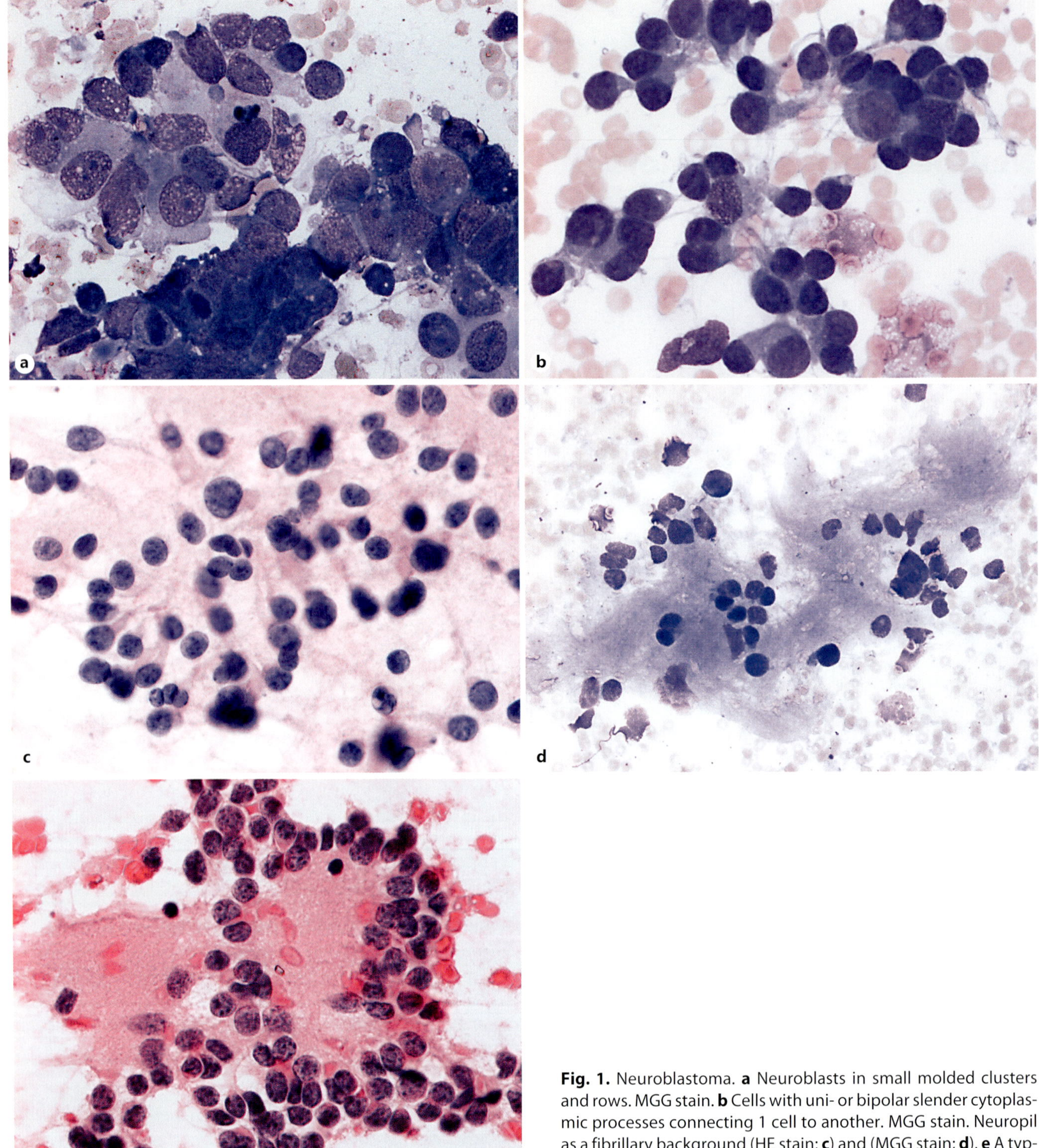

Fig. 1. Neuroblastoma. **a** Neuroblasts in small molded clusters and rows. MGG stain. **b** Cells with uni- or bipolar slender cytoplasmic processes connecting 1 cell to another. MGG stain. Neuropil as a fibrillary background (HE stain; **c**) and (MGG stain; **d**). **e** A typical rosette structure with a central neuropil. HE stain.

- Cells with uni- or bipolar slender cytoplasmic processes
- Cells connected to each other by the cytoplasmic processes
- Variable presence ganglion cells, depending on the degree of differentiation
- Neuropil
- Necrosis, karyorrhexis, calcifications
- Mitotic figures

Ancillary Tests
Immunophenotype
Positive for chromogranin, synaptophysin, and NSE; variable positivity for ALK-1 and glial fibrillary acidic protein (GFAP). Negative for CD99, keratin, epithelial membrane antigen, S100, desmin, MyoD1, and myogenin.

Genetics
Molecular evaluation of neuroblastomas can provide prognostic information and be diagnostically helpful. Sporadic neuroblastomas that display amplifications of the oncogenes ALK or *MYC* are associated with a poor prognosis. Mutations of the *ATRX* gene occur in 17% of children between 1.5 and 12 years of age, and in 44% in children older than 12 years. Familial neuroblastomas are extremely rare but are associated with mutations of the *PHOX2B* and *ALK* genes [5]. These genetic aberrations can be detected with fluorescence in situ hybridization (FISH), polymerase chain reaction (PCR), single nucleotide polymorphism (SNP) array, and next-generation sequencing (NGS) on available fresh or fixed material [5, 6].

Differential Diagnosis
- Alveolar rhabdomyosarcoma
- Ewing sarcoma
- Precursor lymphoma/acute lymphoblastic leukemia
- Wilms tumor

In undifferentiated or poorly differentiated neuroblastoma, rosettes and cytoplasmic processes are absent or rare. In such neoplasms, NSE staining may be focally positive, and chromogranin and synaptophysin negative.

Ganglioneuroma

Ganglioneuroma is a benign neoplasm of neural crest origin arising in sympathetic ganglia, most frequently seated in the posterior mediastinum, retroperitoneum, and occasionally in the adrenal glands. These rare neoplasms occur in children and young adults and are most common between 10 and 30 years of age. Adequate treatment of ganglioneuroma consists of local excision and microscopic examination of tumor tissue is necessary for definitive preoperative evaluation. The typical histologic features of ganglioneuroma include a mixture of fascicles of bland spindle cells (Schwann cells) and randomly distributed single or clustered mature ganglion cells in a fibromyxoid and fibrillary background matrix, and occasional cystic changes, fibrosis, calcification, and lymphoid aggregates. An absence of cell pleomorphism, immature neuroblasts, mitotic activities, and necrosis helps to differ ganglioneuroma from neuroblastoma and ganglioneuroblastoma. Ganglioneuroma is rarely a target for cytologic examination, but correct diagnosis can be rendered from representative FNA smears containing both Schwann cell and ganglion cell components in a typical fibromyxoid background (Fig. 2) [2, 7–14].

Cytologic Features
- Variable cellularity
- Small, loosely cohesive clusters and dispersed bland, uniform spindle cells (Schwann cells) with oval and spindle-shaped nuclei with finely dispersed chromatin
- Dispersed single and clustered ganglion cells with an abundant granular cytoplasm and uniform round nuclei with prominent nucleoli
- Fibromyxoid and fibrillary background matrix
- Absence of immature neuroblasts, necrosis, and mitoses

Ancillary Tests
Immunophenotype
Positive for S100 protein in the Schwann cell component, and synaptophysin in ganglion cells.

Genetics
No diagnostic recurrent genetic abnormalities that distinguish ganglioneuromas from composite paragangliomas or pheochromocytomas are known [15]. In rare cases, ganglioneuromas can be part of the *MEN2* (multiple endocrine neoplasia type 2) familial syndrome, and consequently activation of the *RET* proto-oncogene has been detected [16]. These rare and indicative changes can be detected by PCR and NGS on available material.

Differential Diagnosis
- Schwannoma
- Neurofibroma
- Ganglioneuroblastoma

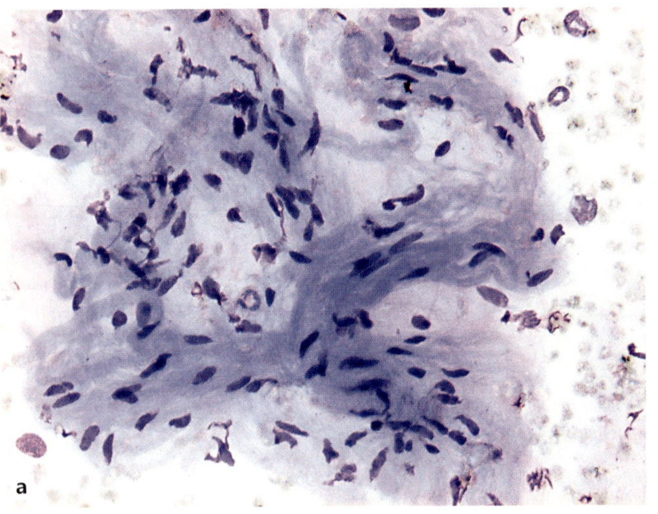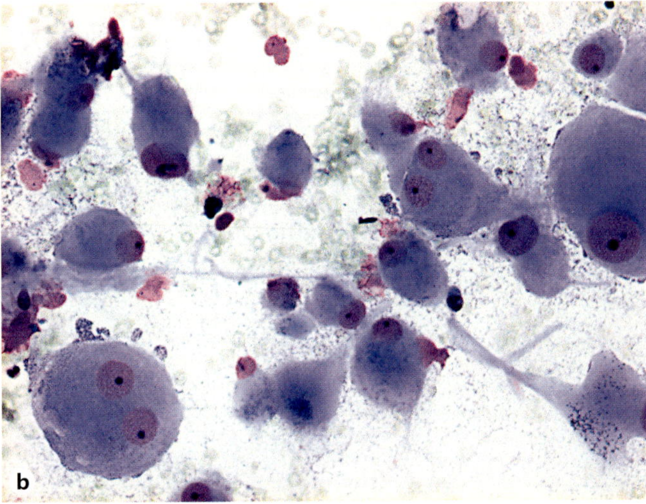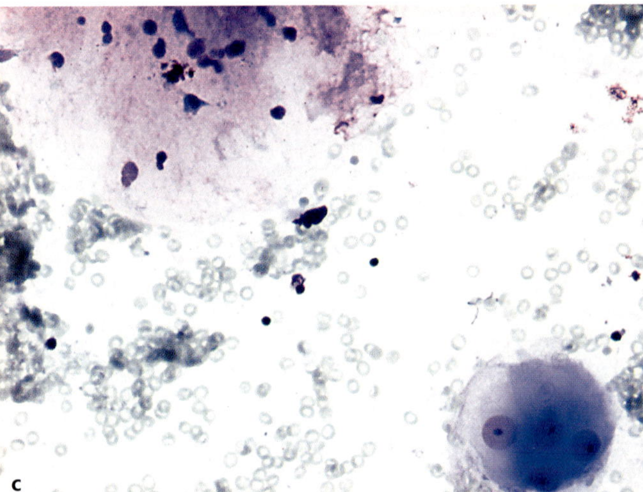

Fig. 2. Ganglioneuroma. **a** Schwannoma-like loosely cohesive cluster of bland, uniform, spindle cells in a fibrillary background matrix. MGG stain. **b** Dispersed single and clustered ganglion cells with an abundant granular cytoplasm and uniform round nuclei with prominent nucleoli. MGG stain. **c** Multinucleated ganglion cell and a loosely cohesive group of Schwann cells in a myxoid/fibrillary background. MGG stain.

The main differential diagnosis of ganglioneuroma is ganglioneuroblastoma, a malign neuroectodermal neoplasm with a similar clinical presentation and showing maturation toward ganglioneuroma. Immature neural elements and immature neuroblasts in smears of ganglioneuroblastoma help to distinguish this neoplasm from ganglioneuroma. FNA smears from benign nerve sheath neoplasms such as Schwannoma and neurofibroma may be similar to that of ganglioneuroma in cases of suboptimal sampling and in the absence of ganglion cells. Access to complete clinical and radiologic data is important; most cases of ganglioneuroma present clinically as a large, deeply seated mediastinal or retroperitoneal mass.

Extraskeletal Ewing Sarcoma

Extraskeletal tumors of the Ewing's sarcoma family are primitive small blue round cell neoplasms characterized by specific *EWRS1* mutations. Although the tumors in the Ewing sarcoma/primitive neuroectodermal tumor family show a varying degree of neuroectodermal differentiation with a somewhat variable morphology, these neoplasms represent a continuous morphologic spectrum with an overlapping immunophenotype and the common denominator that is their cytogenetic aberration, t(11;22)(q24;q12). While Ewing sarcoma is the second most common sarcoma of bone in children and young adults, the extraskeletal Ewing sarcoma accounts for less than 20% of cases. This highly malignant neoplasm occurs most often in children, adolescents,

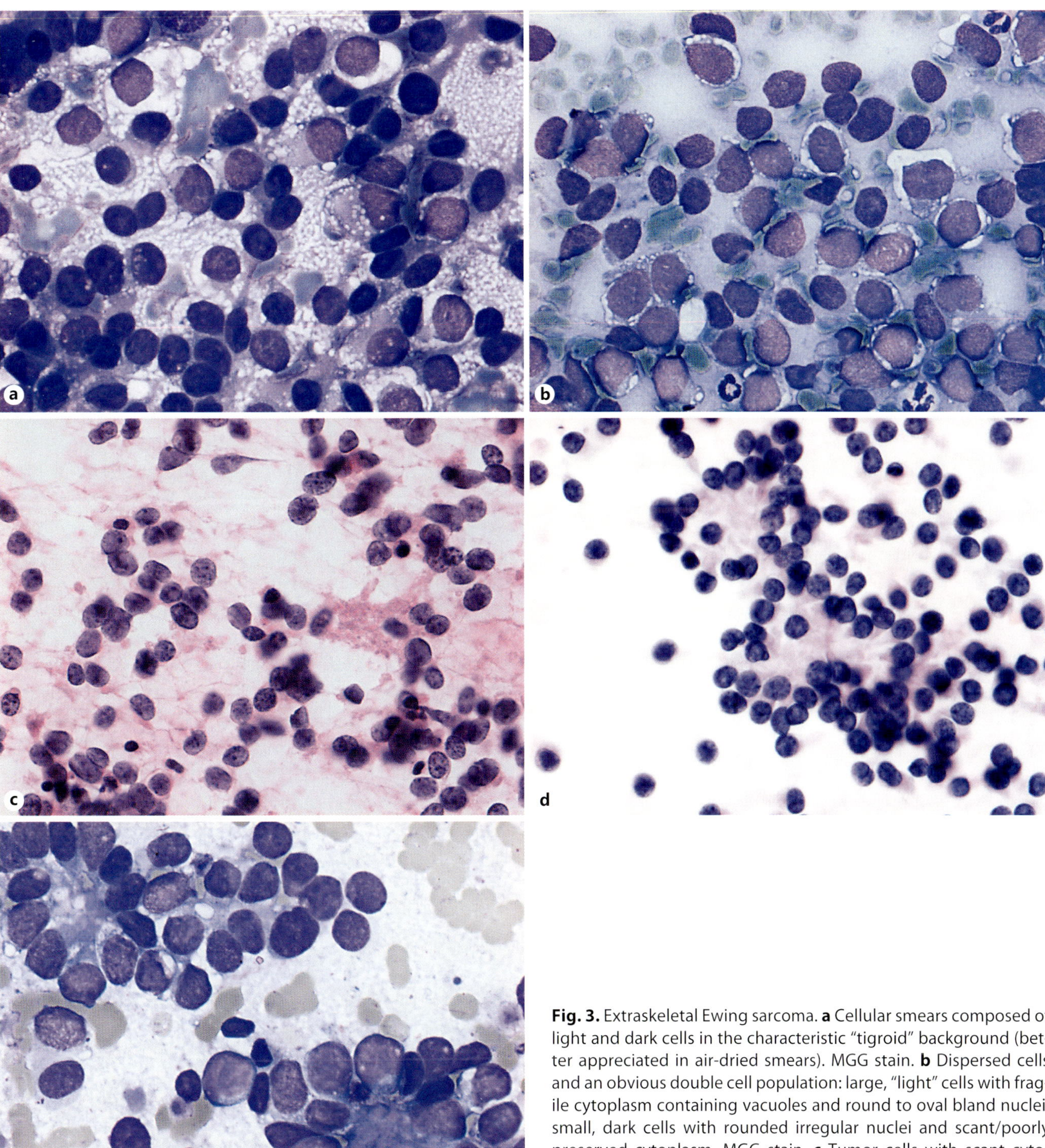

Fig. 3. Extraskeletal Ewing sarcoma. **a** Cellular smears composed of light and dark cells in the characteristic "tigroid" background (better appreciated in air-dried smears). MGG stain. **b** Dispersed cells and an obvious double cell population: large, "light" cells with fragile cytoplasm containing vacuoles and round to oval bland nuclei; small, dark cells with rounded irregular nuclei and scant/poorly preserved cytoplasm. MGG stain. **c** Tumor cells with scant cytoplasm and moderately cellular and nuclear pleomorphism. HE stain. **d**, **e** Rosette-like structures with more or less evident fibrillary centers. HE and MGG stains.

and young adults, arising predominantly in the deep soft tissues with a predilection for the thigh, pelvis, trunk, and foot, but can arise in almost any location. Most smears of Ewing's sarcoma are hypercellular with dispersed cells and numerous naked nuclei as well as scattered cohesive cell clusters in a "tigroid" background. In air-dried smears there is a less or more prominent mixture of larger, "light" viable cells, often with a preserved cytoplasm containing small, irregular vacuoles that contain glycogen and smaller "dark" apoptotic cells with a poorly preserved cytoplasm and round to oval nuclei with smudged chromatin (Fig. 3) [3, 17–21].

Cytologic Features
- Rich yield as a rule
- Mixture of clustered cells and dispersed cells
- High nuclear:cytoplasmic ratio
- Stripped nuclei and a cytoplasmic "tigroid" background is common (best appreciated in air-dried smears)
- Double cell population: large, "light" cells with a fragile cytoplasm containing vacuoles and round to oval bland nuclei with inconspicuous nucleoli; small, dark cells with rounded irregular nuclei and scant/poorly preserved cytoplasm
- The dark cells are often arranged in small molded groups within the cell clusters
- Occasional moderately cellular and nuclear pleomorphism
- Occasional presence of cells with thin cytoplasmic processes
- Rosette-like structures with more or less evident fibrillary centers

Ancillary Tests
Immunophenotype
Strong, diffuse, and membranous positivity for CD99; positive for FLI-1 (nuclear); in about 30% of cases focal expression of keratin, S100, and CD117. Negative for SMA, desmin, MyoD1, myogenin, WT1, CD45, TdT, CD56, and TLE1.

Histochemistry
Periodic acid-Schiff-positive intracytoplasmic glycogen.

Genetics
The most common mutation in Ewing sarcoma is the translocation t(11;22)(q24;q12), which fuses the *EWSR1* gene on chromosome 22 and the *FLI1* gene on chromosome 11. It is present in 85% of cases [22]. The resulting fusion protein has an oncogenic effect as an aberrant transcription factor leading to uncontrolled growth and proliferation [23]. Other translocations fusing the *EWSR1* gene with other *FLI1*-related genes exist but are less common [24]. These genetic changes are useful diagnostic traits that can be detected with cytogenetics, FISH, PCR, and NGS on available material [3, 17, 18, 25–28].

Differential Diagnosis
- Alveolar rhabdomyosarcoma
- Neuroblastoma
- Precursor lymphoma/acute lymphoblastic leukemia
- Poorly differentiated synovial sarcoma
- Desmoplastic small round cell tumor

Cells of Ewing sarcoma lack the eosinophil cytoplasm and rhabdoid features of rhabdomyosarcoma. Compared to Ewing sarcoma, a subset of neuroblastoma cells in FNA smears often show uni- or bipolar slender cytoplasmic processes. In addition, smears of Ewing sarcoma lack a neuropil of neuroblastomas. Molecular genetic examinations as well as immunocytochemistry should be a part of the FNA cytology examination of small blue round cell tumors. However, it should be remembered that rearrangements of the *EWS* gene also occur in desmoplastic small round cell tumor, clear cell sarcoma, and myxoid liposarcoma. The 2 latter tumors are not differential diagnostic problems as their cytology is obviously different from that of Ewing sarcoma. Desmoplastic small round cell tumor may be a diagnostic pitfall in FNA of abdominal and retroperitoneal tumors, especially when the yield is poor and the typical double cell population is absent. In such cases, FISH examination should be supplemented by immunocytochemistry in the differential diagnosis between Ewing sarcoma and desmoplastic small round cell tumor.

References

1 Cole CD, Wu HH: Fine-needle aspiration in pediatric patients 12 years of age and younger: a 20-year retrospective study from a single tertiary medical center. Diagn Cytopathol 2014;42:600–605.
2 Klijanienko J, Couturier J, Brisse H, Pierron G, Freneaux P, Berger F, Maciorowski Z, Sastre-Garau X, Michon J, Schleiermacher G: Diagnostic and prognostic information obtained on fine-needle aspirates of primary neuroblastic tumors: proposal for a cytology prognostic score. Cancer Cytopathol 2011;119:411–423.
3 Pohar-Marinsek Z: Difficulties in diagnosing small round cell tumours of childhood from fine needle aspiration cytology samples. Cytopathology 2008;19:67–79.

4 Frostad B, Tani E, Kogner P, Maeda S, Bjork O, Skoog L: The clinical use of fine needle aspiration cytology for diagnosis and management of children with neuroblastic tumours. Eur J Cancer 1998;34:529–536.

5 Cheung NK, Dyer MA: Neuroblastoma: developmental biology, cancer genomics and immunotherapy. Nat Rev Cancer 2013;13:397–411.

6 Mandelia A, Agarwala S, Sharma A, Iyer VK, Bhatnagar V: Assessment of fine needle aspiration cytology samples for molecular genetic analysis in neuroblastoma. Pediatr Surg Int 2013;29:1131–1138.

7 Bhadarge PS, Poflee SV: Aspiration cytology in the preoperative diagnosis of ganglioneuroma presenting as a neck mass. J Cytol 2014;31:57–58.

8 Kolte SS: Ganglioneuroma presenting as a neck mass diagnosed by fine needle aspiration cytology. Cytopathology 2011;22:205–206.

9 Dim DC, Nugent SL, Peng HQ: Ganglioneuroma presenting as a paraesophageal mass lesion diagnosed by endoscopic ultrasound-guided fine needle aspiration cytology: a case report. Acta Cytol 2010;54:321–324.

10 Catalina-Fernandez I, Saenz-Santamaria J, Lopez-Presa D: Fine needle aspiration cytology of ganglioneuroma. Acta Cytol 2008;52:380–381.

11 Domanski HA: Fine-needle aspiration of ganglioneuroma. Diagn Cytopathol 2005;32:363–366.

12 Rodriguez-Parets JO, Abad M, Garcia MC, Bullon A: Pelvic ganglioneuroma: cytological findings by fine needle aspiration. Cytopathology 2000;11:133–134.

13 Jain M, Shubha BS, Sethi S, Banga V, Bagga D: Retroperitoneal ganglioneuroma: report of a case diagnosed by fine-needle aspiration cytology, with review of the literature. Diagn Cytopathol 1999;21:194–196.

14 Yen H, Cobb CJ: Retroperitoneal ganglioneuroma: a report of diagnosis by fine-needle aspiration cytology. Diagn Cytopathol 1998;19:385–387.

15 Shawa H, Elsayes KM, Javadi S, Morani A, Williams MD, Lee JE, Waguespack SG, Busaidy NL, Vassilopoulou-Sellin R, Jimenez C, Habra MA: Adrenal ganglioneuroma: features and outcomes of 27 cases at a referral cancer centre. Clin Endocrinol 2014;80:342–347.

16 Lora MS, Waguespack SG, Moley JF, Walvoord EC: Adrenal ganglioneuromas in children with multiple endocrine neoplasia type 2: a report of two cases. J Clin Endocrinol Metab 2005;90:4383–4387.

17 Kumar R, Gautam U, Srinivasan R, Lal A, Sharma U, Nijhawan R, Kumar S: Primary Ewing's sarcoma/primitive neuroectodermal tumor of the kidney: report of a case diagnosed by fine needle aspiration cytology and confirmed by immunocytochemistry and RT-PCR along with review of literature. Diagn Cytopathol 2012;40(suppl 2):E156–E161.

18 Klijanienko J, Couturier J, Bourdeaut F, Freneaux P, Ballet S, Brisse H, Lagace R, Delattre O, Pierron G, Vielh P, Sastre-Garau X, Michon J: Fine-needle aspiration as a diagnostic technique in 50 cases of primary Ewing sarcoma/peripheral neuroectodermal tumor. Institute Curie's experience. Diagn Cytopathol 2012;40:19–25.

19 Kalra S, Gupta R, Singh S, Gupta K, Kudesia M: Primary cutaneous Ewing's sarcoma/primitive neuroectodermal tumor: report of the first case diagnosed on aspiration cytology. Acta Cytol 2010;54:193–196.

20 Geramizadeh B, Makarempour A, Foroughi AA: Fine needle aspiration of a breast mass caused by metastatic Ewing's sarcoma. Acta Cytol 2010;54:237–239.

21 Gautam U, Srinivasan R, Rajwanshi A, Bansal D, Marwaha RK: Comparative evaluation of flow-cytometric immunophenotyping and immunocytochemistry in the categorization of malignant small round cell tumors in fine-needle aspiration cytologic specimens. Cancer 2008;114:494–503.

22 Turc-Carel C, Aurias A, Mugneret F, Lizard S, Sidaner I, Volk C, Thiery JP, Olschwang S, Philip I, Berger MP, et al: Chromosomes in Ewing's sarcoma. I. An evaluation of 85 cases of remarkable consistency of t(11;22)(q24;q12). Cancer Genet Cytogenet 1988;32:229–238.

23 Smith R, Owen LA, Trem DJ, Wong JS, Whangbo JS, Golub TR, Lessnick SL: Expression profiling of EWS/FLI identifies *NKX2.2* as a critical target gene in Ewing's sarcoma. Cancer Cell 2006;9:405–416.

24 Patocs B, Nemeth K, Garami M, Arato G, Kovalszky I, Szendroi M, Fekete G: Multiple splice variants of *EWSR1-ETS* fusion transcripts co-existing in the Ewing sarcoma family of tumors. Cell Oncol 2013;36:191–200.

25 Gautam U, Srinivasan R, Rajwanshi A, Bansal D, Marwaha RK, Vasishtha RK: Reverse transcriptase-polymerase chain reaction as an ancillary molecular technique in the diagnosis of small blue round cell tumors by fine-needle aspiration cytology. Am J Clin Pathol 2010;133:633–645.

26 Kang SH, Perle MA, Nonaka D, Zhu H, Chan W, Yang GC: Primary Ewing sarcoma/PNET of the kidney: fine-needle aspiration, histology, and dual color break apart FISH Assay. Diagn Cytopathol 2007;35:353–357.

27 Sanati S, Lu DW, Schmidt E, Perry A, Dehner LP, Pfeifer JD: Cytologic diagnosis of Ewing sarcoma/peripheral neuroectodermal tumor with paired prospective molecular genetic analysis. Cancer 2007;111:192–199.

28 Jambhekar NA, Bagwan IN, Ghule P, Shet TM, Chinoy RF, Agarwal S, Joshi R, Amare Kadam PS: Comparative analysis of routine histology, immunohistochemistry, reverse transcriptase polymerase chain reaction, and fluorescence in situ hybridization in diagnosis of Ewing family of tumors. Arch Pathol Lab Med 2006;130:1813–1818.

Domanski HA, Walther CS: FNA Cytology of Soft Tissue and Bone Tumors. Monogr Clin Cytol.
Basel, Karger, 2017, vol 22, pp 132–138 (DOI: 10.1159/000475105)

Principles in the Examination and Management of Bone Neoplasms; Normal Elements and the Cytologic Features of Reactive Changes in the Bone

Primary bone tumors are relatively uncommon. Osteosarcoma is the most frequent primary bone sarcoma, followed by chondrosarcoma, Ewing sarcoma, and chordoma. Among benign bone neoplasms, the most common are osteochondroma, giant cell tumor, chondroma, osteoid osteoma, and metaphyseal fibrous defect.

Regarding the distribution of malignant and benign bone tumors respectively by histologic type and by age of patient, it is obvious that the majority of benign bone tumors, osteosarcoma, and Ewing sarcoma, arise in children and young adults, while chondrosarcoma and chordoma occur most frequently in the elderly. Generally, skeletal sarcomas have a bimodal age distribution, with the highest risk of development during the second decade of life and the second peak of incidence after the age of 60 years.

Patients with bone tumors usually have some symptoms that bring them to a medical consultation. These include pain, a palpable tumor mass, pathologic fracture, or reduced function of a joint or extremity. In addition, many benign and some malignant bone lesions may be discovered as incidental findings.

Fine-needle aspiration cytology (FNAC) has been used for many years in the diagnosis of skeletal lesions, after Coley and Ellis applied this sampling method as early as 1931 [1]. To date, several large series of cases have been published [2–16]. FNAC can be relatively easily applied to selected groups of neoplasm, such as metastatic deposition to the bone or to confirm the recurrence of a bone sarcoma. FNAC may also be used as the first-line approach or as a complementary tool to core-needle biopsy in the diagnosis of a primary bone neoplasm [3, 17–20]. In addition to FNA, methods for percutaneous sampling, such as core-needle biopsy and drill biopsy have, in recent years, emerged as an important diagnostic substitute for open biopsy.

Different imaging modalities, such as plain radiography, ultrasonography, computed tomography (CT), magnetic resonance imaging, scintigraphy, and positron emission tomography, all play important roles in the evaluation of bone lesions. FNA of nonpalpable bone lesions can be guided by radiologic findings. In cases of obvious bone destruction, the needling can be performed under fluoroscopic guidance. CT-guided aspiration biopsy should be the method of choice for deep lesions. Radiographic examinations give abundant diagnostic information and comprise the necessary modality in the evaluation of bone lesions. The most important task for the radiologist is to evaluate the extent of the tumor rather than the tissue diagnosis. In many cases of benign bone lesions, radiography may be diagnostic, obviating the need for any biopsy. In the majority of benign and malignant bone neoplasms, radiography may exclude or establish malignancy and limits the diagnostic options to 1 diagnosis or a few differential diagnoses. Morphologic examinations, however, are considered to be a necessary part of the diagnostic work-up of malignant and many benign bone neoplasms since therapeutic regiments differ significantly for both malignant and benign/locally aggressive neoplasms. The microscopic diagnosis should confirm the radiologic findings and, in cases of discordance between radiologic imaging and cytologic/histologic diagnosis, the findings must be reevaluated. In this aspect, cooperation between the radiologist and pathologist/cytopathologist is mandatory.

Similar to FNAC of soft tissue lesions, the best approach to a successful diagnostic evaluation of a bone neoplasm is to combine clinical data and imaging with the morphologic interpretation of cells and tissue, complemented by ancillary techniques. The various examination methods and clinical information used to define bone lesions supplement each other.

For example, the position of a tumor in the long bones is an important diagnostic sign. The metaphysis is the most common site for primary bone tumors. This is likely due to the fast turnover of growing cells adjacent to the growth plate. Osteosarcoma typically arises in the metaphyseal region. Benign cysts, which are well demarcated and show a geographic growth pattern, are usually located centrally in the metaphysis. Giant cell tumors are located eccentrically in the metaphysis-epiphysis, often grow close to the subchondral area of a joint (most often around the knee), and display a geographic growth pattern. A diaphyseal location is very common in Ewing sarcoma. Tumor growth in the epiphysis is rare, and the most common type of lesion in the epiphysis is chondroblastoma. Intracortical tumors most often represent metastatic depositions. Destructive lesions of the sacrum may be extensive, with a soft tissue component ventrally as well as dorsally. The suggested diagnosis is chordoma, but the same clinical presentation and radiologic appearance may be seen in giant cell tumors or metastases in the sacrum. In such cases, the patient's age is of importance. In a 60-year-old male, the most likely diagnosis is metastasis or chordoma, while in a 20-year-old female the most probable diagnosis is a giant cell tumor. Although all patients with a suspicion of skeletal lesion do not need to be referred to large medical centers, it is recommended that patients with a suspected primary skeletal neoplasm should be referred to multidisciplinary centers with access to expertise in orthopedic surgery and musculoskeletal oncology, allowing adequate evaluation and therapy, as well as the follow-up of patients with a bone neoplasm.

Biopsy Techniques: Image-Guided Fine-Needle Aspiration of Bone Lesions

An appropriate biopsy technique is critical in the evaluation and treatment of a bone neoplasm. Open biopsy and histopathologic assessment of tissue samples has for many years been considered the "golden standard" in the diagnosis of bone tumors/lesions. However, open biopsy has a number of disadvantages. The patient must be hospitalized and general anesthesia is required. The open biopsy may break compartments and there is a risk for hematoma and infection. Mankin et al. [21] discussed the hazards of core-needle biopsy and open biopsy in patients with primary malignant bone neoplasm where major errors in biopsy diagnosis occurred in 15% of cases, and in an additional 10% of biopsies nonrepresentative or technically poor specimens were obtained.

As a result of destructive growth and soft tissue extensions, primary malignant and locally aggressive bone neoplasms are suitable for FNA. Destroyed cortical bone can be easily penetrated by a thin needle. The equipment used for FNA of bone lesions is the same as for needling other sites. A syringe holder permitting aspiration with 1 hand is essential, and a 22-G (0.7 mm) needle is sufficient in most cases. The length of the needle depends on the location of the lesion. Needles with a stylet are recommended for deep-seated lesions. The stylet strengthens the needle and prevents the aspiration of cells from surrounding tissues. Percutaneous puncture of palpable lesions can be performed in outpatient clinics with or without local anesthesia and without radiologic guidance. Image-guided FNA is necessary for the examination of nonpalpable deep and intraosseous lesions, as well as lesions with areas of different tissue characteristics, such as tumor matrix calcifications, and necrosis versus viable tumor. In addition, image guidance of bone FNA is preferred in the majority of cases examined for a more exact needle placement.

As an intact cortical bone can be difficult or impossible to penetrate with thin needles, when the cortex of the bone is intact, trocar with a drill is necessary in most cases to penetrate the cortical bone. Biopsy instruments for penetrating cortical bone exist, such as the coaxial biopsy system with an eccentric drill invented by Ahlström and Ångström [22]. There are several other alternatives on the market using a cannula with a trocar or a drill. After cortical penetration, FNA samples can be taken from the target lesion using a coaxial technique supporting the use of a single needle-insertion point, even when performing several punctures (Fig. 1a, b). In cases of operative treatment of bone malignancies, subsequent surgical removal of the needle tract can be facilitated by tattooing the site of needle insertion so that it can be identified later.

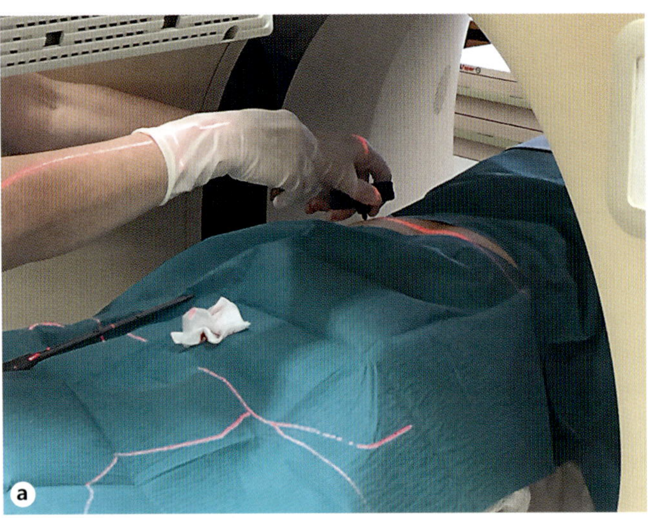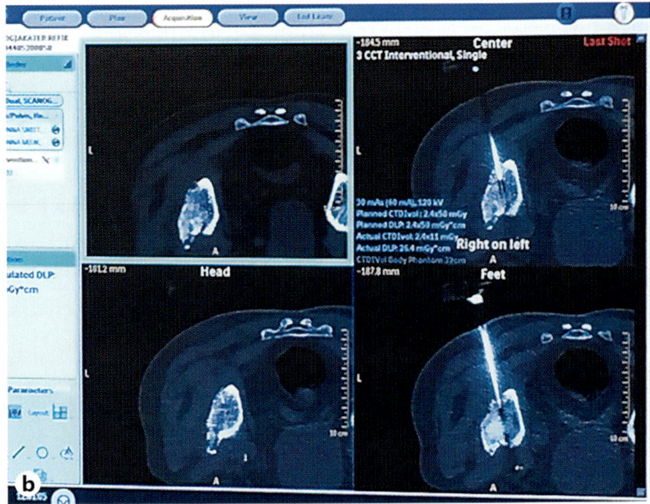

Fig. 1. a Recurrence of non-Hodgkin lymphoma in the pelvic skeleton. The lesion was biopsied through a trocar guided by the CT scanner. **b** Control of the trocar position at the CT screen before performing FNA and core biopsy of the lesion.

Table 1. FNAC of bone tumors: diagnostic accuracy and sufficiency summarized from 8 series comprising 2,152 patients

Study	Publication year	Cases, *n*	Insufficient yield, %	Diagnostic accuracy, %
Kreicbergs et al. [12]	1996	300	8	95
Bommer et al. [10]	1997	450	14	98
Åkerman et al. [24]	1998	333	6	98
Jorda et al. [8]	2000	314	31	95
Agarwal et al. [9]	2000	226	–	83
Wedin et al. [6]	2000	110	8	93
Kilpatrick et al. [5]	2001	49	8	93
Söderlund et al. [14]	2004	370	3	95 (99 with radiologic correlation)

Reporting the Diagnosis

A standardized reporting of bone FNA has been suggested by Åkerman and Domanski [23]:

- Sarcoma (histologic type of sarcoma or sarcoma not otherwise specified)
- Benign tumor (histologic type or benign tumor not otherwise specified)
- Metastasis (suggestion of primary or descriptive diagnosis)
- Lymphohematologic malignancy (exact subtype or general classification)
- Nonneoplastic lesion (infectious, reactive)
- Nondiagnostic (including insufficient)

Advances and Limitations of Fine-Needle Aspiration Cytology in the Diagnosis of Bone Neoplasm

Advances and limitations of FNAC in the diagnosis of bone lesions are basically the same as in the cytologic examinations of soft tissue neoplasms (see Chapter 1 of this volume).

Diagnostic Accuracy, Pitfalls, and Complications

It is essential to point out that there is a relatively limited group of primary bone neoplasms and nonneoplastic conditions that are frequent targets of FNAC examination, and there are well-established diagnostic cytologic criteria in several published series and case reports. These neoplasms can be diagnosed by FNAC in the appropriate clinical and radiologic setting. Some benign and uncommon malignant bone neoplasms are very rarely examined by FNA and only single small series and case reports describing cytologic features of those lesions exist. The reported diagnostic accuracy of bone FNA has varied depending on the era of the study, whether or not using radiology-cytology correlation and reporting terminology used at different centers. Earlier studies reported a lower diagnostic accuracy, while accuracies of up to 98% have been reported in later studies. The results of 8 large series comprising a total of 2,152 patients are summarized in Table 1. In these series, the diagnostic accuracy regarding benign versus malignant was between 83 and 98%, and the rate of insufficient material for diagnosis was variable, ranging from 3 to 31% in 7 studies.

In our experience the common limitations of FNA diagnosis of bone tumors are:

- Inability to aspirate sufficient material for evaluation. Cytologic specimens are often limited when sampled from intramedullary and sclerotic lesions and sclerotic lesions with significant ossifications. Cystic lesions such as simple bone cysts and aneurysmal bone cysts often yield insufficient material.

- Sampling error when aspirating large, heterogeneous tumors, and the aspirated material may not correspond to the diagnostic tumor tissue. An example of this pitfall is the aspiration of giant cell-rich osteosarcoma when the smears lack pleomorphic tumor cells and osteoid, and are dominated by benign osteoclast, giving the false impression of giant cell tumor.

- Extensive necrosis and/or hemorrhage are limiting factors leading to suboptimal material.

- Misinterpretation of the optimal cytologic material. Well-known difficulties include distinguishing benign cartilaginous tumors from well-differentiated chondrosarcoma, and reactive osteoblastic proliferation from osteoblastic neoplasm. Radiologic and clinical correlations are always required.

Severe complications of skeletal FNA that have been documented in single cases include pneumothorax following the needling of lesions in the ribs, and neurologic sequelae to the needling of lesions in the vertebrae.

In more than 40 years of experience of FNA in the diagnosis of bone tumors/lesions in patients referred to the Sarcome Center in Lund, we have never experienced any severe complications. Patients have, at most, complained of brief pain at needling, but we have never seen complications caused by FNA such as infection, neurologic sequelae, or tumor cell seeding in the needle track.

Specimen Preparation and Ancillary Techniques

Regarding the preparation of an FNA specimen for microscopic examinations and for ancillary techniques, the same principles apply for bone aspirates as for FNA specimens of soft tissue lesions (see Chapter 2 of this volume). Essentially, the same ancillary studies applied to tissue samples are applicable on fine-needle aspirates. The current ancillary methods commonly used in the examination of bone lesions are cytochemistry, immunocytochemistry, cytogenetic and molecular genetic examinations, flow cytometry in lymphohematologic lesions, and to some extent electron microscopic examination. Immunocytochemistry and molecular genetic analyses are the most valuable ancillary techniques to facilitate the specific diagnosis in the FNA of bone neoplasms. These techniques are essential in the cytologic evaluation of small round cell neoplasms and indispensable to suggesting the site of origin in the workup of bone metastasis. With regard to cytochemistry, alkaline phosphatase staining is very useful in the demonstration of osteoblastic differentiation of tumor cells in aspirates from osteosarcoma, as tumor cells from all subtypes of osteosarcoma contain abundant cytoplasmic alkaline phosphatase [24].

During recent years, cytogenetic and molecular genetic investigations have emerged as very powerful diagnostic tools in the diagnosis of soft tissue sarcoma. Genetic changes identified within specific tumor types can provide additional diagnostic, prognostic, and therapeutic information. With regard to bone neoplasms, the main use of these techniques is in the diagnosis of Ewing sarcoma/primitive neuroectodermal tumor. In our experience and that of others, performing conventional karyotyping is less suitable on fine-needle aspirates because the number of tumor cells obtained is often insufficient for tissue culture. Fine-needle aspirates have proven to be very suitable for molecular genetic investigations such as reverse polymerase chain reaction and fluorescence in situ hybridization. Electron microscopic examinations are most useful in the diagnosis of Langerhans cell histiocytosis (Birbeck granule) and selected cases of osteosarcoma (osteoid).

Normal Elements and the Cytologic Features of Reactive Changes in Bone

The normal cells that may be present in bone aspirates are osteoblasts, osteoclasts, chondrocytes, bone marrow cells, and mesothelial cells.

Osteoblasts

Osteoblasts appear in smears as small sheets and single uniform rounded to oval or triangular cells with an abundant

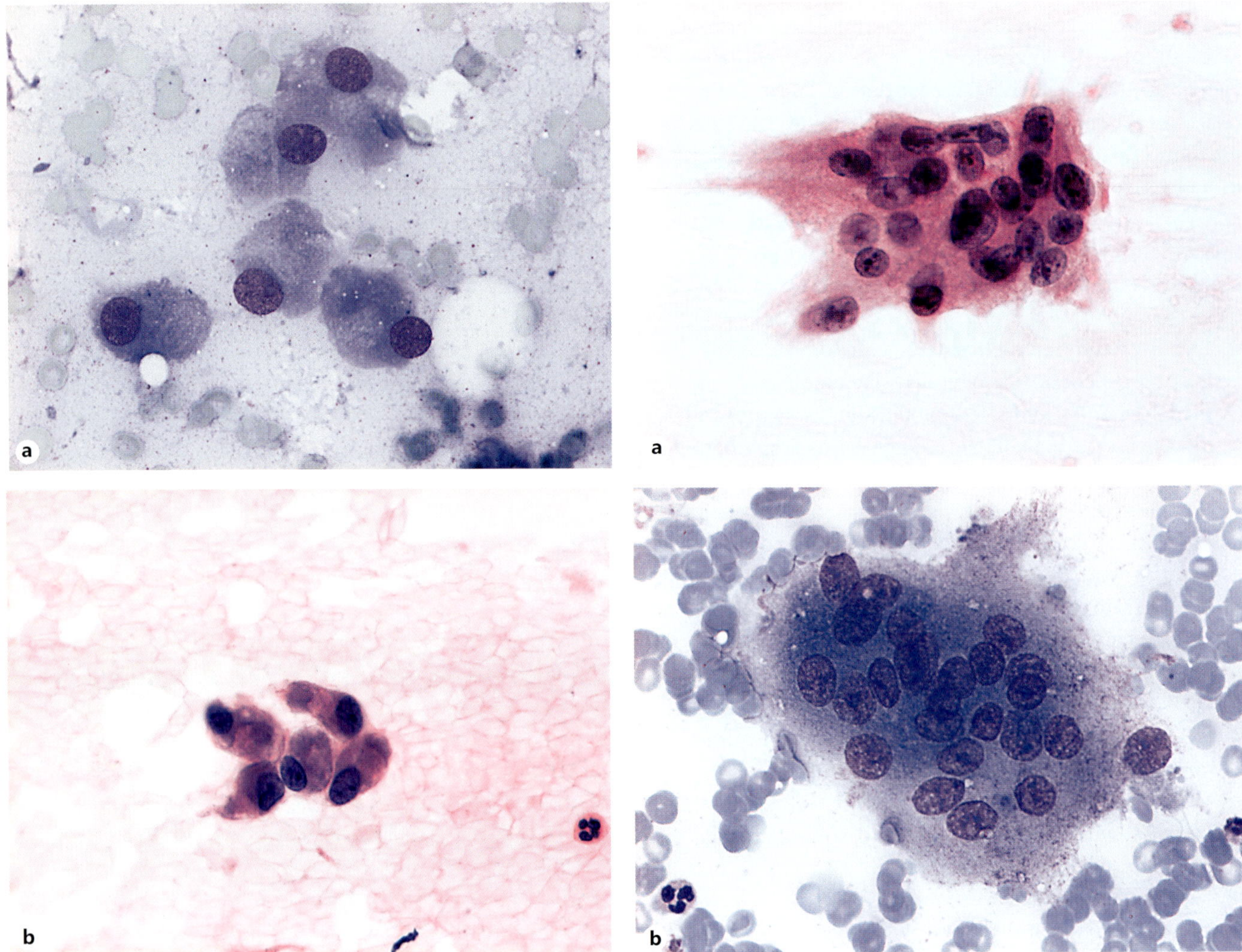

Fig. 2. a, **b** Osteoblasts. Triangular or rounded to oval cells with eccentric nuclei, an abundant cytoplasm, and perinuclear clear "Hof" visible in most cells. MGG and HE stains.

Fig. 3. a Osteoclasts. Large cells with an abundant cytoplasm, 12–20 uniform, round to oval nuclei. HE stain. **b** Fine red granulation is often visible in air-dried and DiffQuick or MGG-stained smears.

cytoplasm, typically containing a clear area or "Hof" adjacent to the nucleus. The nuclei are rounded with central nucleoli and are characteristically eccentrically situated close to the cytoplasmic membrane, almost protruding through it (Fig. 2a, b).

Osteoclasts

Osteoclasts always appear as single large cells with an abundant cytoplasm and multiple, uniform rounded nuclei with small nucleoli. A fine red cytoplasmic granulation is seen in air-dried smears stained with May-Grünwald-Giemsa (MGG) or DiffQuick stain (Fig. 3a, b).

Cartilage and Chondrocytes

Fragments of cartilage and normal chondrocytes are sometimes seen in bone aspirates from lesions near joints and costochondral junctions. However, chondrocytes are a rare finding in FNA smears of normal cartilage. Cartilaginous tissue fragments represent hyaline cartilage, which stains blue or reddish-blue to violet with DiffQuick and MGG stains, and pink or pinkish-violet with hematoxylin and eosin (HE) stain (Fig. 4a, b). The cartilage appears fibrillary and greyish-red in Papanicolaou-stained smears. Chondrocytes have a poorly demarcated cytoplasm and small rounded nuclei, and are usually visible in lacunae within cartilaginous fragments. The texture of chondrocytes is best seen in wet-fixed smears (Fig. 4c).

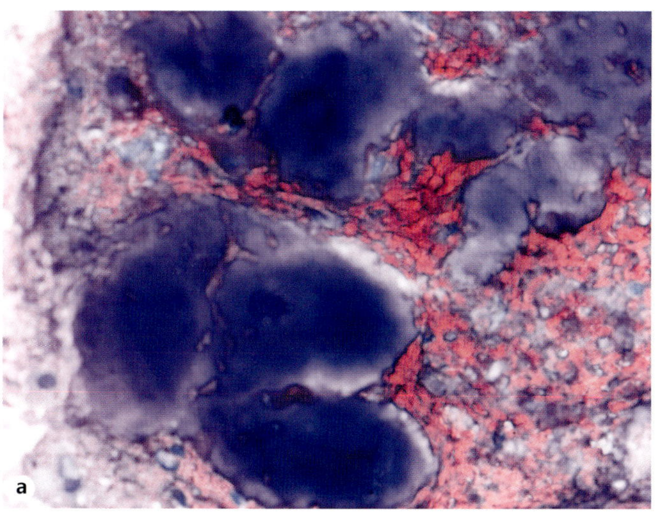
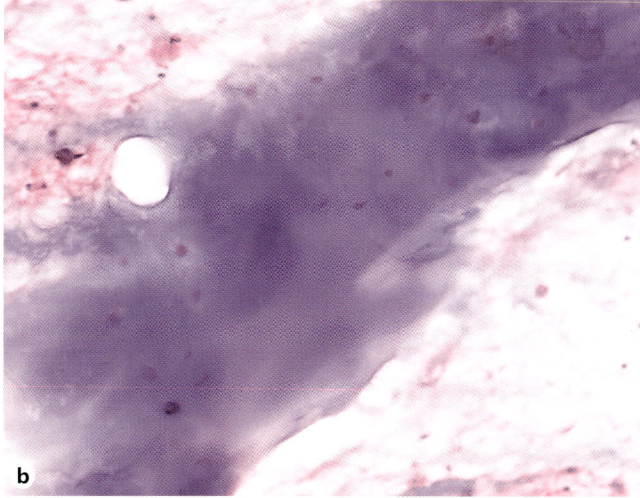
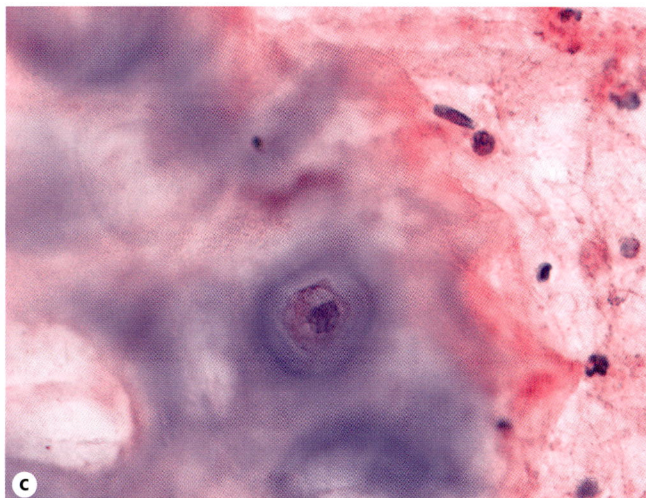

Fig. 4. FNA smears of normal cartilage. Fragments of hyaline cartilage stain blue or reddish-blue to violet with DiffQuick and MGG stain (**a**) and pink or pinkish-violet with HE stain (**b**). **c** Chondrocytes are a rare finding in FNA smears of normal cartilage and are usually visible in lacunae within cartilaginous fragments. HE stain.

Bone Marrow Cells

Bone marrow cells are not an uncommon finding in aspirates from ribs, vertebrae, and the sacrum. There is most commonly a mixture of erythropoietic and myelopoietic cells, and an admixture of megakaryocytes. It is important not to misinterpret scattered megakaryocytes as malignant cells (Fig. 5).

Mesothelial Cells

Sheets of mesothelial cells are occasionally found in the smears when vertebral lesions are needled and the needle misses the target and penetrates through the vertebra. It is important not to misdiagnose reactive mesothelial cells as well-differentiated adenocarcinoma.

Reactive Changes

Reactive changed osteoblasts are usually a component of FNA smears from fracture callus, myositis ossificans, and proliferative periosteitis. The reactive osteoblasts resemble their normal counterparts and have eccentric nuclei and a cytoplasmic "Hof," but their size is variable and anisokaryosis with occasional prominent nucleoli are common findings (Fig. 6).

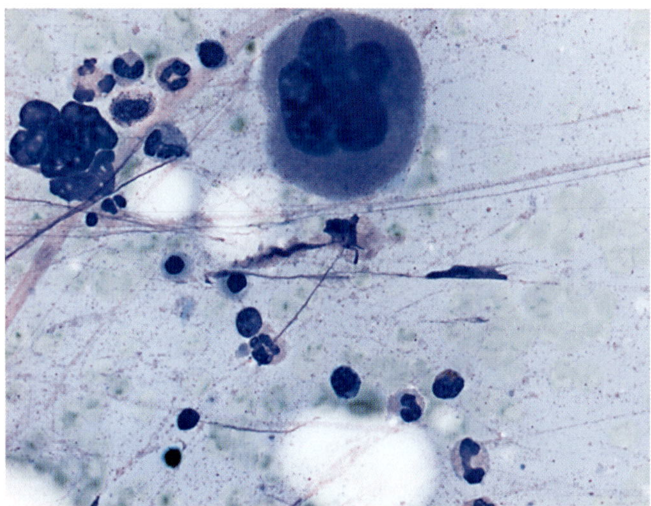 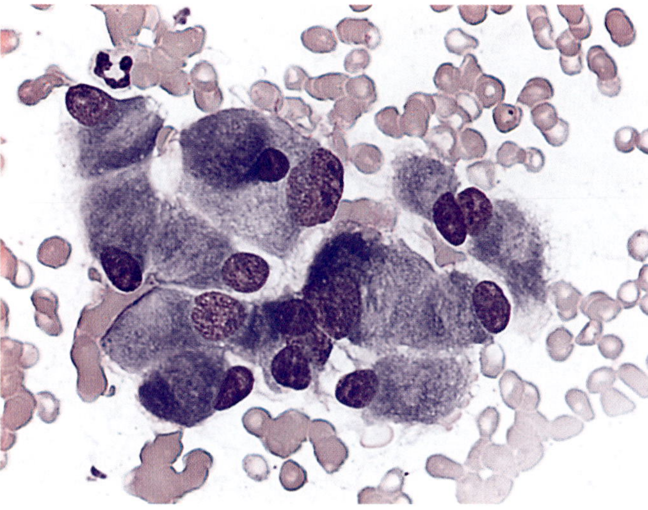

Fig. 5. Bone marrow cells. Erythropoietic cells, myelopoietic cells, and megakaryocytes occasionally appear in FNA smears from skeletal lesions. MGG stain.

Fig. 6. Myositis ossificans. Clusters of reactive osteoblasts with anisokaryosis and somewhat hyperchromatic nuclei. MGG stain.

References

1 Martin HE, Ellis EB: Biopsy by needle puncture and aspiration. Ann Surg 1930;92:169–181.
2 Layfield LJ, Schmidt RL, Sangle N, Crim JR: Diagnostic accuracy and clinical utility of biopsy in musculoskeletal lesions: a comparison of fine-needle aspiration, core, and open biopsy techniques. Diagn Cytopathol 2014;42:476–486.
3 Khalbuss WE, Teot LA, Monaco SE: Diagnostic accuracy and limitations of fine-needle aspiration cytology of bone and soft tissue lesions: a review of 1,114 cases with cytological-histological correlation. Cancer Cytopathol 2010;118:24–32.
4 Nnodu OE, Giwa SO, Eyesan SU, Abdulkareem FB: Fine needle aspiration cytology of bone tumours – the experience from the National Orthopaedic and Lagos University Teaching Hospitals, Lagos, Nigeria. Cytojournal 2006;3:16.
5 Kilpatrick SE, Cappellari JO, Bos GD, Gold SH, Ward WG: Is fine-needle aspiration biopsy a practical alternative to open biopsy for the primary diagnosis of sarcoma? Experience with 140 patients. Am J Clin Pathol 2001;115:59–68.
6 Wedin R, Bauer HC, Skoog L, Soderlund V, Tani E: Cytological diagnosis of skeletal lesions: fine-needle aspiration biopsy in 110 tumours. J Bone Joint Surg Br 2000;82:673–678.
7 Ward WG Sr, Kilpatrick S: Fine needle aspiration biopsy of primary bone tumors. Clin Orthop Relat Res 2000;373:80–87.
8 Jorda M, Rey L, Hanly A, Ganjei-Azar P: Fine-needle aspiration cytology of bone: accuracy and pitfalls of cytodiagnosis. Cancer 2000;90:47–54.
9 Agarwal S, Agarwal T, Agarwal R, Agarwal PK, Jain UK: Fine needle aspiration of bone tumors. Cancer Detect Prev 2000;24:602–609.
10 Bommer KK, Ramzy I, Mody D: Fine-needle aspiration biopsy in the diagnosis and management of bone lesions: a study of 450 cases. Cancer 1997;81:148–156.
11 Agarwal PK, Goel MM, Chandra T, Agarwal S: Predictive value of fine needle aspiration cytology of bone lesions. Acta Cytol 1997;41:659–665.
12 Kreicbergs A, Bauer HC, Brosjo O, Lindholm J, Skoog L, Soderlund V: Cytological diagnosis of bone tumours. J Bone Joint Surg Br 1996;78:258–263.
13 Willén H: Fine needle aspiration in the diagnosis of bone tumors. Acta Orthop Scand Suppl 1997;273:47–53.
14 Söderlund V, Skoog L, Kreicbergs A: Combined radiology and cytology in the diagnosis of bone lesions: a retrospective study of 370 cases. Acta Orthop Scand 2004;75:492–499.
15 Åkerman M, Berg NO, Persson BM: Fine needle aspiration biopsy in the evaluation of tumor-like lesions of bone. Acta Orthop Scand 1976;47:129–136.
16 Stormby N, Åkerman M: Cytodiagnosis of bone lesions by means of fine-needle aspiration biopsy. Acta Cytol 1973;17:166–172.
17 Cardona DM, Dodd LG: Bone cytology: a realistic approach for clinical use. Surg Pathol Clin 2012;5:79–100.
18 Santini-Araujo E, Olvi LG, Muscolo DL, Velan O, Gonzalez ML, Cabrini RL: Technical aspects of core needle biopsy and fine needle aspiration in the diagnosis of bone lesions. Acta Cytol 2011;55:100–105.
19 Layfield LJ: Cytologic diagnosis of osseous lesions: a review with emphasis on the diagnosis of primary neoplasms of bone. Diagn Cytopathol 2009;37:299–310.
20 Wahane RN, Lele VR, Bobhate SK: Fine needle aspiration cytology of bone tumors. Acta Cytol 2007;51:711–720.
21 Mankin HJ, Mankin CJ, Simon MA: The hazards of the biopsy, revisited. J Bone Joint Surg Am 1996;78:656–663.
22 Aström KG, Sundström JC, Lindgren PG, Ahlström KH: Automatic biopsy instruments used through a coaxial bone biopsy system with an eccentric drill tip. Acta Radiol 1995;36:237–242.
23 Åkerman M, Domanski HA: The cytology of soft tissue tumours. Monogr Clin Cytol 2003;16:1–112.
24 Åkerman M, Domanski HA: Fine needle aspiration (FNA) of bone tumours: with special emphasis on definitive treatment of primary malignant bone tumours based on FNA. Curr Diagn Pathol 1998;5:82–92.

Domanski HA, Walther CS: FNA Cytology of Soft Tissue and Bone Tumors. Monogr Clin Cytol.
Basel, Karger, 2017, vol 22, pp 139–146 (DOI: 10.1159/000475106)

Osteogenic Tumors

Osteoid Osteoma and Osteoblastoma

Osteoid osteoma and osteoblastoma are benign osteoblastic tumors with overlapping radiographic and microscopic features. Osteoid osteoma most often arises in the cortex of diaphyseal and metaphyseal regions of long tubular bones, commonly in the femur and the posterior part of vertebrae. Osteoid osteoma has distinctive clinical features and because of the reactive, sclerotic bone surrounding the osteoma nidus, the lesion is not suitable for fine-needle aspiration (FNA) and almost never referred for FNA cytology.

Osteoblastoma is a benign bone-forming tumor morphologically similar to osteoid osteoma but larger than 2 cm per definition. This rare bone neoplasm accounts for less than 1% of all bone tumors and is more common in males than females (2.5:1). Most occur in children and young adults, and the majority of patients are between 10 and 30 years of age. Predilection sites are the spine and sacrum (approximately 50% of cases). Of other sites, the proximal and distal femur and proximal tibia are most frequently involved. The vast majority of osteoblastomas are intraosseous tumors that are very rarely examined by FNA cytology.

Cytologic Features of Osteoblastoma
- Sparse to moderate cellularity
- Single cells or small clusters of osteoblast-like cells
- Mono- and binucleated cells with eccentric, bland, round to oval nuclei
- A clear cytoplasmic "Hof" present in many cells
- Large osteoclast-like multinucleated giant cells
- Small clusters or groups of spindle cells

Ancillary Tests
Immunocytochemical and genetic/molecular examinations do not support a radiologic and microscopic diagnosis.

Genetics
Too few cases of these tumors have been genetically evaluated to provide useful diagnostic information.

Differential Diagnosis
- Osteosarcoma

Only few cases of FNA cytology of osteoblastoma have been reported to date [1–5], and our experience is limited to single cases [5]. We consider, however, that an overall benign pattern of smears of conventional osteoblastomas, including bland osteoblasts (Fig. 1a–c), helps to establish a benign diagnosis. Cytologic criteria have not been defined for the diagnosis of aggressive (epithelioid) osteoblastoma. A primary bone tumor displaying large, atypical osteoblasts with prominent nucleoli should be diagnosed as inconclusive as to whether it is benign or malignant, irrespective of the radiologic features. In such cases, a core biopsy or open biopsy should be a necessary part of the diagnostic workup.

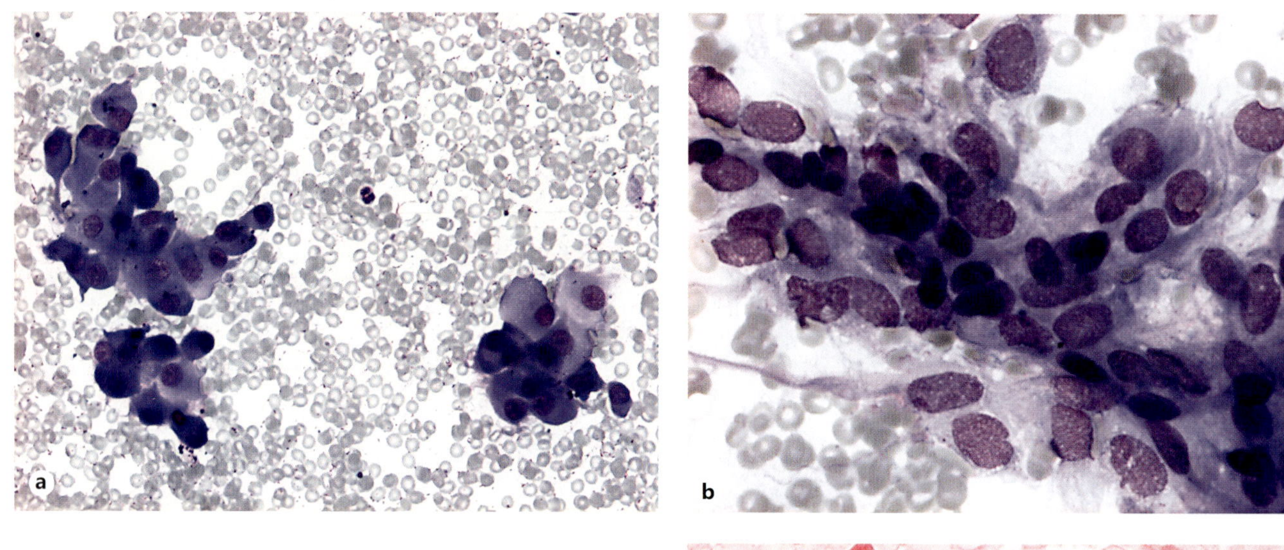

Fig. 1. Osteoblastoma. **a** Small sheets of uniform osteoblasts with eccentric nuclei and an abundant cytoplasm. MGG stain. **b** A loosely cohesive cluster of bland round to oval cells with mild anisokaryosis. MGG stain. **c** A loosely cohesive sheet of osteoblasts and a multinucleated osteoclastic giant cell. HE stain.

Fig. 2. High-grade osteoblastic osteosarcoma. **a** Cellular smears composed of tight clusters and dispersed epithelioid, polygonal, and spindle-shaped pleomorphic tumor cells. MGG stain. **b** High-grade osteoblastic osteosarcoma. Poorly cohesive clusters and some single pleomorphic malignant cells and an admixture of osteoclasts; nuclei show coarse chromatin, nucleoli, and mitoses. HE stain. **c–l** High-grade osteosarcoma. **c, d** Under high magnification, tumor cells show an occasional epithelioid morphology and resemble atypical osteoblasts. Most tumor cells display prominent anisokaryosis, irregular nuclei with coarse chromatin, and macronucleoli indicative of high-grade malignancy. HE stain. **e–g** Multinucleated tumor cells and mitoses are common findings while calcifications are only occasionally seen in smears of high-grade osteosarcoma. MGG and HE stains. **h** FNA smears from soft tissue extensions showing a mixture of pleomorphic malignant cells and damaged muscle cells. HE stain. **i, j** Clusters of loosely cohesive tumor cells with intracellular strands of pinkish-violet-grey matrix, corresponding to osteoid. MGG stain. **k, l** The architecture of the tumor tissue, calcifications, and osteoid is better appreciated on cell block sections. HE stain. **m, n** Chondroblastic osteosarcoma. Atypical tumor cells resembling an osteoblast mixture with the cartilaginous matrix (**m**) or dispersed in the myxoid and chondroid background matrix (**n**). MGG stain. **o** Small cell osteosarcoma. Dispersed small- to medium-sized tumor cells with rounded nuclei and a scanty cytoplasm resembling those of Ewing sarcoma. HE stain. **p, q** Smears of high-grade osteosarcoma stained with ALP staining: positive ALP staining indicative of osteoblastic differentiation of tumor cells, whereas osteoclast-like giant cells are unstained (**p**); in smears from chondroblastic osteosarcoma, it can be difficult to distinguish a chondroid matrix from osteoid; ALP stains red the cytoplasm of cells with osteoblastic differentiation, whereas cartilage is unstained (**q**).

(For Figure see next pages.)

    FNA Cytology of Soft Tissue and Bone Tumors

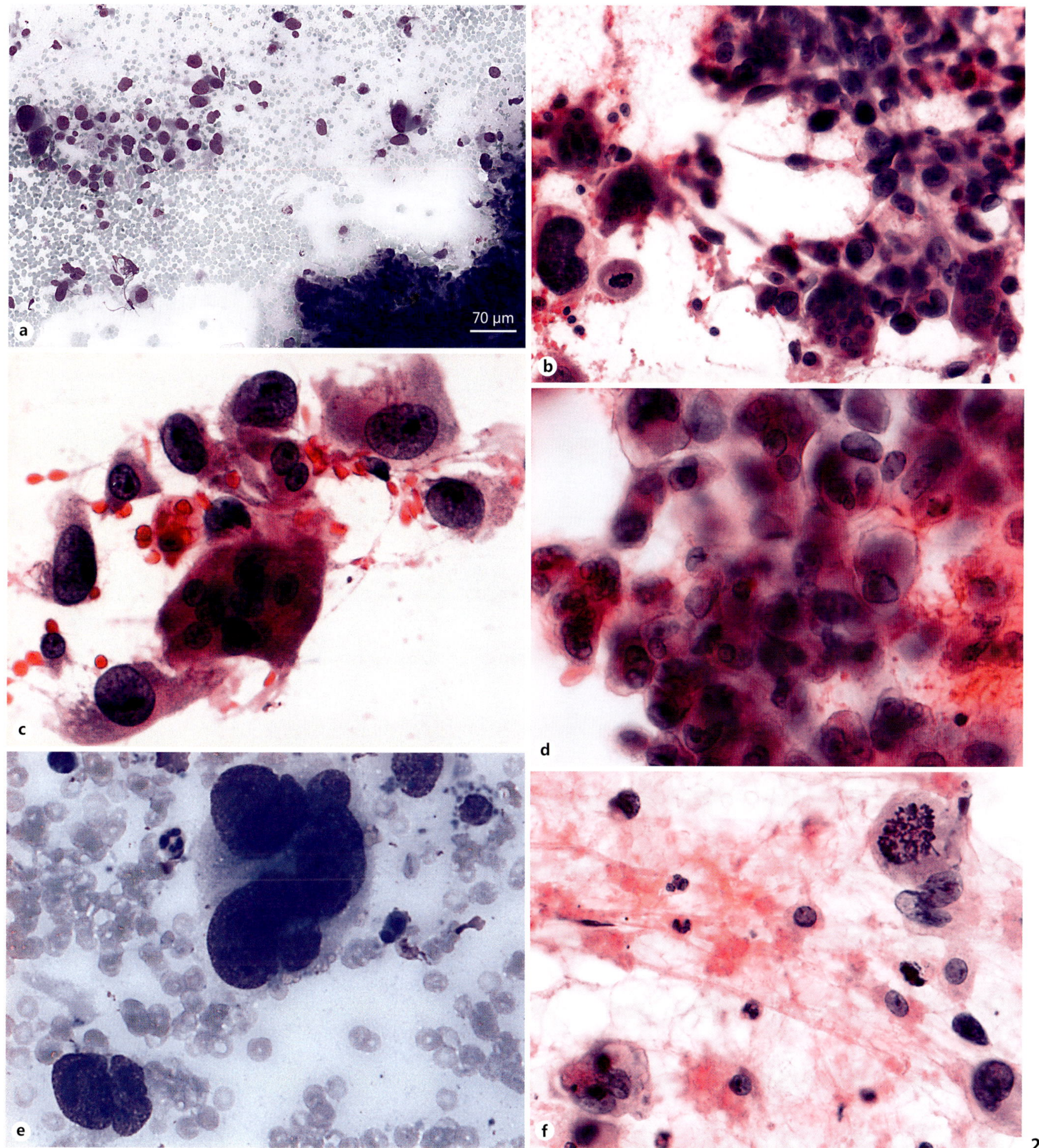

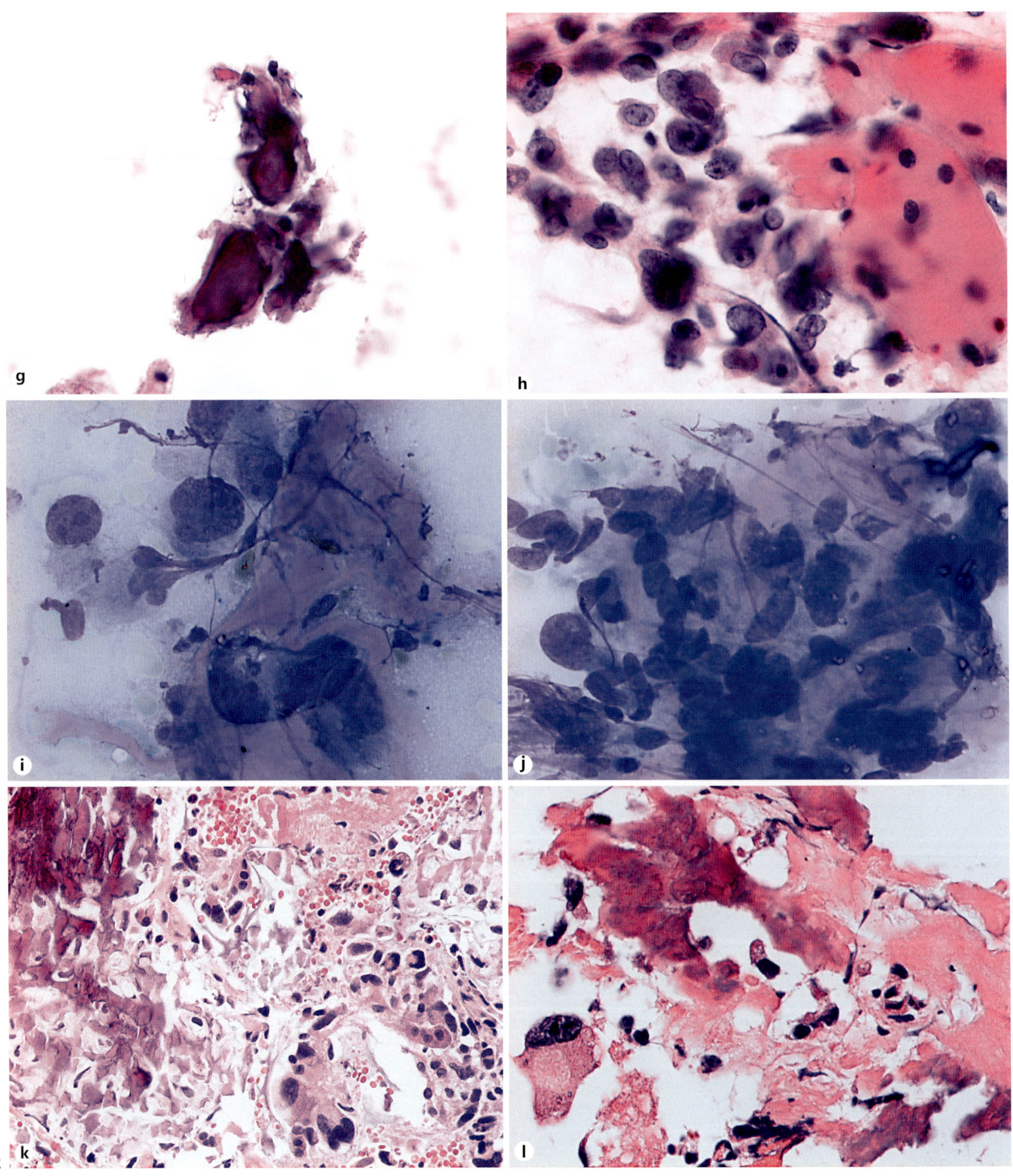

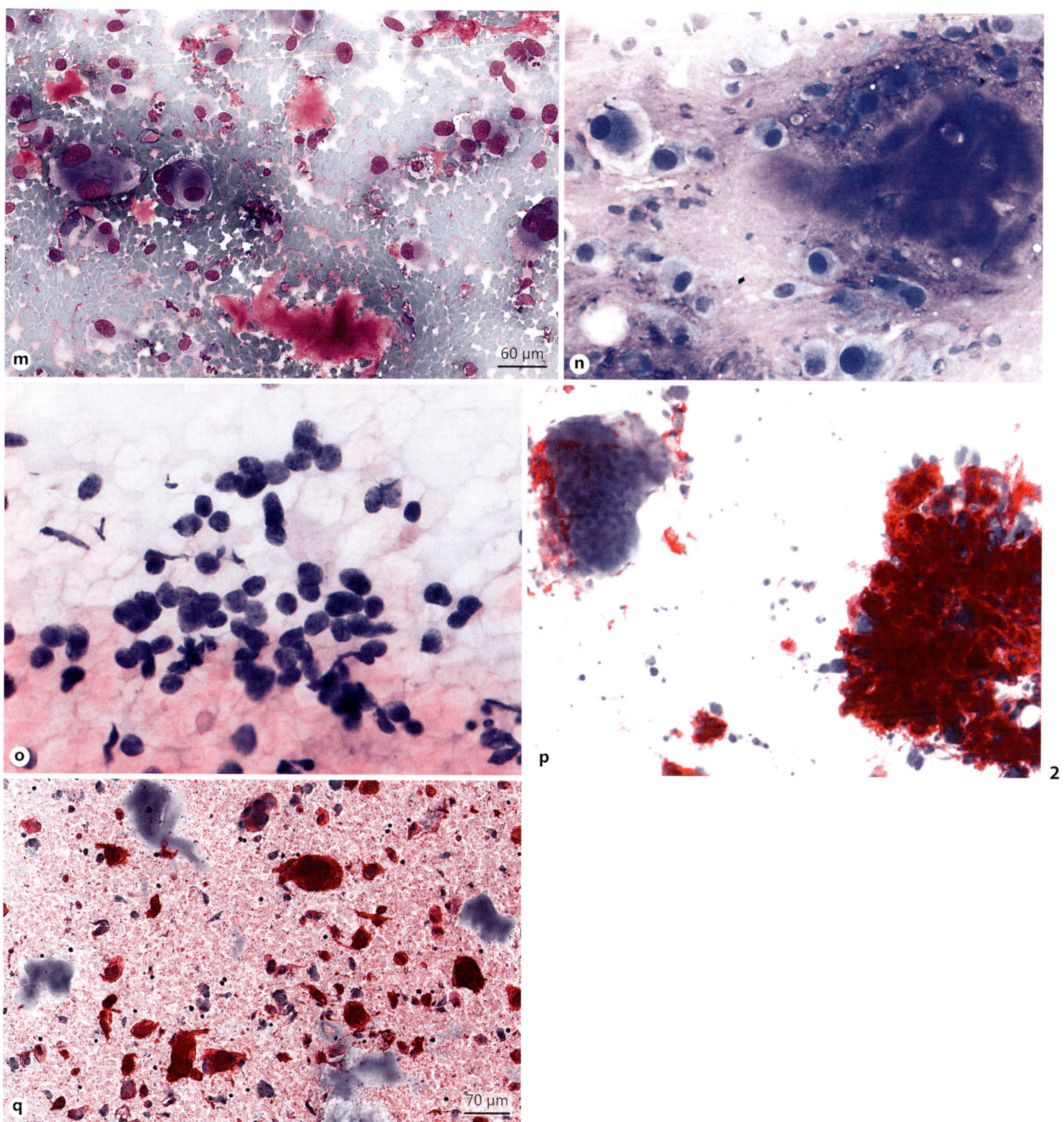

Osteosarcoma

Osteosarcoma is a primary bone tumor composed of cells producing osteoid and tumoral bone. Osteosarcoma is the most frequent primary nonhematopoietic malignant bone tumor and accounts for approximately 20% of all primary bone sarcomas. The majority of patients are older children, adolescents, and young adults, but up to 30% of osteosarcomas occur in patients older than 40 years, with a second peak at the age of 60 years. Osteosarcoma is rare in infants.

Male patients are affected slightly more frequently than females, with an equal distribution among races. The most common symptoms are pain and a palpable bone mass, often with a soft tissue extension.

Most osteosarcomas arise around the knee, followed by the humerus and pelvic bones. Approximately 7–10% arise in the craniofacial bones (mandible and maxilla). In addition, osteosarcoma may arise in any bone but rarely so in the spine or in the small bones of the hands and feet. The most frequent site of osteosarcoma in the long bones is the metaphysis (in approximately 90% of cases) followed by the diaphysis and rarely the epiphysis.

Osteosarcomas show a wide variety of microscopic features, biologic potential, and relation to bone, either intramedullary or surface. The most common type is the conventional, high-grade osteosarcoma and its osteoblastic and chondroblastic subtypes, which account for 75–85% of all osteosarcomas. The high-grade conventional type is also the most common target for FNA examination [6–16]. Less common variants are periosteal, parosteal, and juxtacortical osteosarcoma, central low-grade osteosarcoma, high-grade surface osteosarcoma, and small cell osteosarcoma [17].

Infrequent secondary osteosarcomas are associated with severe Paget disease, previous bone infarction, chronic osteomyelitis, metallic bone implants, and preexisting numerous benign bone neoplasms, such as enchondroma, osteochondroma, giant cell tumor (GCT), fibrous dysplasia, osteoblastoma, and bone cysts [18]. Osteosarcoma may be associated with some genetic syndromes, such as Rothmund-Thomson, Bloom, Werner, Li-Frumani, and Bilateral retinoblastoma [19].

FNA cytology is an efficient technique in the diagnosis of high-grade osteosarcoma in conjunction with imaging and appropriate clinical data [6–8]. FNA is less useful in the evaluation of low-grade osteosarcoma, often providing nonspecific or aspiration smears insufficient for a diagnosis. FNA smears of the osteoblastic subtype of osteosarcoma display variable cellularity but are often hypercellular. A mixture of single cells and loosely or somewhat cohesive clusters of moderately to highly pleomorphic rounded, ovoid, and polygonal tumor cells in a hemorrhagic background is a common pattern in smears (Fig. 2a–e). Most tumor cells have a moderate or abundant amount of well demarcated cytoplasm, often containing small vacuoles. The nuclei have a coarse chromatin and 1 or more often prominent macronucleoli. The nuclei may be eccentrically placed and such tumor cells resemble atypical osteoblasts (Fig. 2c, d). In the chondroblastic subtype, the most common cell types are similar to those of osteoblastic osteosarcoma, but nuclei are

often central and the nucleoli smaller and less prominent. A variable number of pleomorphic, often multinucleated tumor cells is almost always visible in smears irrespective of subtype. Osteoclast-like cells and mitoses are also frequent findings, while necrosis and calcifications are occasional findings in smears of high-grade osteosarcomas (Fig. 2b–g). When soft tissue extensions are sampled, tumor cells may be mixed with fragments of collagenous tissue and muscle cells indicative of infiltrative growth (Fig. 2h). A background matrix is present in most of the smears and strands of tumor matrix stained pinkish-violet-grey and red-violet-grey in DiffQuick and May-Grünwald-Giemsa (MGG) stains are considered to represent osteoid. This matrix also occurs as thin strands separating cells that lay in clusters (Fig. 2i, j). The architecture of the tumor tissue, calcifications, and osteoid is better appreciated on cell block sections, which makes the diagnosis easier, especially when both malignant cells and strands of osteoid or fragments of cartilage are present in the cell block sections (Fig. 2k, l). Smears of chondroblastic subtype display a chndromyxoid background matrix surrounded by single tumor cells and small fragments of acellular cartilage or cartilage containing atypical chondrocytes (Fig. 2m, n). Smears of fibroblastic osteosarcomas are dominated by atypical spindle cells with ovoid or fusiform nuclei showing coarse chromatin and small nucleoli. Smears of teleangiectatic osteosarcoma are bloody and hypocellular with scattered pleomorphic tumor cells. Aspirates from rare small cell osteosarcomas are hypercellular and tumor cells resemble those of Ewing sarcoma (Fig. 2o).

Low-grade osteosarcomas irrespective of subtype are difficult to evaluate cytologically with respect to malignancy and the histologic type of neoplasm. FNA smears from these neoplasms are usually hypocellular and show limited cytologic atypia of the tumor cells.

Cytologic Features of Conventional High-Grade Osteosarcoma

- Often hemorrhagic aspirates with variable cellularity
- Pleomorphic osteoblast-like tumor cells
- Epithelioid cells with distinct cytoplasmic borders and rounded irregular nuclei with prominent nucleoli
- Multinucleated pleomorphic tumor giant cells
- Strands of osteoid matrix in the background or between tumor cells in clusters
- Mitoses, often atypical
- Osteoclast-like giant cells; numerous in "giant cell-rich" osteosarcoma
- Occasional necrosis and calcifications

High-Grade Chondroblastic Osteosarcoma
- An admixture of dispersed atypical chondroblast-like tumor cells in addition to a similar cell population as in osteoblastic osteosarcoma
- Myxoid background matrix
- Fragments of hyaline cartilage with atypical cells

Ancillary Tests
Ancillary tests have a limited role in diagnosing osteosarcomas, which are largely diagnosed by synthesis of imaging and routinely stained histologic sections or FNA smears.

Immunophenotype
Osteosarcoma cells express a broad immunoreactivity that lacks diagnostic specificity. Many osteosarcomas express at least focally vimentin, osteonectin, osteocalcin, S100 protein, keratins, epithelial membrane antigen (EMA), desmin, muscle-specific actin, smooth muscle actin, and CD99.

Histochemistry
Tumor cells of osteosarcoma display strong and diffuse cytoplasmic alkaline phosphatase (ALP) staining, either in air-dried FNA smears or imprint preparation of biopsy specimens. This helps to establish osteogenic differentiation in smears that lack osteoid (Fig. 2n, o).

Genetics
The genetic changes in osteosarcoma are often complex and comprehensive, resulting in highly rearranged karyotypes. There are different subtypes with specific changes that can be helpful in the subclassification of the disease, but in the conventional type alterations such as the loss of chromosomes 3q, 6q, 9, 10, 13, 17p, and 18q, and gains of portions of chromosomes 1p, 1q, 6p, 8q, and 17p are recurrent [20, 21]. Mutations in the *TP53* gene are also thought to be of importance in the development of osteosarcoma and are a result of changes to the gene situated at 17p13.1 [20]. These alterations can be detected with cytogenetics, fluorescence in situ hybridization, single nucleotide polymorphism array, polymerase chain reaction, and next-generation sequencing on available material.

Differential Diagnosis
- Reactive osteoblastic proliferations such as fracture callus and myositis ossificans
- GCT
- Epithelioid (aggressive) osteoblastoma
- High-grade sarcomas arising in bone
- High-grade chondrosarcoma
- Metastasis of malignant melanoma
- Metastasis of carcinomas
- Skeletal manifestation of large-cell anaplastic lymphoma
- Epithelioid vascular neoplasm

Due to their destructive growth and extension to the surrounding soft tissues, the majority of high-grade osteosarcomas are easily accessible for FNA. When the cortex is intact but an FNA sampling technique is desired, trocar with a drill is necessary to penetrate the cortical bone. After cortical penetration, FNA samples can be taken from the target lesion using a coaxial technique supporting the use of a single needle-insertion point, even when performing several punctures.

Reactive osteoblastic proliferations such as fracture callus and pseudomalignant myositis ossificans are the most important benign mimics of osteosarcoma in FNA smears [22–24]. The correlation of cytologic features with imaging studies and clinical history is very important in such cases, as is applying distinctive cytomorphologic criteria in the evaluation of smears, as in the vast majority of cases smears of high-grade osteosarcomas display firm signs of malignancy compared to smears of callus fracture and myositis ossificans. Other benign mimics of osteosarcoma are GCT and osteoblastoma/epithelioid osteoblastoma. Smears of bone GCT display a double-cell population of clustered spindle cells and multinucleated osteoclastic cells, but osteoclastic giant cells are randomly distributed in the smears in osteosarcoma, whereas in GCT giant cells are often situated in the periphery of cohesive clusters of spindle cells. The radiographic appearances and cytologic features of osteoblastomas, including osteoblast-like cells containing round to oval, eccentric nuclei with a fine chromatin pattern and smooth nuclear membrane, an admixture of bland spindle cells, and an absence of significant atypia and mitoses, helps in distinguishing these neoplasm from osteosarcoma. An important differential diagnosis of high-grade chondroblastic osteosarcoma is high-grade chondrosarcoma [25, 26]. Similar to chondrosarcoma, smears of chondroblastic osteosarcoma may contain an abundance of atypical cartilage in addition to more undifferentiated pleomorphic malignant cells. Some tumor cells, however, usually show features of atypical osteoblasts, making the possibility of chondroblastic osteosarcoma more likely than high-grade chondrosarcoma (Fig. 2j). In addition, a strong cytoplasmic positivity of ALP and osteoid present in air-dried smears or cell block sections facilitates the diagnosis of chondroblastic osteosarcoma (Fig. 2o, p). Undifferentiated pleomorphic sarcoma, leiomyosarcoma, and less frequently other subtypes of sarcoma arising primarily in bone, as well as metastatic depositions of malignant melanomas, carcinomas, and the manifestation of large-cell anaplastic lymphoma constitutes other differential diagnoses of osteosarcoma. Antibodies to keratin, EMA, melanoma markers, CD45, CD30, and ALK are thus not always entirely specific, which may help to render the correct diagnosis. As mentioned previously, clinical data, imaging, and ALP staining are all important adjuncts in the examination of smears of osteosarcoma. The clue to the cytologic diagnosis of conventional high-grade osteosarcoma in routinely stained smears is the presence of intercellular osteoid and osteoblast-like tumor cells. Osteoid is best appreciated in MGG-stained smears. Differentiating osteoid from collagenous matrix can occasionally be difficult.

Electron microscopic examination is a well-established method of defining osteoid in fine-needle aspirates. We believe, however, that ALP staining has been underestimated in many studies of FNA of osteosarcoma. Strong intracytoplasmic ALP staining in intact tumor cells confirms their osteoblastic differentiation.

The optimal use of the FNA technique as a diagnostic tool in the evaluation of osteosarcomas requires the referral of patients to specialized orthopedic-oncologic centers with multidisciplinary expertise in the examination and treatment of bone sarcoma. In the experience of our institution, cases of intraosseous osteosarcomas without destruction of the cortical bone are difficult to examine by FNA alone. In such cases we complement FNA with core-needle or less often surgical biopsies in order to obtain sufficient material.

References

1 Venugopal SB, Prasad S: Cytological diagnosis of osteoblastoma of cervical spine: a case report with review of literature. Diagn Cytopathol 2015;43:218–221.

2 Gupta N, Kaur J, Srinivasan R, Das A, Mohindra S, Rajwanshi A, Nijhawan R: Fine needle aspiration cytology in lesions of the nose, nasal cavity and paranasal sinuses. Acta Cytol 2011;55:135–141.

3 Rhode MG, Lucas DR, Krueger CH, Pu RT: Fine-needle aspiration of spinal osteoblastoma in a patient with lymphangiomatosis. Diagn Cytopathol 2006;34:295–297.

4 Mondal A, Misra DK: CT-guided needle aspiration cytology (FNAC) of 112 vertebral lesions. Indian J Pathol Microbiol 1994;37:255–261.

5 Akerman M, Domanski HA: The cytology of soft tissue tumours. Monogr Clin Cytol 2003;16:1–112.

6 VandenBussche CJ, Sathiyamoorthy S, Wakely PE Jr, Ali SZ: Chondroblastic osteosarcoma: cytomorphologic characteristics and differential diagnosis on FNA. Cancer Cytopathol 2016;124:493–500.

7 Sathiyamoorthy S, Ali SZ: Osteoblastic osteosarcoma: cytomorphologic characteristics and differential diagnosis on fine-needle aspiration. Acta Cytol 2012;56:481–486.

8 Klijanienko J, Caillaud JM, Orbach D, Brisse H, Lagace R, Sastre-Gareau X: Cyto-histological correlations in primary, recurrent, and metastatic bone and soft tissue osteosarcoma. Institut Curie's experience. Diagn Cytopathol 2007;35:270–275.

9 Domanski HA, Akerman M: Fine-needle aspiration of primary osteosarcoma: a cytological-histological study. Diagn Cytopathol 2005;32:269–275.

10 Soderlund V, Skoog L, Unni KK, Bertoni F, Brosjo O, Kreicbergs A: Diagnosis of high-grade osteosarcoma by radiology and cytology: a retrospective study of 52 cases. Sarcoma 2004;8:31–36.

11 Dodd LG, Scully SP, Cothran RL, Harrelson JM: Utility of fine-needle aspiration in the diagnosis of primary osteosarcoma. Diagn Cytopathol 2002;27:350–353.

12 Kilpatrick SE, Ward WG, Bos GD, Chauvenet AR, Gold SH: The role of fine needle aspiration biopsy in the diagnosis and management of osteosarcoma. Pediatr Pathol Mol Med 2001;20:175–187.

13 Nicol KK, Ward WG, Savage PD, Kilpatrick SE: Fine-needle aspiration biopsy of skeletal versus extraskeletal osteosarcoma. Cancer 1998;84:176–185.

14 Bhatia A, Ashokraj G: Cytological diversity of osteosarcoma. Indian J Cancer 1992;29:56–60.

15 Walaas L, Kindblom LG: Light and electron microscopic examination of fine-needle aspirates in the preoperative diagnosis of osteogenic tumors: a study of 21 osteosarcomas and two osteoblastomas. Diagn Cytopathol 1990;6:27–38.

16 White VA, Fanning CV, Ayala AG, Raymond AK, Carrasco CH, Murray JA: Osteosarcoma and the role of fine-needle aspiration: a study of 51 cases. Cancer 1988;62:1238–1246.

17 Park SH, Kim I: Small cell osteogenic sarcoma of the ribs: cytological, immunohistochemical, and ultrastructural study with literature review. Ultrastruct Pathol 1999;23:133–140.

18 Hakky M, Kolbusz R, Reyes CV, Chinoy MJ: Fine needle aspiration cytology in a case of osteogenic sarcoma in Paget's disease. Cytopathology 1990;1:183–186.

19 Jhala DN, Eltoum I, Carroll AJ, Lopez-Ben R, Lopez-Terrada D, Rao PH, Pettenati MJ, Siegal GP: Osteosarcoma in a patient with McCune-Albright syndrome and Mazabraud's syndrome: a case report emphasizing the cytological and cytogenetic findings. Hum Pathol 2003;34:1354–1357.

20 Martin JW, Squire JA, Zielenska M: The genetics of osteosarcoma. Sarcoma 2012;2012:627254.

21 Yen CC, Chen WM, Chen TH, Chen WY, Chen PC, Chiou HJ, Hung GY, Wu HT, Wei CJ, Shiau CY, Wu YC, Chao TC, Tzeng CH, Chen PM, Lin CH, Chen YJ, Fletcher JA: Identification of chromosomal aberrations associated with disease progression and a novel 3q13.31 deletion involving LSAMP gene in osteosarcoma. Int J Oncol 2009;35:775–788.

22 Mokhtari M, Kumar PV, Rezazadeh S: Confusing cytological findings in myositis ossificans. Acta Cytol 2012;56:565–570.

23 Koh JS, Chung JH, Kweon MS, Lee SS, Lee SY, Lee JH: Fine needle aspiration cytology of late-stage callus in stress fracture: a case report. Acta Cytol 2001;45:445–448.

24 Rooser B, Herrlin K, Rydholm A, Akerman M: Pseudomalignant myositis ossificans. Clinical, radiologic, and cytologic diagnosis in 5 cases. Acta Orthop Scand 1989;60:457–460.

25 Gupta N, Rajwanshi A, Gupta P, Vaiphei K, Gupta AK: Chondroblastic osteosarcoma of the temporal region: a diagnostic dilemma. Diagn Cytopathol 2011;39:377–379.

26 Chhabra S, Chopra R, Handa U, Punia RS, Mohan H: Cytomorphologic features of chondroid neoplasms: a comparative study. Acta Cytol 2010;54:1101–1110.

Domanski HA, Walther CS: FNA Cytology of Soft Tissue and Bone Tumors. Monogr Clin Cytol.
Basel, Karger, 2017, vol 22, pp 147–160 (DOI: 10.1159/000475107)

Cartilaginous Tumors

Cartilaginous tumors of bone constitute the most common group of primary bone neoplasms with a broad spectrum of entities of different biologic potential and clinical course, but that occasionally display an overlapping histo- and cytomorphology. The most common targets for fine-needle aspiration (FNA) among cartilage-forming neoplasms are conventional low-grade and high-grade chondrosarcomas and benign chondromas. Experience of FNA of chondroblastoma, chondromyxoid fibroma, clear cell chondrosarcoma, and some other rare cartilaginous lesions is limited, and at most is based on single cases or short series.

Osteochondroma

Osteochondroma is the most common benign neoplasm of the bone, accounting for up to 35% of all benign bone neoplasms. Most cases of osteochondroma are solitary lesions present in the first 3 decades of life with a slight male predominance. About 15% of patients present with multiple osteochondromas associated with the autosomal dominant hereditary multiple osteochondromas syndrome. Most solitary osteochondromas arise in the metaphysis of the distal femur, proximal tibia, fibula, and humerus, while flat bones are less often involved. The majority of patients present with a solitary asymptomatic slowly growing mass which is found incidentally. Some of the lesions may cause pain due to fracture, arthritis, and impingement of adjacent tendons, nerves and blood vessels. Rapid growth of preexisting osteochondroma with pain and enlarging of the cartilage cap, which is normally 1.0–1.5 up to 2.0 cm thick, may raise suspicion of

malignant transformation. FNA smears from osteochondroma usually contain fragments of cartilage sampled from the cartilaginous cap [1] (Fig. 1a). Typical osteochondroma is rarely sampled by FNA cytology as its radiologic appearances are diagnostic. FNA cytology may help to establish the diagnosis in rare cases of malignant transformation of osteochondroma. The risk of malignant transformation to chondrosarcoma is estimated at about 1% for solitary and 5% for multiple osteochondromas. The presence of significant cellular and nuclear pleomorphism and a myxoid matrix in FNA smears may suggest malignant transformation; however, the morphology of malignant transformation may be quite subtle. Correlation with radiology is essential, and core biopsy or surgical biopsy remains necessary to confirm the malignant diagnosis.

Ancillary Tests
Immunophenotype
Immunocytochemical examinations serve little roll in the cytologic diagnosis of osteochondromas.

Genetics
Cytogenetic changes at 8q22–24.1 involving the *EXT1* gene can be found in both sporadic and hereditary osteochondroma cases [2]. In hereditary multiple osteochondromas, mutations in the *EXT1* or *EXT2* genes result in a defective protein with disturbed cell growth [3]. These changes can be detected by cytogenetics, fluorescence in situ hybridization (FISH), single nucleotide polymorphism (SNP) array, polymerase chain reaction (PCR), and next-generation sequencing (NGS) on available material.

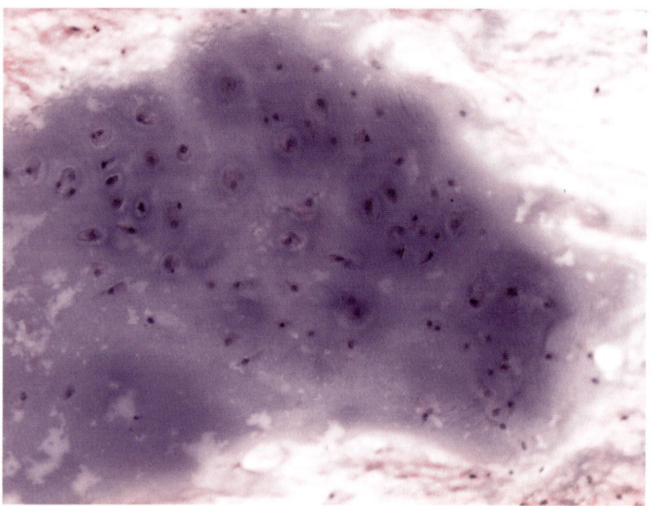

Fig. 1. Osteochondroma. FNA smears contain large fragments of cartilage with uniformed chondrocytes in lacunae. HE stain.

Chondroma

Chondromas are benign tumors of hyaline cartilage that account for approximately 10% of all benign bone neoplasms. Enchondromas are the most common subtype of chondromas arising in the medullary bone with a wide age distribution, although the majority of patients are 20–40 years of age. Almost 50% of surgically removed enchondromas occur in the small bones of the hands and feet. The second most common sites are the proximal part of the humerus and the proximal and distal femur. Enchondromas of the hands and feet are typically palpable and sometimes painful tumors. However, these tumors are often discovered when a mild to moderate trauma causes a fracture. Multiple enchondromas are designated as enchondromatosis or Ollier disease. Periosteal chondromas are less common than enchondromas. They represent about 20% of all chondromas and commonly arise in the long bones.

Cytologic Features
- Smears of low to moderate cellularity
- Cartilaginous tissue fragments, blue or red-purple in May-Grünwald-Geiemsa (MGG) and DiffQuick stains, and pale, faintly pink in wet-fixed smears
- Uniform, small chondrocytes in lacunae within cartilage fragments
- Uncommon single cells

- Cellular smears with occasional anisokaryosis and binucleation of chondrocytes in chondromas of the hands and feet

Ancillary Tests
Immunophenotype
Chondrocytes show immunoreactivity for S100 protein.

Genetics
Cytogenetic changes at 8q22 involving the *EXT1* and *EXT2* genes have been detected [2]. Mutation of the *EXT1* gene results in a dysfunctional protein. These changes can be detected by cytogenetics, FISH, SNP array, PCR, and NGS on available material.

Differential Diagnosis
- Low-grade chondrosarcoma

Combined evaluation of radiologic and cytologic features of chondromas is mandatory in order to avoid a false positive diagnosis of low-grade malignant chondrosarcoma [1, 4]. This is especially important in enchondromas of the hands and feet [1, 5]. Radiologically, enchondromas are well circumscribed, often with lobulated contour, cortical expansion, and endosteal erosions. There are varying degrees of calcifications within the lesion. In microscopic examinations, most chondromas are rather paucicellular tumors with an abundant hyaline cartilage matrix and small, bland chondrocytes with small nuclei, sometimes with small nucleoli (Fig. 2a, b). Occasional binucleated chondrocytes may be seen in smears (Fig. 2c). Typically, smears of chondromas of the hands and feet are more cellular and may exhibit a cellular pleomorphism with relatively marked anisokaryosis (Fig. 2b).

It is unwise to suggest a chondrosarcoma diagnosis (even in tumors with a marked cellular pleomorphism) when radiologic features are unequivocally in favor of chondroma. The presence of benign acellular cartilage or cartilaginous matrix containing chondrocytes with no or little cytologic atypia in FNA smears of lesions showing clinical and radiographic features of chondroma confirms a benign diagnosis and excludes chondrosarcoma.

Chondroblastoma

Chondroblastomas are rare bone tumors (representing approximately 1% of all bone tumors) that affect children and young adults, with a 2:1 male predominance and the majority occurring in the second decade of life. Most chondroblastomas occur in the epiphyseal regions of the long tubular bones with common involvement of the humerus and tibia. Small tubular bones of the hands and the ribs are rarely involved, and unusual sites are the calcaneus, talus, patella, and the temporal bone. Many patients complain of mild pain, sometimes for many years. Chondroblastomas adjacent to joints may cause a joint effusion with swelling and pain. In approximately 30% of cases, chondroblastomas are associated with secondary aneurysmal bone cysts. This may cause confusion and diagnostic difficulties in cases examined by small samples such as FNA and core biopsies. On imaging, chondroblastomas are usually well demarcated, lytic lesions with a thin sclerotic rim. Sometimes small calcifications are seen within the lytic lesion, and in those instances the information garnered from the radiologic image is an important aid to the diagnosis. In histologic sections, the chondroblasts are arranged in sheets containing numerous randomly distributed giant cells of osteoclastic type. There is a varying amount of chondroid or fibrochondroid matrix (Fig. 3a, b). A typical finding is a network of pericellular "chicken wire" calcifications. Chondroblastoma cells are uniform, rounded to polygonal, with well-defined cell borders and rounded or ovoid nuclei. The nuclei often display grooves or clefts and contain small nucleoli. Some nuclei can be enlarged and hyperchromatic. The cytoplasm is clear or faintly eosinophilic. Mitoses are often observed in histologic sections but rarely in smears.

Cytologic Features
- Moderate to hypercellular smears
- A mixture of loosely clustered and dispersed tumor cells
- Fragments of chondroid matrix
- Rounded to oval mononuclear cells with well-defined borders and rounded nuclei with fine chromatin and small nucleoli
- Often indented or lobulated nuclei exhibiting longitudinal grooves
- Multinucleated giant cells of osteoclastic type
- Slight anisokaryosis and binucleation may be seen

Ancillary Tests
Immunophenotype
Tumor cells express S100 in about 75% of cases.

Genetics
No diagnostic or specific rearrangements have been found. However, several cases have displayed aberrations on chromosomes 5 and 8, which can be detected by cytogenetics, FISH, SNP array, and NGS on available material [6].

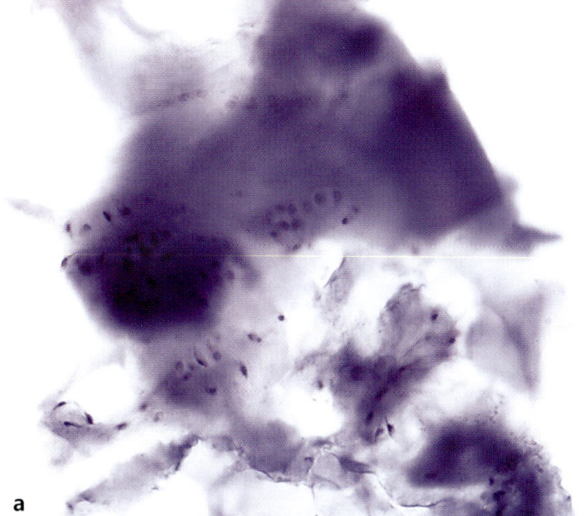

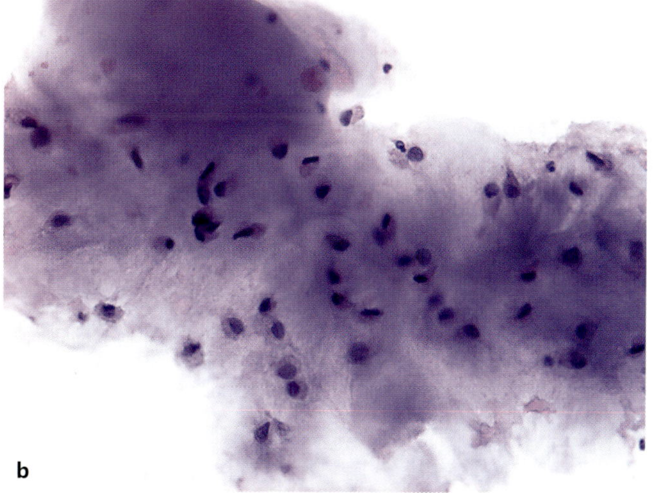

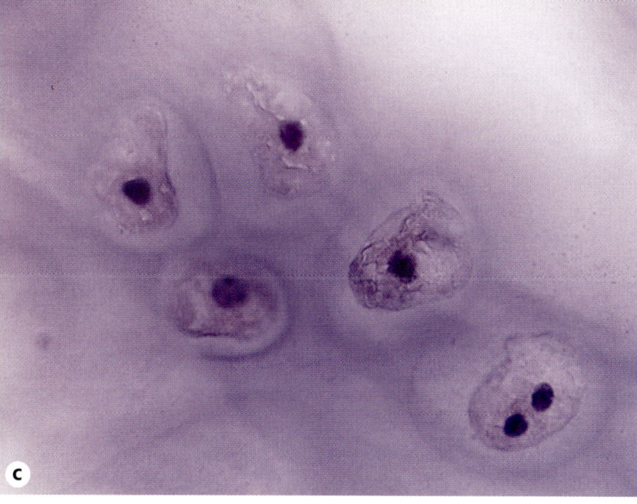

Fig. 2. Chondroma. **a** Fragments of cartilage with areas of random scattered uniform chondrocytes, some in lacunar spaces. Some chondrocytes shows slight atypia (**b**) and binucleation (**c**). HE stain.

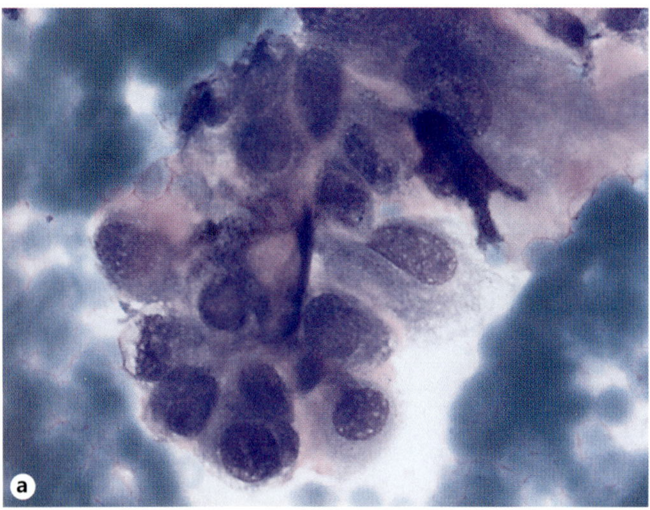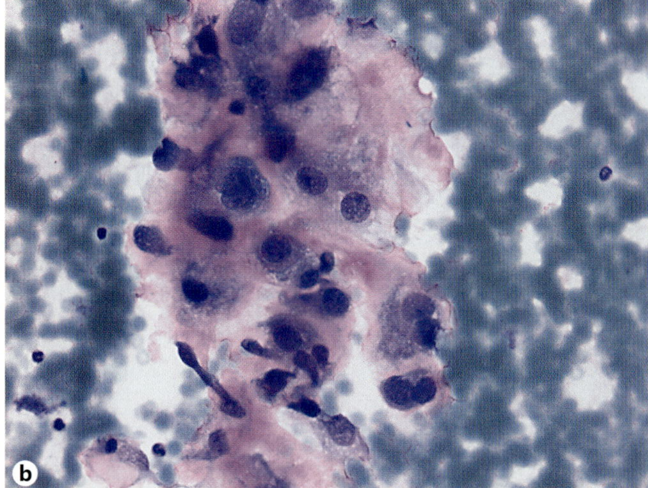

Fig. 3. Chondroblastoma. **a** Mononuclear rounded cells with a rather abundant, well-defined cytoplasm embedded in the chondroid matrix. **b** Nuclei may vary in size and binucleated cells may be present. MGG stain.

Differential Diagnosis
- Chondromyxoid fibroma
- Aneurysmal bone cyst
- Giant cell tumor
- Clear cell chondrosarcoma

The cytology of chondroblastoma has been described in a few series and some case reports [1, 4, 7–16]. In our own experience, the most important cytologic feature has been the chondroblasts with their indented, lobulated or grooved nuclei, and the presence of chondroid or fibrochondroid matrix and osteoclast-like giant cells. According to Kilpatrick et al. [17], the presence of typical chondroblasts in an epiphyseal bone tumor with classic radiographic features of chondroblastoma is sufficient to suggest the diagnosis even without fragments of matrix and giant cells. Chondromyxoid fibroma occurs in the same age group as chondroblastoma but is situated in the metaphysis. Aneurysmal bone cyst may be associated with chondroblastoma. In such cases, the radiologic features may be interpreted as an aneurysmal bone cyst. Cytologically, however, these combined lesions have no malignant features and are diagnosed as benign bone tumors with numerous giant cells. The mono- and binucleated stromal cells of giant cell tumors are smaller than tumor cells in chondroblastomas and do not exhibit either nuclear grooves or indentations of chondroblasts, or fragments of chondroid matrix. The cytologic appearance of clear cell chondrosarcoma in FNA smears is not sufficiently defined, but tumor cells of this neoplasm are evidently malignant.

Chondromyxoid Fibroma

Chondromyxoid fibroma is an uncommon, benign, intramedullary comprising 1–2% of benign bone tumors and about 2% of all cartilaginous tumors. Most tumors appear in the second and third decades of life, with a 2:1 male predominance. The most frequent site is the distal femur and the proximal tibia. Other common sites are the flat bones, especially the ileum, but the distribution of chondromyxoid fibromas is widespread and less commonly includes pelvic, foot, and cranial bones. Chondromyxoid fibromas are typically eccentrically located in the metaphysis in the long bones.

Imaging of these tumors displays osteolytic, predominantly lucent lesions, usually without matrix calcifications. The tumors may be elongated and vary in size up to 10 cm in length. The cortex over the lesion is often expanded with endosteal sclerosis. A complete penetration of the cortex may be seen as a hemispherical osseous defect but with intact periosteum.

The typical chondromyxoid fibroma grows in a lobular pattern with characteristically hypocellular centers and increased cellularity in the periphery of lobules. Tumor lobules containing spindly and stellate cells are embedded in the abundant myxoid matrix. The tumor cells often have cytoplasmic extensions and in many cases there are single cells with enlarged, hyperchromatic, and somewhat pleomorphic nuclei. Foci of hyaline cartilage are present in

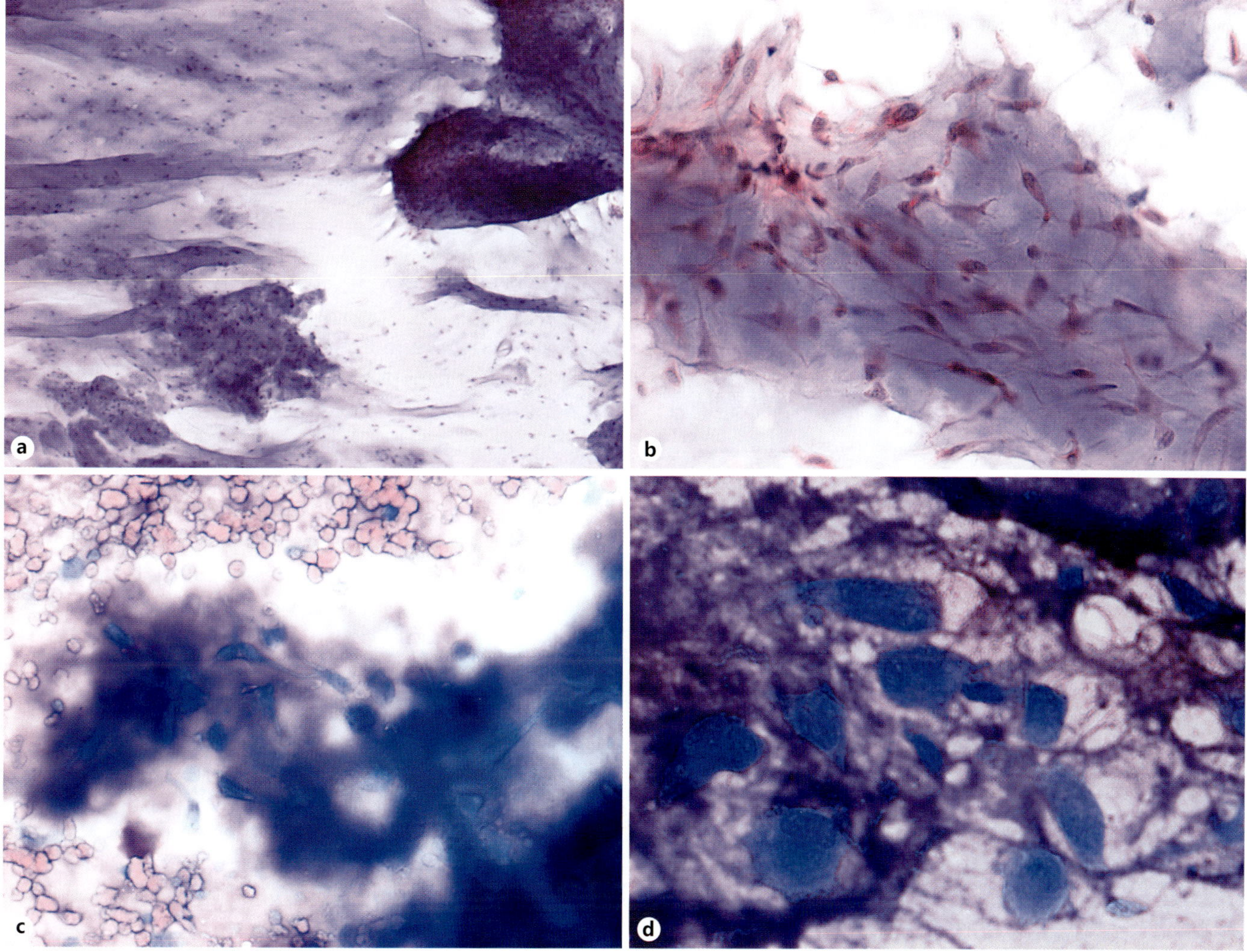

Fig. 4. Chondromyxoid fibroma. **a** Cellular smears with fragments of cartilaginous-myxoid tissue and an abundant myxoid matrix in the background. HE stain. **b**, **c** Fusiform, stellate, or spindle cells embedded in cartilaginous tissue fragments. HE and MGG stains. **d** Chondroblast- or chondrocyte-like cells occur in the myxoid background. MGG stain.

some tumors and osteoclast-like giant cells may be seen at the periphery of the tumor lobules. Cytologic smears of chondromyxoid fibroma display moderate to high cellularity (Fig. 4a) showing similar features to the histologic sections, such as a mixture of round to ovoid chondroid cells, bland spindle cells, and stellate cells with cytoplasmic extensions in a myxoid/chondromyxoid background matrix (Fig. 4b–d). FNA smears occasionally contain osteoclastic giant cells.

Cytologic Features
- Moderate to hypercellular smears
- Chondroid cells
- Spindle-shaped or stellate cells, dispersed or clustered
- Myxoid/chondromyxoid background matrix
- Occasional osteoclastic giant cells

Ancillary Tests
Immunophenotype
Tumor cells express S100 and the extracellular matrix is immunopositive for collagen II and SOX9.

Genetics
Different anomalies of chromosome 6 can be found, including translocations and inversions. However, different parts and subregions of chromosome 6 can be affected [18]. The

changes can be detected with cytogenetics, FISH, SNP array, and NGS on available material.

Differential Diagnosis
- Chondrosarcoma
- Chondroblastoma
- Chondroma

FNA and cytologic features of chondromyxoid fibroma have been described in single case reports and a few small series [1, 19–26]. Our experience is limited to a few cases [5]. The spindly and stellate cells may vary in size and may exhibit occasional moderately pleomorphic nuclei with hyperchromasia and prominent nucleoli. Chondroblast-like cells may also show occasional pleomorphism and binucleation. Compared to chondrosarcoma, smears of chondromyxoid fibroma do not display fragments of dense hyaline cartilage containing atypical chondrocytes in the lacunar spaces, which is a consistent finding in smears of chondrosarcomas. In addition, characteristic clinical/radiographic features of chondromyxoid fibromas help to distinguish these neoplasms from other cartilaginous neoplasms.

Chondrosarcoma

Chondrosarcomas constitute a heterogeneous group of cartilaginous malignant tumors. These neoplasms are the second most common primary bone sarcomas, representing up to 27% of cases in the published series. The vast majority of chondrosarcomas are primary, conventional intramedullary tumors. Primary periosteal (juxtacortical) chondrosarcomas are very rare. The term "secondary chondrosarcoma" is reserved for those tumors that arise in patients with Ollier disease and Maffucci syndrome. Special variants of chondrosarcoma include dedifferentiated, mesenchymal, and clear cell tumors. Roughly 90% of chondrosarcomas are of primary, conventional type.

Conventional Chondrosarcoma

Most chondrosarcomas are of the conventional hyaline cartilage type arising in an intramedullary location in adults with a broad age distribution ranging from 20 to 80 years, with a peak of incidence in the fourth to sixth decades of life. Tumor predilection sites are the large bones of the axial skeleton, with the majority of chondrosarcomas occurring in the pelvic bone, femur, humerus, and ribs. Uncommon sites are the acral and extraskeletal regions. In the long bones, chondrosarcomas are metadiaphyseal, with the tumor matrix containing calcifications suggestive of a cartilage tumor at radiography. Chondrosarcomas show permeative growth with infiltration of the medullary cavity and erosion of the cortex, but without or only very rarely with a periosteal reaction.

Results from several studies confirm that the grading of chondrosarcomas is important in predicting the prognosis. Most low-grade chondrosarcomas have a clinical course and prognosis comparable with benign chondromas.

Conventional chondrosarcomas are common targets for cytologic examinations and FNA often provides a rich yield with fragments or "microbiopsies" of tumor tissue in smears (Fig. 5a). Fragments of the cartilage and myxochondroid matrix stain strongly red-blue and violet in MGG and DiffQuick stains, and pale pink in hematoxylin and eosin (HE) stain (Fig. 5b, c). The heavy staining in air-dried preparations makes the study of cellular and nuclear details difficult compared to alcohol-fixed and HE- or Papanicolaou-stained smears.

Cytologic Features
- Often abundant smears but variable cellularity depending on the malignancy grade
- Low cellularity in low-grade and high cellularity in higher-grade tumors
- Mixture of dispersed cells with fragments of hyaline cartilage
- Number of dispersed cells and degree of pleomorphism increase in higher-grade tumors
- Mononuclear and binuclear tumor cells often in lacunae
- Large round individual cells with well-defined, often vacuolated cytoplasm and irregular, lobulated nuclei
- Hyperchromatic nuclei with coarse chromatin in higher-grade tumors
- Myxoid or myxochondroid matrix in higher-grade tumors
- Presence of noncartilaginous pleomorphic or spindle cell sarcoma suggesting dedifferentiation

Specific for Low-Grade Chondrosarcomas
- Often abundant smears with fragments of hyaline cartilage of variable size
- Variable but often low cellularity in the fragments
- Low number of dispersed single cells
- Mononuclear and less common binuclear rounded tumor cells with a well-defined cytoplasm, often in lacunae
- Slight to moderate atypia
- Mitoses absent or very rare

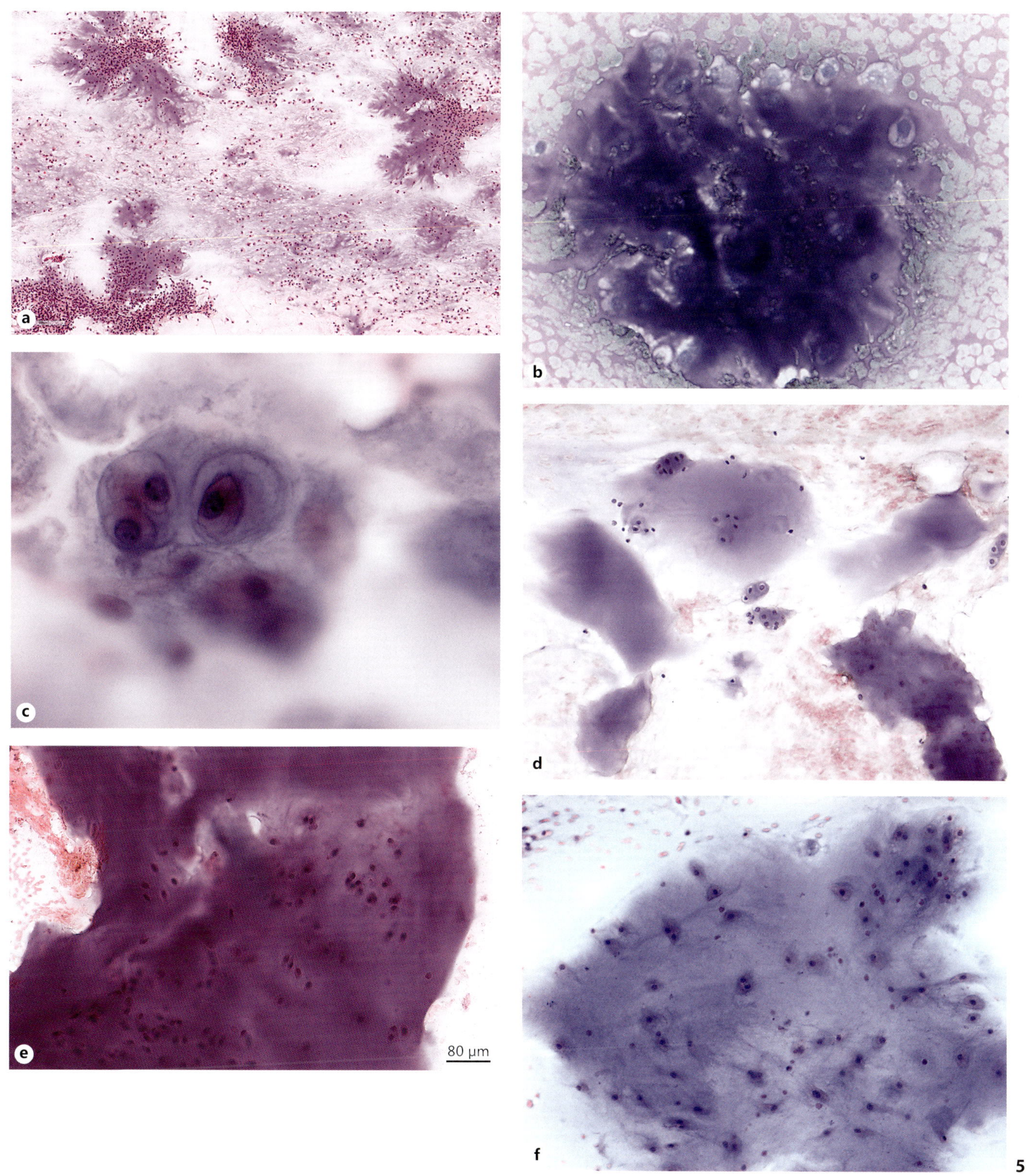

(Figure continued on next pages.)

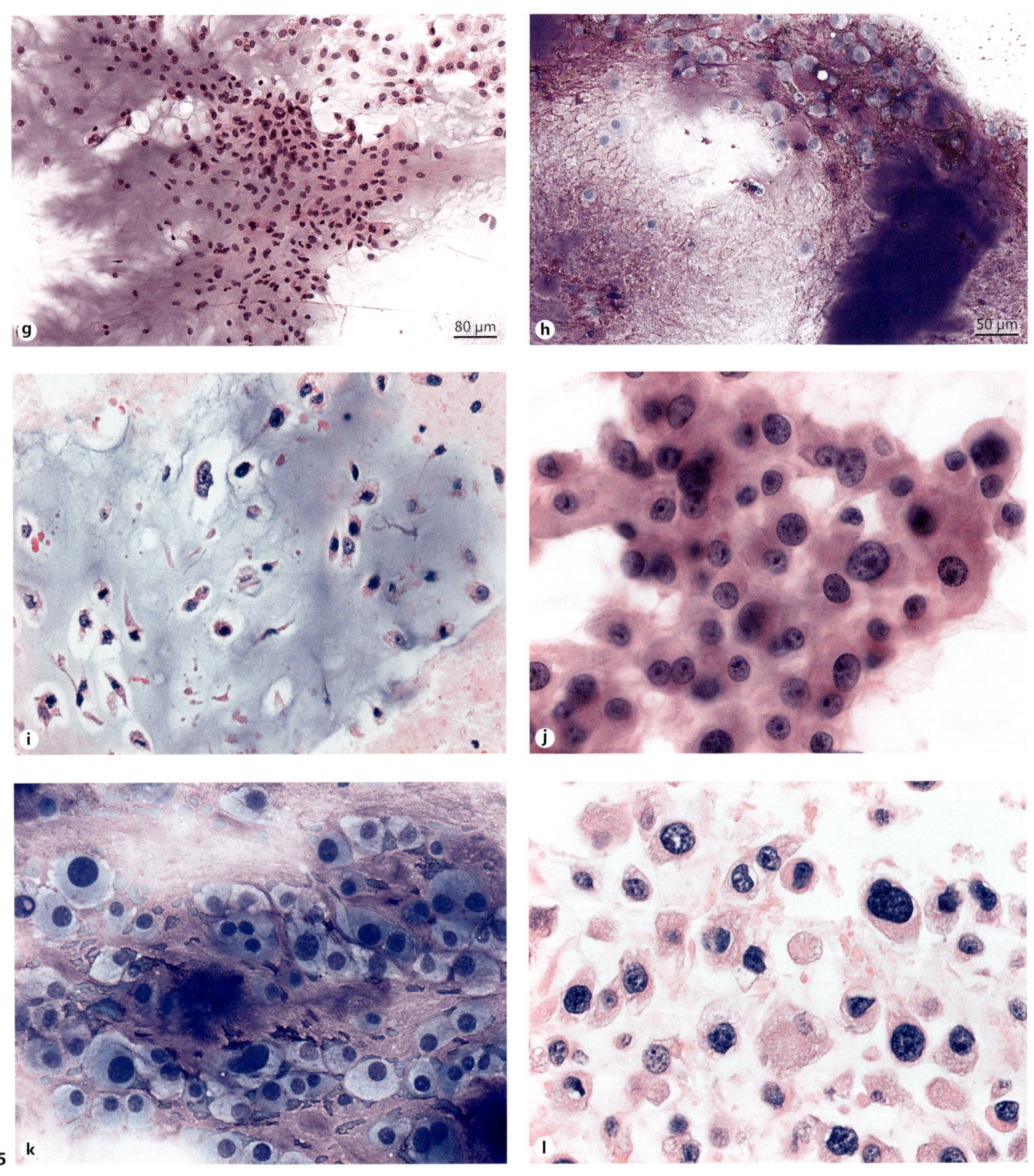

(For legend see next page.)

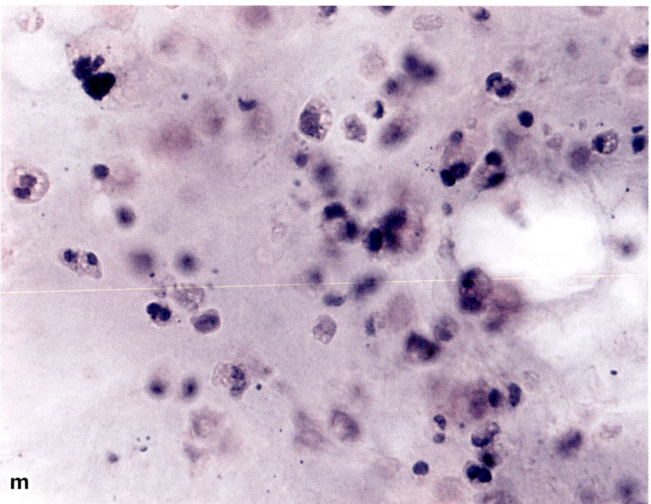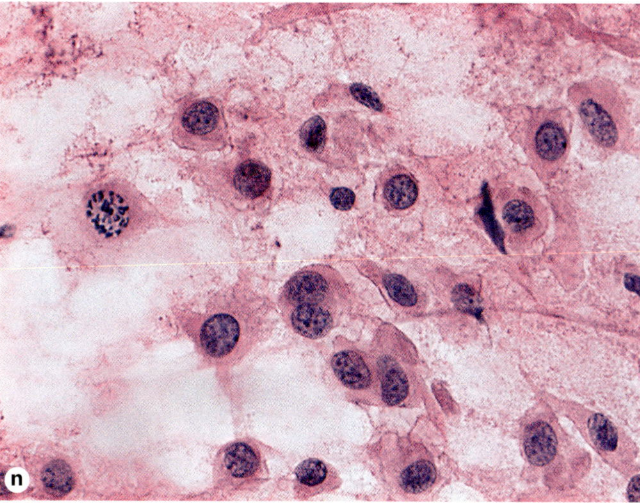

Fig. 5. Chondrosarcoma. **a** FNA of conventional chondrosarcomas often provides a rich yield with fragments or "microbiopsies" of tumor tissue in smears. Fragments of the cartilage and myxochondroid matrix stain strongly red-blue and violet in MGG and DiffQuick stains (**b**) and pink or pale pink in HE stain (**c**). **d–f** Grade 1 chondrosarcoma: cartilaginous fragments containing randomly distributed uniform or slightly atypical and occasionally binucleated cells, many of them in lacunar spaces. Low cellularity and lack of dispersed single cells or very few single cells indicate a grade 1 tumor. HE and MGG stains. **g**, **h** Grade 2 chondrosarcoma: these aspirates from 2 cases of conventional grade 2 chondrosarcoma show the difficulty of malignancy grading in FNA smears; rather uniform tumor cells with slight to moderate nuclear atypia, increased cellularity and dispersed tumor cells as well as a myxoid background indicate grade 2 chondrosarcoma. HE and MGG stains. **i** The corresponding cell block section shows moderately atypical chondrocytes and slightly myxoid areas indicating a malignancy grade higher than 1. HE stain. **j**, **k** Grade 3 chondrosarcoma: compared to grade 1 or 2 chondrosarcomas, there is marked cellular and nuclear atypia, predominantly dispersed single tumor cells, and a prominent myxoid background. HE and MGG stains. **l** The corresponding cell block section shows increased nuclear atypia and hyperchromasia. HE stain. Necrosis (**m**) and occasional mitosis (**n**) indicative of a higher malignancy grade. HE stain.

Specific for High-Grade Chondrosarcomas
- Abundant myxoid background matrix
- Relatively few fragments of hyaline cartilage
- Often high cellularity in the cartilage fragments
- High number of dispersed single cells
- Marked cellular and nuclear pleomorphism, prominent nucleoli
- Occasional mitoses

Ancillary Tests
Immunophenotype
Cartilaginous tumor cells express S100 in well-differentiated chondrosarcoma, while in poorly differentiated neoplasms the immunoreactivity for S100 is weak or absent. The immunoreactivity for vimentin is uniformly positive.

Genetics
Chondrosarcomas show complex karyotypes with both structural and numerical aberrations [27]. Mutations in the *IDH1* and *IDH2* genes are found in the majority of cases and are considered early tumorigenic events [28]. These changes can be detected by cytogenetics, FISH, SNP array, PCR, and NGS on available material.

Differential Diagnosis
- Chondroma
- Chondroblastic osteosarcoma
- Chordoma

The cytology of chondrosarcoma has been described in some rather large series and case reports [1, 29–35]. The cytologic features are closely related to the grade of malignancy. Low-grade chondrosarcomas yield tumor cells in fragments of variable size, and a dispersed cell pattern is an infrequent finding. Variable cellularity occurs in the fragments of cartilaginous tissue, with many cells lying in lacunar spaces. Individual tumor cells display a slight to moderate atypia and some of them are binucleated (Fig. 5d–f).

Smears from higher-grade tumors are generally hypercellular with cellular cartilage fragments and often a prominent myxoid background matrix (Fig. 5g–i). As a rule, the number of cartilage fragments is lower than in low-grade neoplasm, and dispersed tumor cells are much more com-

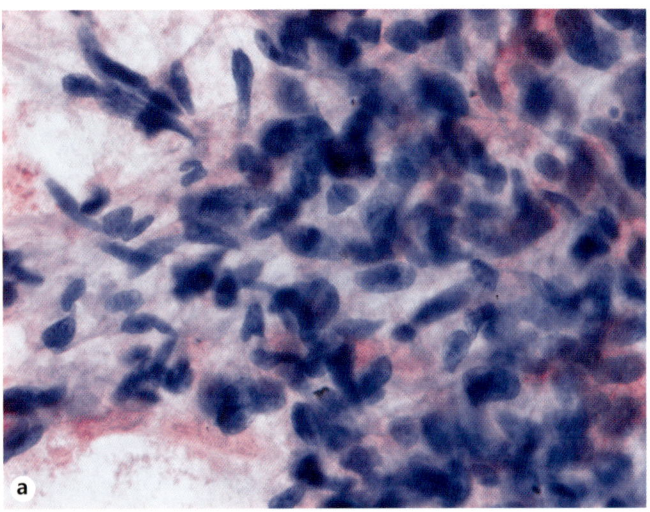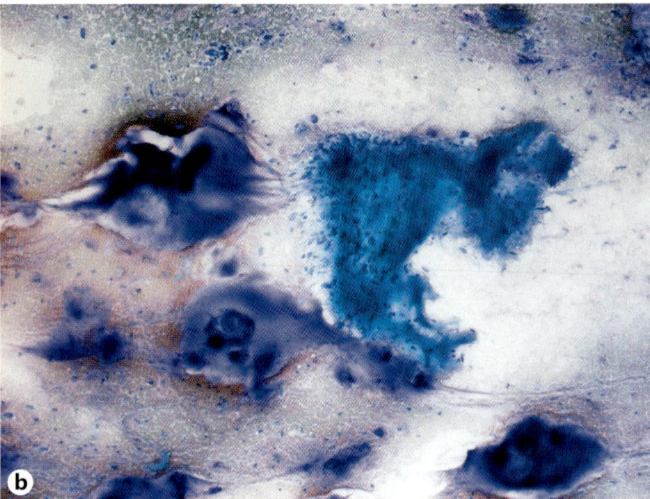

Fig. 6. Dedifferentiated chondrosarcoma. **a** Sampling only the high-grade component of dedifferentiated chondrosarcoma is a common pitfall in the FNA cytology of this bimorphic sarcoma. HE stain. **b** FNA smears display a high-grade sarcomatous component adjacent to the low-grade chondromatous component. MGG stain.

mon and occasionally the only component of smears (Fig. 5j, k). The cellular and nuclear pleomorphism is marked, and occasional mitoses and necrosis may be seen in smears, especially in grade 3 tumors (Fig. 5j–n). The accuracy of the grading of chondrosarcoma in FNA material was investigated by Lerma et al. [36], who found that concordance with the histologic grade was high in grade 2 and 3 tumors. Grade 1 chondrosarcomas are usually difficult to distinguish from benign chondromas in FNA smears, but a similar diagnostic dilemma is present in the examination of small biopsy samples, especially core-needle biopsies. This is not a very serious problem from a clinical point of view. In a retrospective analysis of the behavior of low-grade chondrosarcomas, Bauer et al. [37] demonstrated a similar long-term prognosis regarding recurrence rates and metastatic potential in 40 enchondromas and 40 low-grade chondrosarcomas, and concluded that the distinction between those neoplasms was of little clinical significance. The problem of distinguishing high-grade chondrosarcoma from chondroblastic osteosarcoma is addressed in Chapter 18 of this volume.

Smears from sacrum and spine chordomas may occasionally be difficult to distinguish from those of high-grade chondrosarcomas [38]. The structure of the myxoid matrix in chordoma is, however, different from that in chondrosarcoma. The matrix of chordoma is typically fibrillar and forms a network of thin strands encircling individual cells, either singly or in groups. Furthermore, the large, cytoplasm-rich, and vacuolated physaliferous cells with central nuclei are present in smears of every case of chordoma, but not in chondrosarcoma [38]. In addition, the immunocytochemical demonstration of epithelial markers and brachyury positivity is useful in distinguishing chordoma from chondrosarcoma [39, 40].

Dedifferentiated Chondrosarcoma

Dedifferentiated chondrosarcoma progresses in approximately 10–15% of chondrosarcomas and has a very aggressive clinical course. The transition from a low-grade chondrosarcoma component to a high-grade noncartilaginous pleomorphic or spindle cell sarcoma area is usually abrupt, and the proportions of 2 components are very variable. A dedifferentiated chondrosarcoma diagnosis is hard to render from FNA specimens alone [41–43]. Sampling only 1 of the components is a common pitfall in the FNA cytology diagnosis of this high-grade bimorphic sarcoma (Fig. 6a, b)

Clear Cell Chondrosarcoma

Clear cell chondrosarcoma is a rare variant of low-grade chondrosarcoma, commonly arising in the epiphyses of long bones. However, other bones of the skeleton, including the skull, spine, and hand and foot bones, may be affected.

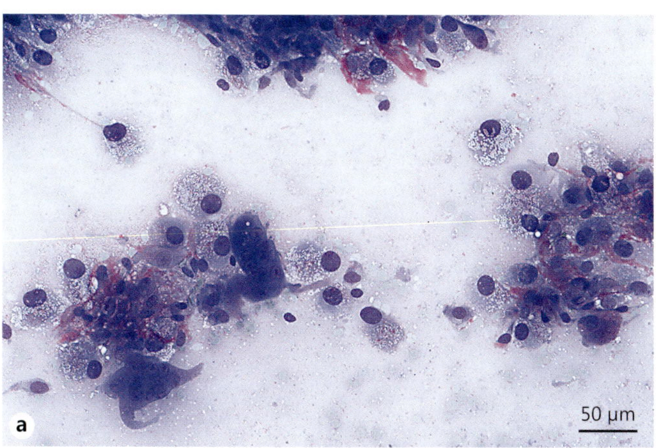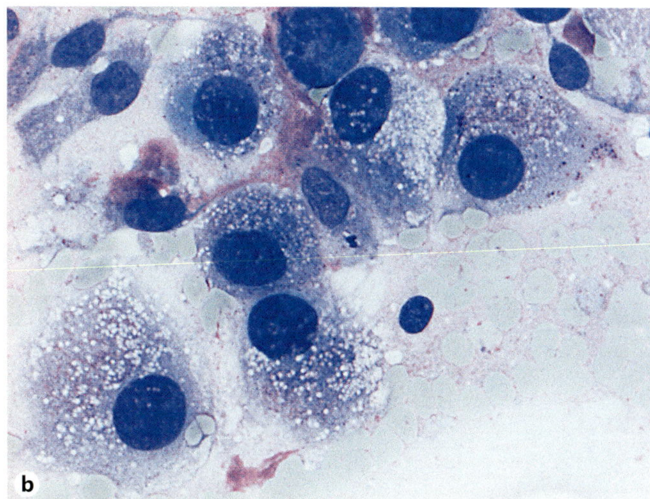

Fig. 7. Clear-cell chondrosarcoma. **a**, **b** The FNA smears are cellular and dominated by large epithelioid tumor cells with an abundant, finely vacuolated cytoplasm, round to oval eccentric or central nuclei, fragments of cartilage, and occasional osteoclast-like giant cells. MGG stain.

Clear cell chondrosarcoma comprises about 2% of all chondrosarcomas and arises in a younger age group than conventional chondrosarcoma, with a peak of incidence in the third decade of life and a male:female ratio of 2:1.

The FNA smears are cellular and dominated by large epithelioid tumor cells with an abundant, finely vacuolated cytoplasm and round to oval eccentric or central nuclei (Fig. 7a, b). Fragments of cartilage and occasional osteoclast-like cells are also present [44]. The main differential diagnoses include chondroblastoma and metastatic carcinoma, especially clear cell renal cell carcinoma [43].

Cytologic Features
- Hypercellular smears
- Small cartilaginous fragments in a background of myxoid matrix
- Large (epithelioid) tumor cells with a well demarcated, abundant vacuolated cytoplasm
- Hyperchromatic nuclei with central nucleoli
- Occasional osteoclast-like giant cells

Ancillary Tests
Immunophenotype
Positive for S100 in the chondroblastoma-like cells.

Genetics
Cytogenetically, extra copies of chromosome 20 and loss or rearrangements of 9p have been detected [45]. *TP53* overexpression can be found in the absence of other mutations [46]. These changes can be detected by cytogenetics, FISH, SNP array, PCR, and NGS on available material.

Differential Diagnosis
- Chondroblastoma
- Metastatic adenocarcinoma

Only one small series and single cases of clear cell chondrosarcoma have been reported. The most important differential diagnosis is chondroblastoma. Compared to chondroblastoma, tumor cells in FNA smears of clear cell chondrosarcoma lack nuclear grooves of chondroblasts and generally show a somewhat more prominent nuclear pleomorphism and hyperchromatic nuclei with prominent nucleoli. Compared to metastatic carcinomas, cells of clear cell chondrosarcoma show strong immunoreactivity for S100 protein and negativity for keratins.

Mesenchymal Chondrosarcoma

Mesenchymal chondrosarcoma is a rare, high-grade bimorphic malignant tumor composed of islands of low-grade hyaline cartilage and malignant small round cells. Mesenchymal chondrosarcomas account for less than 3% of all primary chondrosarcomas. Most cases occur in the second and third decades of life. The craniofacial bones (jawbones), ribs, vertebrae, and the ilium are the most common sites.

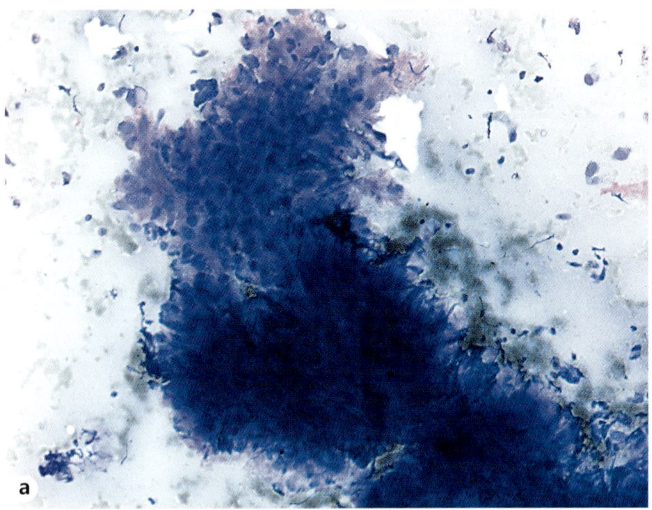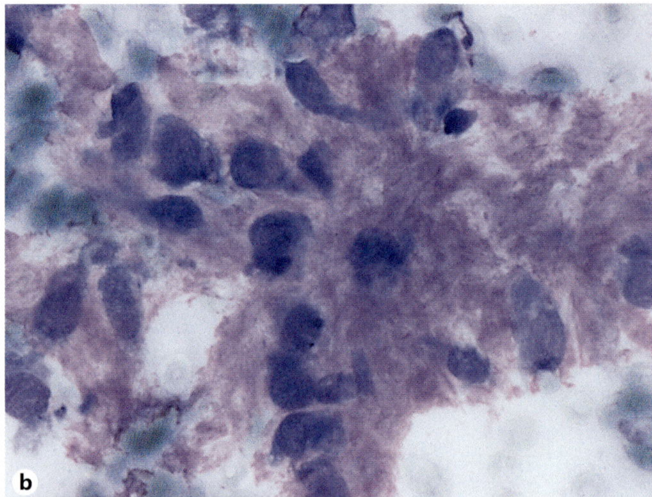

Fig. 8. Mesenchymal chondrosarcoma. **a, b** Clusters of small cells with round to oval, irregular nuclei and a sparse cytoplasm embedded in a blue-violet collagenous or cartilaginous matrix. MGG stain.

Approximately 30% of mesenchymal chondrosarcomas arise primarily in extraskeletal sites, commonly in meninges and somatic soft tissues.

The cytologic features of mesenchymal chondrosarcoma in FNA smears have been reported in a small series and a few case reports [47–53]. Smears contain small, blue, round (Ewing sarcoma-like) tumor cells in cohesive clusters, some embedded in a fibrillar matrix (Fig. 8a, b). Fragments of cartilaginous matrix may be found as well as osteoclast-like giant cells. The main differential diagnoses include Ewing sarcoma, small cell osteosarcoma, and non-Hodgkin lymphoma.

Cytologic Features
- Hypercellular smears
- Clusters of small cells with sparse cytoplasm and rounded, ovoid, sometimes elongated nuclei
- Coarse nuclear chromatin and small nucleoli
- Variable presence of fibrillar myxoid matrix associated with the cell clusters
- Variable presence of cartilaginous matrix and osteoclastic giant cells

Ancillary Tests
Immunophenotype
The small cell component shows positive reactivity for CD99, SOX9, variable positivity for desmin, and negative immunoreactivity for FLI-1 and CD45. The cartilaginous component shows variable immunoreactivity for S100 protein.

Genetics
A recurrent and specific *HEY1-NCOA2* gene fusion is found in this subtype of chondrosarcoma and it is notably missing in the other variants of the disease. The pathogenetic mechanism of the fusion is not fully elucidated but it could upregulate transcription [54]. The *IDH1* and *IDH2* mutations seen in the conventional chondrosarcomas are usually missing [28]. These changes can be detected by FISH, SNP array, PCR, and NGS on available material.

Differential Diagnosis
- Ewing sarcoma
- Small cell osteosarcoma
- Non-Hodgkin lymphoma

A biphasic pattern of cartilaginous fragments and small blue round cells support the diagnosis mesenchymal chondrosarcoma in FNA smears. When a biphasic pattern is not obvious and smears only show a small round cell population, the differential diagnosis includes other small cell malignancies, and correlations to clinical and radiographic data as well as ancillary techniques are necessary for a correct diagnosis. The typical immunophenotype of mesenchymal chondrosarcoma is S100 protein positivity in the cartilaginous component and CD99 and SOX9 positivity in the small cell population. Negative staining for FLI-1 and CD45 help in distinguishing mesenchymal chondrosarcoma from Ewing sarcoma and non-Hodgkin lymphoma. Small cell osteosarcoma may exhibit CD99 membrane positivity in some cases, which may cause a problem in distinguishing it from mesenchymal chondrosarcoma.

References

1 Chhabra S, Chopra R, Handa U, Punia RS, Mohan H: Cytomorphologic features of chondroid neoplasms: a comparative study. Acta Cytol 2010;54: 1101–1110.
2 Bridge JA, Nelson M, Orndal C, Bhatia P, Neff JR: Clonal karyotypic abnormalities of the hereditary multiple exostoses chromosomal loci 8q24.1 (EXT1) and 11p11–12 (EXT2) in patients with sporadic and hereditary osteochondromas. Cancer 1998;82:1657–1663.
3 Jennes I, Pedrini E, Zuntini M, Mordenti M, Balkassmi S, Asteggiano CG, Casey B, Bakker B, Sangiorgi L, Wuyts W: Multiple osteochondromas: mutation update and description of the multiple osteochondromas mutation database (MOdb). Hum Mutat 2009;30:1620–1627.
4 Walaas L, Kindblom LG, Gunterberg B, Bergh P: Light and electron microscopic examination of fine-needle aspirates in the preoperative diagnosis of cartilaginous tumors. Diagn Cytopathol 1990;6: 396–408.
5 Akerman M, Domanski HA: The cytology of soft tissue tumours. Monogr Clin Cytol 2003;16:1– 112.
6 Swarts SJ, Neff JR, Johansson SL, Nelson M, Bridge JA: Significance of abnormalities of chromosomes 5 and 8 in chondroblastoma. Clin Orthop Relat Res 1998;349:189–193.
7 Krishnappa A, Shobha SN, Shankar SV, Aradhya S: Fine needle aspiration cytology of chondroblastoma: a report of two cases with brief review of pitfalls. J Cytol 2016;33:40–42.
8 Cozzolino I, Zeppa P, Zabatta A, Merolla F, Vetrani A, Sadile F: Benign chondroblastoma on fine-needle aspiration smears: a seven-case experience and review of the literature. Diagn Cytopathol 2015;43:734–738.
9 Malukani K, Nandedkar SS, Yeshwante P, Rihal P: Fine needle aspiration cytology of chondroblastoma of the fibula. J Cytol 2014;31:233–235.
10 Akhtar K, Qadri S, Sen Ray P, Sherwani RK: Cytological diagnosis of chondroblastoma: diagnostic challenge for the cytopathologist. BMJ Case Rep 2014;2014:bcr2014204178.
11 Hernandez Martinez SJ, Campa Nunez H, Ornelas Cortinas G, Garza Garza R: Chondroblastoma of the fourth lumbar vertebra diagnosed by aspiration biopsy: case report and review of the literature. Acta Cytol 2011;55:473–477.
12 Gudi N, Venkatesh Reddy VR, Chidanand KJ: Chondroblastoma patella presenting as a pathological fracture. Indian J Orthop 2008;42:100–101.
13 Cabrera RA, Almeida M, Mendonca ME, Frable WJ: Diagnostic pitfalls in fine-needle aspiration cytology of temporomandibular chondroblastoma: report of two cases. Diagn Cytopathol 2006; 34:424–429.
14 Pohar-Marinsek Z, Us-Krasovec M, Lamovec J: Chondroblastoma in fine needle aspirates. Acta Cytol 1992;36:367–370.

15 Ascoli V, Facciolo F, Muda AO, Martelli M, Nardi F: Chondroblastoma of the rib presenting as an intrathoracic mass: report of a case with fine needle aspiration biopsy, immunocytochemistry and electron microscopy. Acta Cytol 1992;36:423–429.
16 Fanning CV, Sneige NS, Carrasco CH, Ayala AG, Murray JA, Raymond AK: Fine needle aspiration cytology of chondroblastoma of bone. Cancer 1990;65:1847–1863.
17 Kilpatrick SE, Pike EJ, Geisinger KR, Ward WG: Chondroblastoma of bone: use of fine-needle aspiration biopsy and potential diagnostic pitfalls. Diagn Cytopathol 1997;16:65–71.
18 Romeo S, Duim RA, Bridge JA, Mertens F, de Jong D, Dal Cin P, Wijers-Koster PM, Debiec-Rychter M, Sciot R, Rosenberg AE, Szuhai K, Hogendoorn PC: Heterogeneous and complex rearrangements of chromosome arm 6q in chondromyxoid fibroma: delineation of breakpoints and analysis of candidate target genes. Am J Pathol 2010;177: 1365–1376.
19 Gupta S, Dev G, Marya S: Chondromyxoid fibroma: a fine-needle aspiration diagnosis. Diagn Cytopathol 1993;9:63–65.
20 Layfield LJ, Ferreiro JA: Fine-needle aspiration cytology of chondromyxoid fibroma: a case report. Diagn Cytopathol 1988;4:148–151.
21 Estrada-Villasenor E, Cedillo ED, Martinez GR, Chavez RD: Periosteal chondromyxoid fibroma: a case study using imprint cytology. Diagn Cytopathol 2005;33:402–406.
22 Daneshbod Y, Khademi B: Chondromyxoid fibroma of the mandible: a diagnostic pitfall on aspiration cytology of parotid. Acta Cytol 2008;52:636–638.
23 Siddiqui B, Faridi S, Faizan M, Sherwani RK: Cytodiagnosis of chondromyxoid fibroma of the metatarsal head: a case report. Iran J Pathol 2016; 11:272–275.
24 Sreedharanunni S, Gupta N, Rajwanshi A, Bansal S, Vaiphei K: Fine needle aspiration cytology in two cases of chondromyxoid fibroma of bone and review of literature. Diagn Cytopathol 2013;41: 904–908.
25 Bergman S, Madden CR, Geisinger KR: Fine-needle aspiration biopsy of chondromyxoid fibroma: an investigation of four cases. Am J Clin Pathol 2009;132:740–745.
26 Hazarika D, Kumar RV, Rao CR, Mukherjee G, Pattabhiraman V, Shekar MC: Fine needle aspiration cytology of chondroblastoma and chondromyxoid fibroma: a report of two cases. Acta Cytol 1994;38:592–596.
27 Bridge JA, Bhatia PS, Anderson JR, Neff JR: Biologic and clinical significance of cytogenetic and molecular cytogenetic abnormalities in benign and malignant cartilaginous lesions. Cancer Genet Cytogenet 1993;69:79–90.

28 Amary MF, Bacsi K, Maggiani F, Damato S, Halai D, Berisha F, Pollock R, O'Donnell P, Grigoriadis A, Diss T, Eskandarpour M, Presneau N, Hogendoorn PC, Futreal A, Tirabosco R, Flanagan AM: *IDH1* and *IDH2* mutations are frequent events in central chondrosarcoma and central and periosteal chondromas but not in other mesenchymal tumours. J Pathol 2011;224:334–343.
29 Wahane RN, Lele VR, Bobhate SK: Fine needle aspiration cytology of bone tumors. Acta Cytol 2007;51:711–720.
30 Dodd LG: Fine-needle aspiration of chondrosarcoma. Diagn Cytopathol 2006;34:413–418.
31 Skoog L, Pereira ST, Tani E: Fine-needle aspiration cytology and immunocytochemistry of soft-tissue tumors and osteo/chondrosarcomas of the head and neck. Diagn Cytopathol 1999;20:131–136.
32 Kreicbergs A, Bauer HC, Brosjo O, Lindholm J, Skoog L, Soderlund V: Cytological diagnosis of bone tumours. J Bone Joint Surg Br 1996;78:258–263.
33 Wakely PE Jr, Geisinger KR, Cappellari JO, Silverman JF, Frable WJ: Fine-needle aspiration cytopathology of soft tissue: chondromyxoid and myxoid lesions. Diagn Cytopathol 1995;12:101–105.
34 Kumar RV, Hazarika D, Mathews T, Rao CR, Satpute S: Fine needle aspiration biopsy cytology of chondrosarcoma. Indian J Pathol Microbiol 1993; 36:436–441.
35 Abdul-Karim FW, Wasman JK, Pitlik D: Needle aspiration cytology of chondrosarcomas. Acta Cytol 1993;37:655–660.
36 Lerma E, Tani E, Brosjo O, Bauer H, Soderlund V, Skoog L: Diagnosis and grading of chondrosarcomas on FNA biopsy material. Diagn Cytopathol 2003;28:13–17.
37 Bauer HC, Brosjo O, Kreicbergs A, Lindholm J: Low risk of recurrence of enchondroma and low-grade chondrosarcoma in extremities: 80 patients followed for 2–25 years. Acta Orthop Scand 1995; 66:283–288.
38 Layfield LJ: Cytologic differential diagnosis of myxoid and mucinous neoplasms of the sacrum and parasacral soft tissues. Diagn Cytopathol 2003;28:264–271.
39 Moriki T, Takahashi T, Wada M, Ueda S, Ichien M, Miyazaki E: Chondroid chordoma: fine-needle aspiration cytology with histopathological, immunohistochemical, and ultrastructural study of two cases. Diagn Cytopathol 1999;21:335–339.
40 Jo VY, Hornick JL, Qian X: Utility of brachyury in distinction of chordoma from cytomorphologic mimics in fine-needle aspiration and core needle biopsy. Diagn Cytopathol 2014;42:647–652.
41 Dee S, Meneses M, Ostrowski ML, Murakami M, Horowitz M, Graf W: Pleomorphic ("dedifferentiated") chondrosarcoma: report of a case initially examined by fine needle aspiration biopsy. Acta Cytol 1991;35:467–471.

42 Faquin WC, Pilch BZ, Keel SB, Cooper TL: Fine-needle aspiration of dedifferentiated chondrosarcoma of the larynx. Diagn Cytopathol 2000;22: 288–292.

43 Akerman M, Domanski HA, Jonsson K: Cytological features of bone tumours in FNA smears II: cartilaginous tumours. Monogr Clin Cytol 2010; 19:31–44.

44 Jiang XS, Pantanowitz L, Bui MM, Esther R, Budwit D, Dodd LG: Clear cell chondrosarcoma: cytologic findings in six cases. Diagn Cytopathol 2014; 42:784–791.

45 Mandahl N, Gustafson P, Mertens F, Akerman M, Baldetorp B, Gisselsson D, Knuutila S, Bauer HC, Larsson O: Cytogenetic aberrations and their prognostic impact in chondrosarcoma. Genes Chromosomes Cancer 2002;33:188–200.

46 Park YK, Park HR, Chi SG, Ushigome S, Unni KK: Overexpression of p53 and absent genetic mutation in clear cell chondrosarcoma. Int J Oncol 2001;19:353–357.

47 Cheim AP Jr, Queiroz TL, Alencar WM, Rezende RM, Vencio EF: Mesenchymal chondrosarcoma in the mandible: report of a case with cytological findings. J Oral Sci 2011;53:245–247.

48 Trembath DG, Dash R, Major NM, Dodd LG: Cytopathology of mesenchymal chondrosarcomas: a report and comparison of four patients. Cancer 2003;99:211–216.

49 Jaetli V, Gupta S: Mesenchymal chondrosarcoma of maxilla: a rare case report. Med Oral Patol Oral Cir Bucal 2011;16:e493–e496.

50 Misra V, Singh PA: Cytodiagnosis of extraosseous mesenchymal chondrosarcoma of meninges: a case report. Acta Cytol 2008;52:366–368.

51 Gonzalez-Campora R, Otal Salaverri C, Gomez Pascual A, Hevia Vazquez A, Galera Davidson H: Mesenchymal chondrosarcoma of the retroperitoneum: report of a case diagnosed by fine needle aspiration biopsy with immunohistochemical, electron microscopic demonstration of S100 protein in undifferentiated cells. Acta Cytol 1995;39: 1237–1243.

52 Doria MI Jr, Wang HH, Chinoy MJ: Retroperitoneal mesenchymal chondrosarcoma: report of a case diagnosed by fine needle aspiration cytology. Acta Cytol 1990;34:529–532.

53 Handa U, Singhal N, Punia RS, Garg S, Mohan H: Cytologic features and differential diagnosis in a case of extraskeletal mesenchymal chondrosarcoma: a case report. Acta Cytol 2009;53:704–706.

54 Wang L, Motoi T, Khanin R, Olshen A, Mertens F, Bridge J, Dal Cin P, Antonescu CR, Singer S, Hameed M, Bovee JV, Hogendoorn PC, Socci N, Ladanyi M: Identification of a novel, recurrent *HEY1-NCOA2* fusion in mesenchymal chondrosarcoma based on a genome-wide screen of exon-level expression data. Genes Chromosomes Cancer 2012;51:127–139.

Domanski HA, Walther CS: FNA Cytology of Soft Tissue and Bone Tumors. Monogr Clin Cytol.
Basel, Karger, 2017, vol 22, pp 161–164 (DOI: 10.1159/000475108)

Ewing Sarcoma

Ewing Sarcoma

Ewing sarcoma is a primitive small round cell neoplasm showing pathognomonic molecular findings. A subset of the neoplasm, traditionally named "peripheral neuroectodermal tumor" (PNET), is defined when the tumor cells display neuroectodermal differentiation. In the World Health Organization's 2013 classification, both neoplasms share the same name of Ewing sarcoma. The term "Ewing family of tumors" has been used to summarize subtypes of Ewing sarcoma showing a slightly variable morphology, variable ultrastructure, and clinical presentation with different sites of involvement. However, several studies demonstrated that all those neoplasms belong to the same group of small round cell tumors defined by *EWSR1-ETS* gene fusions that generate specific chimeric transcripts.

Ewing sarcoma is the third most frequent primary bone sarcoma after osteosarcoma and chondrosarcoma, and the second most common bone sarcoma in children and young adults after osteosarcoma, accounting for 6–8% of all primary sarcoma of bone. These neoplasms are rare before the age of 5 years and after the age of 30 years, and extremely rare in elderly patients. In our files going back to 1980, 1 patient aged 67 years was diagnosed with skeletal Ewing sarcoma, and 1 patient was diagnosed with extraskeletal Ewing sarcoma at the age of 80 years. Approximately 80% of cases arise in patients younger than 20 years of age.

The most common sites are the shafts of the long bones, the pelvic bones, ribs, and spine. However, Ewing sarcoma may arise in almost every bone in the skeleton, including the craniofacial bones and the scapula.

Skeletal Ewing sarcoma is an aggressive tumor characterized by a permeative or moth-eaten growth pattern, periosteal involvement, and a soft tissue component. The tumor is often not very well defined with conventional radiography. Frequently, an extensive spiculated periosteal reaction is evident as "hair-on-end" or several "onion peel"-type layers. Ewing sarcoma is, in most cases, a medullary lesion, but the radiographic signs of malignancy are most prominent in the cortical bone. The soft tissue component is usually prominent with a tumor growth surrounding the entire bone.

Cytologic Features
- Generally a rich yield
- A mixture of clustered cells and dispersed cells
- High N:C ratio
- Stripped nuclei and a cytoplasmic "tigroid" background are common (best appreciated in the air-dried smears)
- Double cell population: large, "light" cells with a fragile cytoplasm containing vacuoles and round to oval bland nuclei with inconspicuous nucleoli; small, dark cells with rounded irregular nuclei and a scant/poorly preserved cytoplasm
- The dark cells are often arranged in small molded groups within the cell clusters
- An occasional moderately cellular and nuclear pleomorphism
- Rosette-like structures with a more or less evident fibrillary center

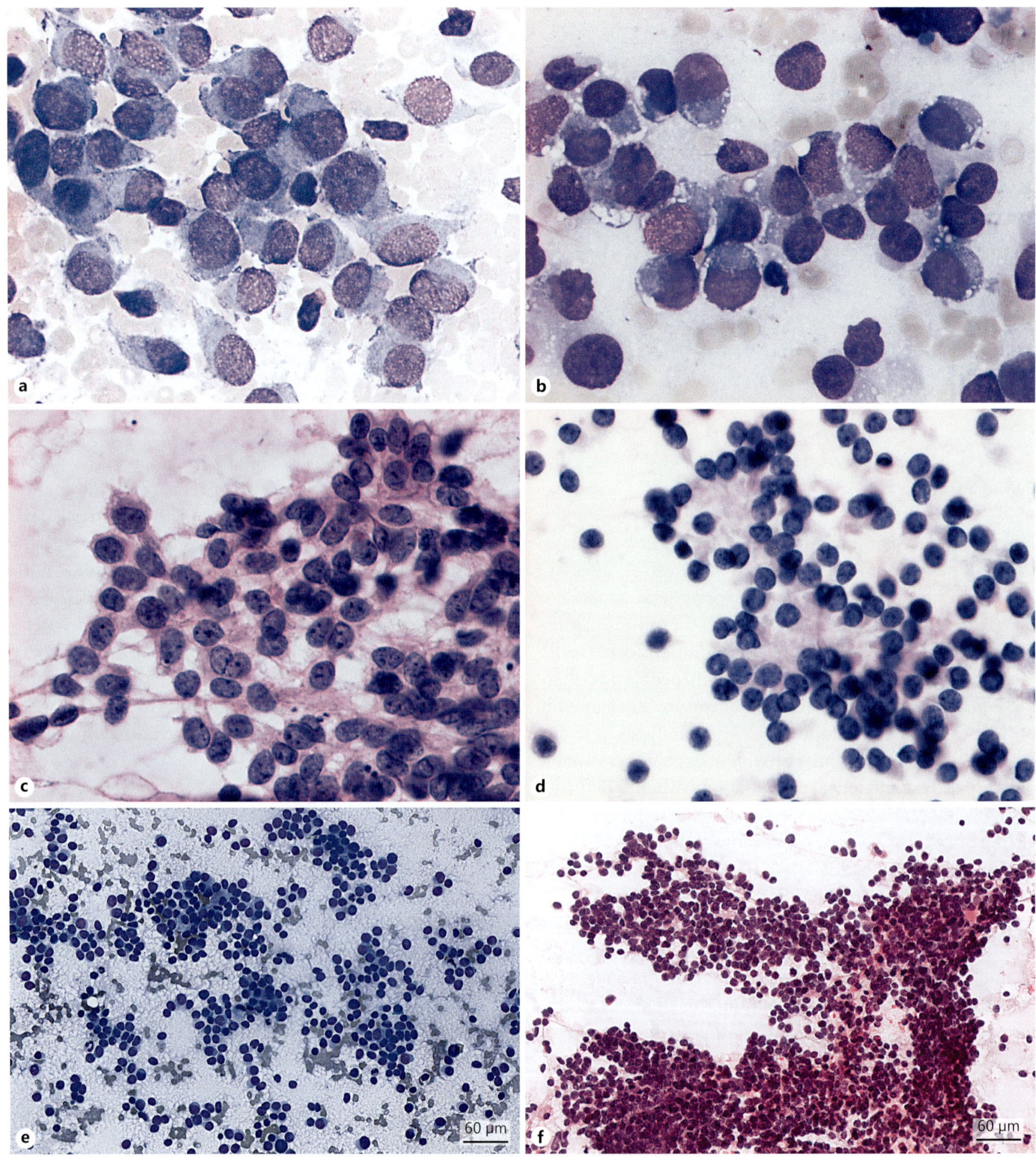

Fig. 1. Ewing sarcoma/PNET. **a** Smears showing dispersed, moderately pleomorphic tumor cells with round to oval nuclei and occasionally cytoplasmic projections. MGG stain. **b** Tumor cells with a rhabdoid morphology may be present in PNET smears. MGG stain. **c** A variable degree of cellular pleomorphism is often observed in smears of PNET. HE stain. **d** Rosette-like structures appear more often in PNET smears than in smears of conventional Ewing sarcoma. MGG stain. **e, f** Typically hypercellular smears of conventional Ewing sarcoma showing small uniform round cells with a high N:C ratio. MGG and HE stains. **g** A diffuse and strong membranous staining pattern for CD99 is considered highly sensitive but not specific for Ewing sarcoma. Cell block, CD99.

(Figure continued on next page.)

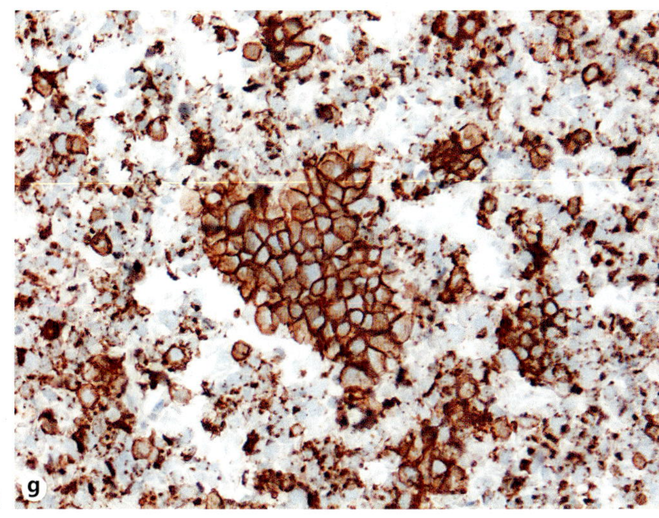

Specific for "PNET"

- The 2 cell types are less evident
- Presence of spindle-shaped cells with cytoplasmic extensions (Fig. 1a)
- Cells with ovoid/fusiform nuclei are common
- Tumor cells with a rhabdoid morphology may be present (Fig. 1b)
- Variable degree of cellular pleomorphism, including anisokaryosis, hyperchromasia, and prominent nucleoli (Fig. 1c)
- Mitoses and rosette-like structures appear more often than in smears of conventional Ewing sarcoma (Fig. 1d)

Ancillary Tests

Immunophenotype

Strong, diffuse, and membranous positivity for CD99 (in more than 90% of cases); positive for FLI-1 (nuclear); in about 30% of cases focal expression of keratin, S100, and CD117. Negative for smooth muscle actin, desmin, MyoD-1, myogenin, WT1, CD45, TdT, CD56, and TLE1. The differentiated subtype (previously termed PNET) expresses neuroectodermal markers such as neuron-specific enolase, chromogranin A, and synaptophysin.

Histochemistry

Cytoplasmic periodic acid-Schiff positivity in classical Ewing sarcoma.

Genetics

The most common mutation in Ewing sarcoma is the translocation t(11;22)(q24;q12), which fuses the *EWSR1* gene on chromosome 22 and the *FLI1* gene on chromosome 11. It is present in 85% of cases [1]. The resulting fusion protein has an oncogenic effect as an aberrant transcription factor leading to uncontrolled growth and proliferation [2]. Other translocations fusing the *EWSR1* gene with other *FLI1*-related genes exist but are less common [3]. These genetic changes are useful diagnostic traits that can be detected with cytogenetics, fluorescence in situ hybridization, polymerase chain reaction, and next-generation sequencing on available material [4–10].

Differential Diagnosis

- Small cell osteosarcoma
- Mesenchymal chondrosarcoma
- Non-Hodgkin lymphoma (precursor lymphoma)
- Neuroblastoma/esthesioneuroblastoma
- Poorly differentiated synovial sarcoma

The cytologic diagnostic criteria of Ewing sarcoma have been established in several publications. A correct diagnosis requires technically satisfactory smears, and preferably both air-dried and wet-fixed smears (Fig. 1e, f). The double-cell population, large light cells with round nuclei and a finely chromatin texture, small nucleoli, and "thin" cytoplasm often containing clear spaces or vacuoles as well as small dark cells with hyperchromatic nuclei and a scanty cytoplasm, are better appreciated in the air-dried smears, as is the "tigroid" background (see "Extraskeletal Ewing Sarcoma" in Chapter 16 of this volume). Nuclear characteristics are better appreciated in wet-fixed smears stained with hematoxylin and eosin (HE) or Papanicolaou stains. When only wet-fixed material is available, Ewing sarcoma may be difficult to determine from other small round cell malignancies. Despite the fact that routinely stained smears often suggest a diagnosis of Ewing sarcoma, ancillary studies remain necessary to confirm the diagnosis. A diffuse and strong membranous staining pattern for CD99 and nuclear staining of FLI-1 are considered highly sensitive but not specific for Ewing sarcoma (Fig. 1g). These markers should be used together with a panel of other antibodies to exclude other small round cell tumors, such as alveolar rhabdomyosarcoma, lymphoblastic lymphoma, and poorly differentiated synovial sarcoma. A distinction between small cell osteosarcoma and Ewing sarcoma is difficult. The presence of osteoid and/or positive alkaline phosphatase staining in fine-needle aspiration smears favors a diagnosis of small cell osteosarcoma. Mesenchymal chondrosarcoma is a differential diagnostic problem in those cases where the small cell population predominates and fragments of hyaline cartilage are difficult to find. Demonstration of the characteristic chromosomal aberration is considered the gold standard for diagnosing Ewing sarcoma with relatively easily obtained results using different molecular techniques. Common soft tissue extension of skeletal Ewing sarcoma can be misinterpreted as a true soft tissue neoplasm prior to a radiologic investigation. The clinical setting of other small round cell tumors determines to some extent which of the possible differential diagnoses are the most relevant in a given case (e.g., esthesioneuroblastoma occurs in the nasopharyngeal space, neuroblastoma occurs in children below the age of 5 years, etc.).

References

1 Turc-Carel C, Aurias A, Mugneret F, Lizard S, Sidaner I, Volk C, Thiery JP, Olschwang S, Philip I, Berger MP, et al: Chromosomes in Ewing's sarcoma. I. An evaluation of 85 cases of remarkable consistency of t(11;22)(q24;q12). Cancer Genet Cytogenet 1988;32:229–238.

2 Smith R, Owen LA, Trem DJ, Wong JS, Whangbo JS, Golub TR, Lessnick SL: Expression profiling of EWS/FLI identifies *NKX2.2* as a critical target gene in Ewing's sarcoma. Cancer Cell 2006;9:405–416.

3 Patocs B, Nemeth K, Garami M, Arato G, Kovalszky I, Szendroi M, Fekete G: Multiple splice variants of *EWSR1-ETS* fusion transcripts co-existing in the Ewing sarcoma family of tumors. Cell Oncol 2013;36:191–200.

4 Gautam U, Srinivasan R, Rajwanshi A, Bansal D, Marwaha RK, Vasishtha RK: Reverse transcriptase-polymerase chain reaction as an ancillary molecular technique in the diagnosis of small blue round cell tumors by fine-needle aspiration cytology. Am J Clin Pathol 2010;133:633–645.

5 Kang SH, Perle MA, Nonaka D, Zhu H, Chan W, Yang GC: Primary Ewing sarcoma/PNET of the kidney: fine-needle aspiration, histology, and dual color break apart FISH Assay. Diagn Cytopathol 2007;35:353–357.

6 Sanati S, Lu DW, Schmidt E, Perry A, Dehner LP, Pfeifer JD: Cytologic diagnosis of Ewing sarcoma/peripheral neuroectodermal tumor with paired prospective molecular genetic analysis. Cancer 2007;111:192–199.

7 Jambhekar NA, Bagwan IN, Ghule P, Shet TM, Chinoy RF, Agarwal S, Joshi R, Amare Kadam PS: Comparative analysis of routine histology, immunohistochemistry, reverse transcriptase polymerase chain reaction, and fluorescence in situ hybridization in diagnosis of Ewing family of tumors. Arch Pathol Lab Med 2006;130:1813–1818.

8 Pohar-Marinsek Z: Difficulties in diagnosing small round cell tumours of childhood from fine needle aspiration cytology samples. Cytopathology 2008;19:67–79.

9 Kumar R, Gautam U, Srinivasan R, Lal A, Sharma U, Nijhawan R, Kumar S: Primary Ewing's sarcoma/primitive neuroectodermal tumor of the kidney: report of a case diagnosed by fine needle aspiration cytology and confirmed by immunocytochemistry and RT-PCR along with review of literature. Diagn Cytopathol 2012;40(suppl 2):E156–E161.

10 Klijanienko J, Couturier J, Bourdeaut F, Freneaux P, Ballet S, Brisse H, Lagace R, Delattre O, Pierron G, Vielh P, Sastre-Garau X, Michon J: Fine-needle aspiration as a diagnostic technique in 50 cases of primary Ewing sarcoma/peripheral neuroectodermal tumor. Institute Curie's experience. Diagn Cytopathol 2012;40:19–25.

Domanski HA, Walther CS: FNA Cytology of Soft Tissue and Bone Tumors. Monogr Clin Cytol.
Basel, Karger, 2017, vol 22, pp 165–170 (DOI: 10.1159/000475109)

Giant Cell Tumor of Bone and Other Giant Cell-Rich Lesions

Giant Cell Tumor

Giant cell tumor (GCT) is a benign but locally aggressive neoplasm comprising approximately 5% of all primary bone tumors. This neoplasm displays a tendency for local recurrences and approximately 2% of GCTs develop pulmonary metastasis, so-called benign metastasizing GCT [1–3]. True malignant transformation occurs in less than 1% of GCTs. Most patients are between 20 and 45 years of age and GCT is very rare in the immature skeleton of patients younger than 15 years of age. The most common locations are the distal femur, proximal tibia, distal radius, and proximal humerus. GCT may less frequently arise in the vertebral bones of the spine, usually in the sacrum, but flat bones are rarely involved, with the exception of pelvic bones, especially the ilium. This tumor always involves the epiphysis or metaphysis. Very rarely the lesion arises in young individuals before closure of the growth plate, and in such cases the location is metaphyseal. The histologic pattern, characterized by a proliferation of mononuclear cells admixed with mononuclear macrophage-like cells and numerous large osteoclastic giant cells, is often modified by hemorrhage, necrosis, or reactive fibrous tissue. Areas resembling aneurysmal bone cyst (ABC) may be present.

At radiography GCTs are lytic, the cortical outline is often thin and may seem destroyed, but the tumor is almost always outlined and defined by the periosteum. GCT typically grows eccentrically, usually close to the subchondral bone and, depending on the size and the thickness of the cortex, there is risk of penetration into the adjacent joint and an increased risk of fractures.

Cytologic Features
- Hypercellular yield with both cohesive cell clusters and dispersed single cells
- Double-cell population: mononuclear spindle or round to ovoid cells and multinucleated osteoclasts
- Classical pattern of smears includes giant cells attached to the periphery of clusters of mononuclear cells
- Mononuclear cells contain nuclei with open chromatin and prominent nucleoli
- The size of nuclei in mononuclear cells is comparable to that in the osteoclastic giant cells
- Usually an absence of osteoid and cartilaginous matrix

Ancillary Tests
Immunophenotype
Mononuclear cells may express CD45, CD33, and CD68, while the giant cells express cathepsin K and vitronectin receptor CD51.

Genetics
About 50% of the tumors show chromosomal end-to-end fusions without loss of material, so-called telomeric association, as well as other structural and numerical aberrations. No clear relationship between cytogenetic changes and the

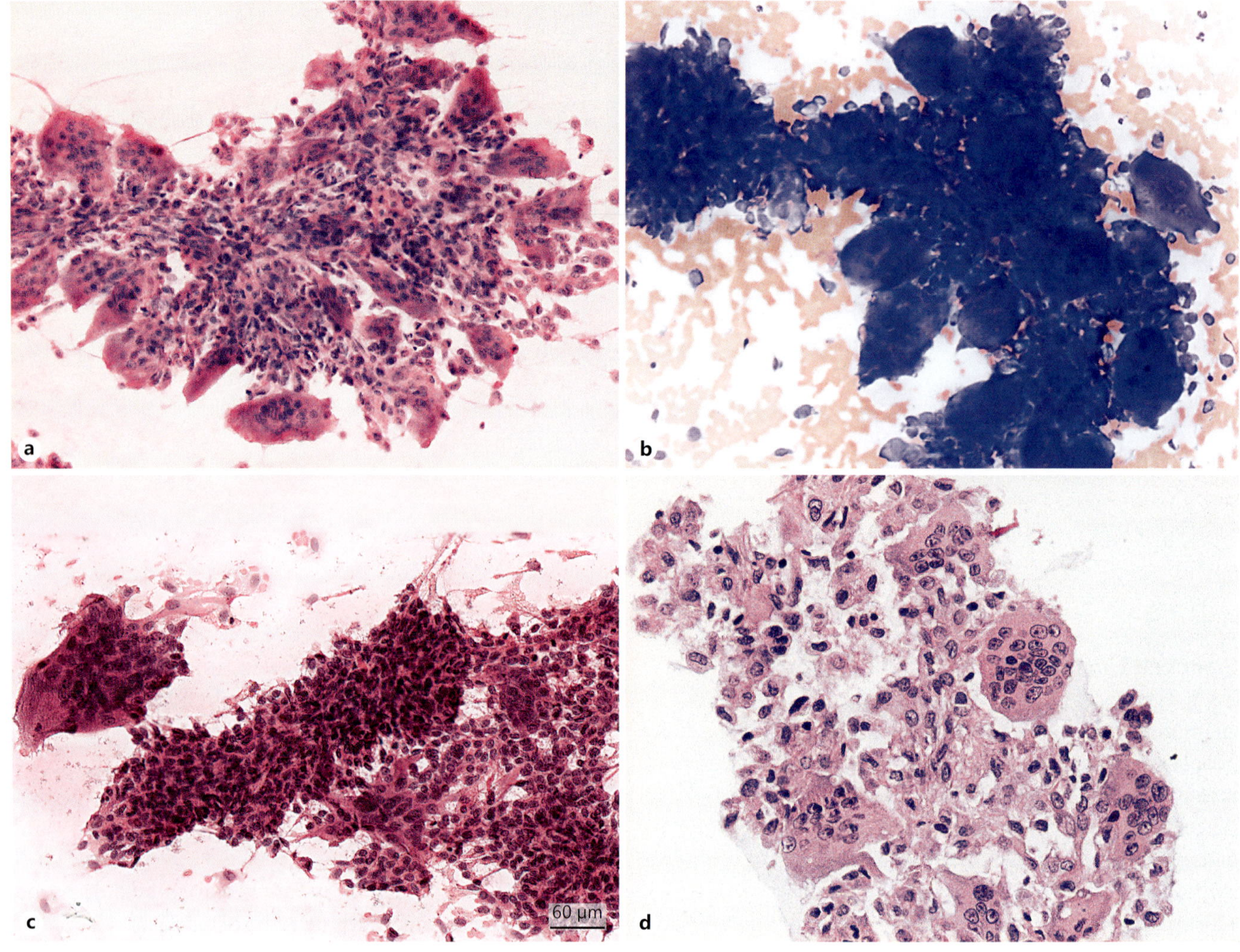

Fig. 1. GCT. **a–b** Cohesive clusters of slightly pleomorphic rounded, ovoid, or spindle cells bordered by multiple multinucleated giant cells. HE and MGG stains. **c** The morphology of GCT may also show overlapping features with other benign giant cell lesions occurring in the skeleton. HE stain. **d** Cell block prepared from the aspirated material corresponds well with cytology. HE stain.

clinical outcome is known [4]. The pathogenetic function of the telomeric fusions are not known [5]. These changes can be detected by cytogenetics, fluorescence in situ hybridization (FISH), single nucleotide polymorphism (SNP) array, and next-generation sequencing (NGS) on available material.

Differential Diagnosis

- ABC
- Brown tumor of hyperparathyroidism
- Reparative giant cell granuloma
- Osteoblastoma
- High-grade osteosarcoma (giant cell-rich osteosarcoma)

Due to their expansive and destructive growth with thinning of the cortical bone, most GCTs are easy to needle and the material is usually abundant. The cytologic features of conventional GCT have been described in some series and case reports [6–13]. Although it has been emphasized that smears of GCT are characterized by clusters of mononuclear cells bordered by giant cells at the periphery (Fig. 1a, b), similar patterns may also be seen in smears from brown tumors of hyperparathyroidism. The morphology of other benign giant cell lesions occurring in the skeleton may also show overlapping features with GCT in fine-needle aspiration (FNA) smears (Fig. 1c, d).

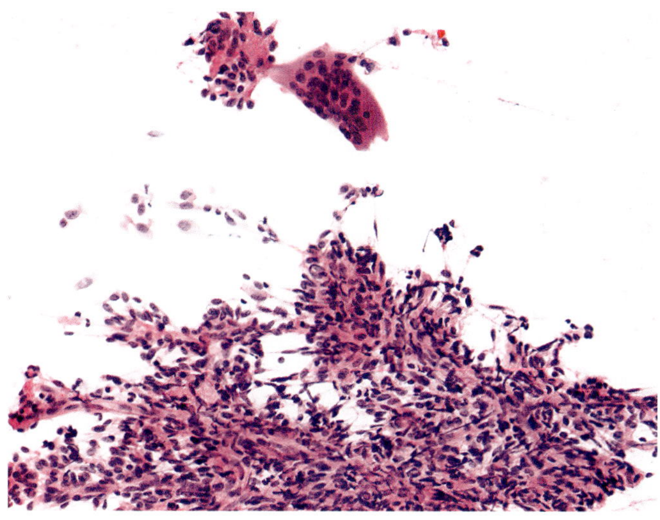

Fig. 2. Giant cell reparative granuloma. A loose cluster of oval and spindle cells with an admixture of some giant cells. HE stain.

From a clinical point of view, the most important differential diagnosis is giant cell-rich osteosarcoma. The marked pleomorphism of the tumor cells in giant cell-rich osteosarcoma helps to distinguish it from GCT. In smears with numerous giant cells and few mononuclear cells, it is wise to complement FNA cytology by core biopsy before reporting a definitive benign diagnosis. With regard to the differential diagnosis of other benign tumors/lesions with smears containing numerous giant cells, knowledge of clinical and radiographic data is essential for a correct diagnosis.

Giant Cell Reparative Granuloma

Giant cell reparative granuloma is a benign reactive tumor-like lesion occurring in the craniofacial bones and the small tubular bones of the hands and feet. The so-called solid variant of ABC and giant cell reparative granuloma likely represent the same process, and they share the same translocation involving the *USP6* gene with classic ABC. Most patients are between 10 and 30 years of age. Giant cell reparative granuloma may occur in normal bone secondary to trauma or hemorrhage, or may be associated with lesions such as brown tumor of hyperparathyroidism. This neoplasm consisting of fibrous tissue with randomly distributed giant cells, reactive bone formations, hemorrhage, and hemosiderin depositions mimics other giant cell lesions in smears, and it is cytomorphologically indistinguishable from GCT

and brown tumor (Fig. 2). Giant cell reparative granulomas are lytic and expansile lesions that involve the metaphysis and diaphysis, but can expand to the epiphysis of tubular bones of the hands and feet. The overlying cortex is thin, but not destroyed. There are no calcifications.

Radiologically, giant cell reparative granuloma may resemble several other entities, including GCT, ABC, brown tumor of hyperparathyroidism, and enchondroma.

Cytologic Features [14]
- Hypercellular yield with sheets and clusters of spindle cells
- Multinucleated giant cells
- Osteoblasts
- Histiocytes
- Lack of significant cytologic atypia

Ancillary Tests
Immunophenotype
Mononuclear cells at least focally express vimentin, CD68, and CD45.

Genetics
No diagnostic genetic changes are known.

Differential Diagnosis
- Conventional GCT
- ABC
- Brown tumor of hyperparathyroidism

From our experience of single cases of giant cell reparative granuloma examined by FNA cytology, it is difficult or impossible to distinguish reparative granuloma from GCT and ABC in FNA smears.

Aneurysmal Bone Cyst

ABC is a multilocular, expansile, locally destructive, benign neoplasm. ABC may affect any bone, but approximately 60% of lesions arise in the vertebral column of any level, including the sacrum, the craniofacial bones, and metaphysis of long tubular bones. The majority (80%) of patients are younger than 20 years of age, but ABC may affect all age groups. Both sexes are equally affected. Approximately 30% of ABC is associated with another tumor/lesion occurring in bone, commonly with GCT, osteoblastoma, chondroblastoma, and chondromyxoid fibroma. The cystic cavities of ABC may present themselves on plain radiography as thin sclerotic tra-

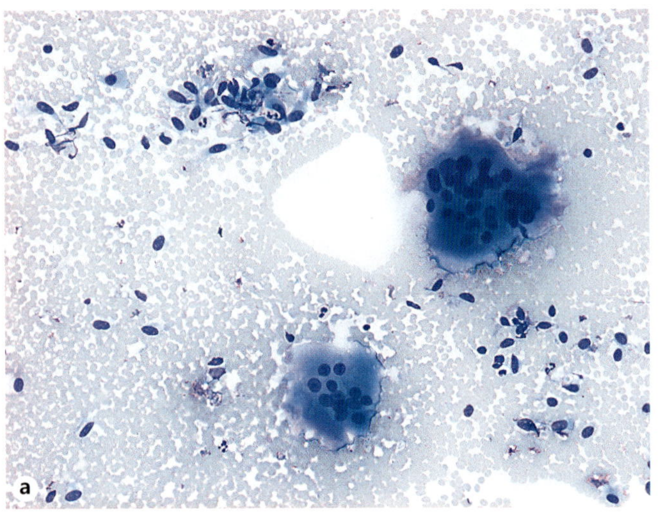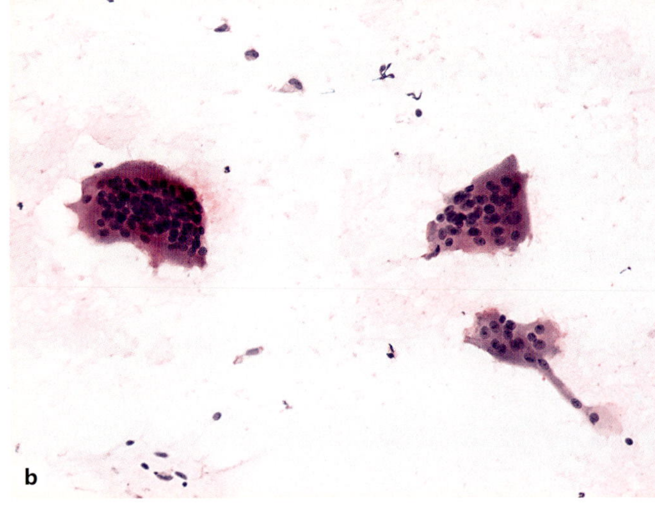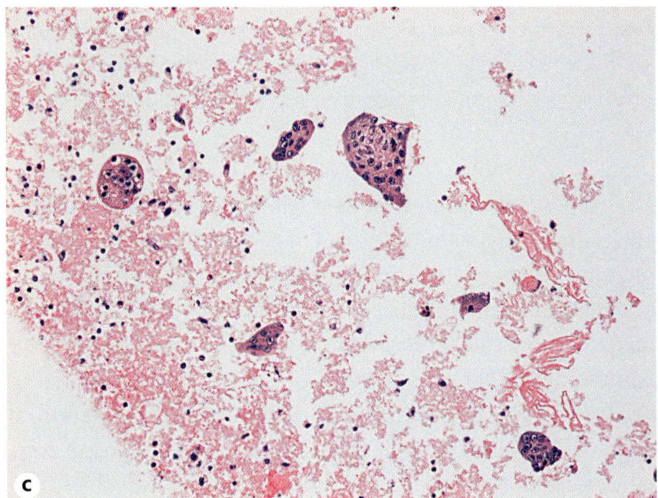

Fig. 3. ABC. **a**, **b** Hypocellular smears showing dispersed spindle or ovoid cells and scattered osteoclastic giant cells. MGG and HE stains. **c** Cell block prepared from the aspirated material shows scattered osteoclast-like giant cells, single spindle cells, and inflammatory cells. HE stain.

beculae. The lesion is eccentrically located, lytic, and surrounded by a rim of sclerosis. The cortical surface of the affected bone is expanded and ballooned, often with loss of cortical definition and extension into the adjacent soft tissue, which may appear as a malignant tumor. Radiologically, the lesion can be confused with a GCT but the localization differs in the long bones. With CT and MRI, characteristic localized fluid levels may be seen within the cystic spaces.

Cytologic Features
- Hemorrhagic aspirates and hypocellular aspirates
- Variable numbers of multinucleated giant cells
- Variable presence of clusters of spindled myofibroblastic cells
- Histiocytes and inflammatory cells
- Lack of significant cytologic atypia

Ancillary Tests
Immunophenotype
Immunocytochemical examinations serve little role in the cytologic diagnosis of ABC.

Genetics
The *USP6* gene at 17p13 is commonly rearranged in these tumors. Different cytogenetic changes, including the translocation t(16;17)(q22;p13), lead to fusions and upregulation of *USP6* [15]. This can be used for diagnostic purposes and detected with cytogenetics, FISH, SNP array, and NGS on available material.

Differential Diagnosis
- Conventional GCT
- Solitary bone cyst

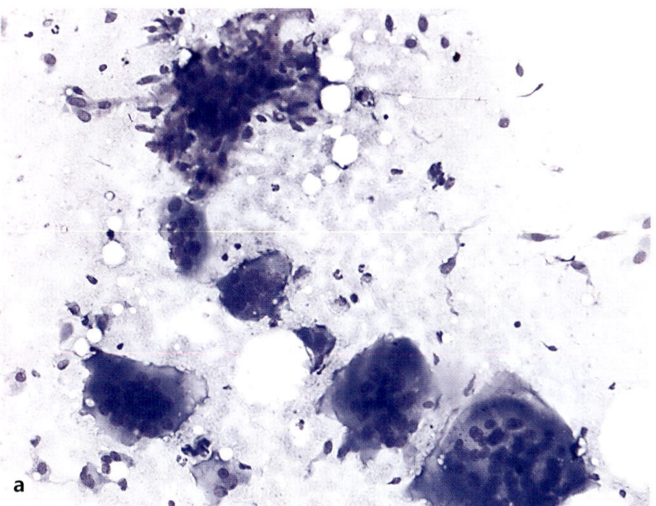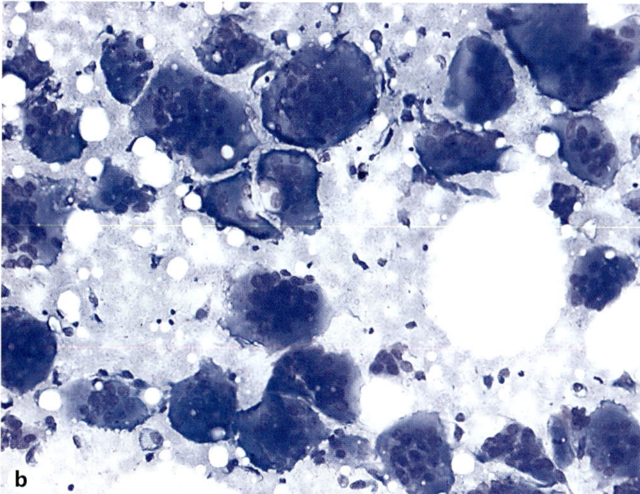

Fig. 4. Brown tumor of hyperparathyroidism. Smears show small clusters and few dispersed spindle cells with an admixture of osteoclast-like giant cells (**a**) or predominantly osteoclastic giant cells and single scattered spindle cells (**b**). MGG stain.

- Brown tumor of hyperparathyroidism
- Giant cell reparative granuloma
- Telangiectatic osteosarcoma

The cytologic features of ABC have been recorded in single series and case reports [16–19]. The cytomorphology of ABC shares many signs with other giant cell lesions and does not permit a precise diagnosis (Fig. 3a–c). In our experience, most ABCs are diagnosed as benign tumors with osteoclast-like giant cells or as solitary bone cysts. Radiologic and clinical data are necessary for making a specific diagnosis. Recently, *USP6* gene rearrangement has been identified in approximately 70% of primary ABC but not in secondary ABC, and only in the spindle cell myofibroblastic component, not in other cell types, such as multinucleated osteoclast-like giant cells.

Brown Tumor of Hyperparathyroidism

Brown tumor, formerly named osteitis fibrosa cystica, is a rare tumor-like lesion occurring in the skeleton and caused by a high level of parathyroid hormone in hyperparathyroidism. Brown tumor is commonly seen in patients with secondary hyperparathyroidism due to chronic renal failure. The predilection sites for this lesion are the facial and pelvic bones, ribs, and femur. The site in the long bones is predominantly diaphyseal or metaphyseal. The bone trabeculae in brown tumor are replaced by fibrous tissue containing variable amounts of osteoclastic giant cells and hemosiderin-laden macrophages secondary to hemorrhage.

Cytologic Features [20, 21]
- Dispersed spindle cells or small- to medium-sized clusters of spindle cells
- Osteoclast-like giant cells
- Hemosiderin-laden macrophages
- Lack of significant cytologic atypia

Ancillary Tests
Immunophenotype
Immunocytochemical examinations serve little role in the cytologic diagnosis of brown tumor.

Genetics
No recurrent diagnostic genetic changes are known.

Differential Diagnosis
- Conventional GCT
- ABC
- Giant cell reparative granuloma

Brown tumors are rare targets for FNA cytology. Single case reports have been published to date describing cytologic findings that are very similar to those in a GCT (Fig. 4a, b). Without knowledge of the clinical history and radiographic features, it may be impossible to distinguish a brown tumor from GCT and other giant cell lesions in FNA smears.

References

1 Cai G, Ramdall R, Garcia R, Levine P: Pulmonary metastasis of giant cell tumor of the bone diagnosed by fine-needle aspiration biopsy. Diagn Cytopathol 2007;35:358–362.

2 van Hoeven KH, Kellogg K, Bavaria JE: Pulmonary metastasis from histologically benign giant cell tumor of bone: report of a case diagnosed by fine needle aspiration cytology. Acta Cytol 1994;38:410–414.

3 Powers CN, Bull JM, Raval P, Schmidt WA: Fine-needle aspiration of a solitary pulmonary nodule following treatment of metastatic giant-cell tumor of bone. Diagn Cytopathol 1991;7:286–289.

4 Gorunova L, Vult von Steyern F, Storlazzi CT, Bjerkehagen B, Folleras G, Heim S, Mandahl N, Mertens F: Cytogenetic analysis of 101 giant cell tumors of bone: nonrandom patterns of telomeric associations and other structural aberrations. Genes Chromosomes Cancer 2009;48:583–602.

5 Gebre-Medhin S, Broberg K, Jonson T, Gorunova L, von Steyern FV, Brosjo O, Jin Y, Gisselsson D, Panagopoulos I, Mandahl N, Mertens F: Telomeric associations correlate with telomere length reduction and clonal chromosome aberrations in giant cell tumor of bone. Cytogenet Genome Res 2009;124:121–127.

6 Witt BL, Garcia CA, Cohen MB: Giant cell tumor of bone presenting in the lumbar spine of a 35-year-old female: cytodiagnosis and other diagnostic considerations. Diagn Cytopathol 2014;42:624–627.

7 Khare P, Kishore B, Gupta RJ, Vanita, Dhal A: GCT of proximal phalanx of ring finger: a case report. Diagn Cytopathol 2012;40(suppl 2):E165–E168.

8 Gupta A, Singh U, Singh P, Kundu ZS, Gupta S, Gupta S: Fine needle aspiration of a huge pelvic mass involving the iliac bone. Cytopathology 2009;20:63–65.

9 Volmar KE, Sporn TA, Toloza EM, Martinez S, Dodd LG, Xie HB: Giant cell tumor of rib masquerading as thymoma: a diagnostic pitfall in needle core biopsy of the mediastinum. Arch Pathol Lab Med 2004;128:452–455.

10 Jain M, Aiyer HM, Singh M, Narula M: Fine-needle aspiration diagnosis of giant cell tumour of bone presenting at unusual sites. Diagn Cytopathol 2002;27:375–378.

11 Saikia B, Goel A, Gupta SK: Fine-needle aspiration cytologic diagnosis of giant-cell tumor of the sacrum presenting as a rectal mass: a case report. Diagn Cytopathol 2001;24:39–41.

12 Vetrani A, Fulciniti F, Boschi R, Marino G, Zeppa P, Troncone G, Palombini L: Fine needle aspiration biopsy diagnosis of giant-cell tumor of bone: an experience with nine cases. Acta Cytol 1990;34:863–867.

13 Sneige N, Ayala AG, Carrasco CH, Murray J, Raymond AK: Giant cell tumor of bone: a cytologic study of 24 cases. Diagn Cytopathol 1985;1:111–117.

14 Kaw YT: Fine needle aspiration cytology of central giant cell granuloma of the jaw: a report of two cases. Acta Cytol 1994;38:475–478.

15 Oliveira AM, Perez-Atayde AR, Inwards CY, Medeiros F, Derr V, Hsi BL, Gebhardt MC, Rosenberg AE, Fletcher JA: *USP6* and *CDH11* oncogenes identify the neoplastic cell in primary aneurysmal bone cysts and are absent in so-called secondary aneurysmal bone cysts. Am J Pathol 2004;165:1773–1780.

16 Creager AJ, Madden CR, Bergman S, Geisinger KR: Aneurysmal bone cyst: fine-needle aspiration findings in 23 patients with clinical and radiologic correlation. Am J Clin Pathol 2007;128:740–745.

17 Yamamoto T, Nagira K, Akisue T, Marui T, Hitora T, Kawamoto T, Yoshiya S, Kurosaka M, Tsukamoto R: Fine-needle aspiration biopsy of solid aneurysmal bone cyst in the humerus. Diagn Cytopathol 2003;28:159–162.

18 Agarwal A, Goel P, Khan SA, Kumar P, Qureshi NA: Large aneurysmal bone cyst of iliac bone in a female child: a case report. J Orthop Surg Res 2010;5:24.

19 Yadavrao KA, Rajaram DS, Vijaykumar WJ, Langade YB: Fine needle aspiration cytology diagnosis of aneurysmal bone cyst: a case report. Indian J Pathol Microbiol 2007;50:425–426.

20 Galed Placed I, Patino-Seijas B, Pombo-Otero J, Alvarez-Rodriguez R: Fine needle aspiration diagnosis of brown tumor of the maxilla. Acta Cytol 2010;54:1076–1078.

21 Pavlovic S, Valyi-Nagy T, Profirovic J, David O: Fine-needle aspiration of brown tumor of bone: cytologic features with radiologic and histologic correlation. Diagn Cytopathol 2009;37:136–139.

Domanski HA, Walther CS: FNA Cytology of Soft Tissue and Bone Tumors. Monogr Clin Cytol.
Basel, Karger, 2017, vol 22, pp 171–174 (DOI: 10.1159/000477315)

Notochordal Tumors

Chordomas

Chordoma, a low-grade malignant tumor arising from remnants of the notochord, accounts for up to 4% of primary bone sarcomas. Chordoma most commonly occurs in the sixth to seventh decades of life and is very rare under the age of 30 years. Chordomas are almost exclusively located in the axial spine, with the sacrococcygeal region being the most common site (35–50% of all chordomas), followed by the spheno-occipital area, cervical spine, and thoracolumbar spine. Sacral chordoma is a slowly growing, locally destructive neoplasm, which tends to expand into soft tissue and into the rectum, occasionally with a palpable mass on rectal examination. Chordomas arising in the base of the skull may grow intracranially, invading the sella turcica, petrous, and sphenoid bones.

Chordomas are often difficult to diagnose by plain radiography due to the fact that bowel gas and content obscure the outlining of the sacrum. Large chordomas with soft tissue involvement may be overlooked due to overlying structures in the pelvis or cranium. CT and MRI are the methods of choice for diagnosing and to outlining these tumors. In the sacrum, the tumor destroys the cortex of the anterior as well as posterior face, often with a large soft tissue component. Calcifications are often found, likely representing residual bone. The radiologic findings of vertebral chordomas are of bone destruction, often with growth into the spinal canal. Chordomas have a lobulated growth pattern and the tumor lobules are separated by fibrous bands. An abundant myxoid matrix is always present. The tumor cells are arranged in sheets or cords, or seen as single elements floating in the background matrix. Typical tumor cells are large with an abundant multivacuolated cytoplasm and rounded or ovoid nuclei (physaliferous cells). The physaliferous cells are admixed with smaller, epithelioid-like or spindle cells. Cellular atypia is usually not prominent although multinucleated tumor giant cells and cells with hyperchromasia and prominent nucleoli may be present.

Cytologic Features
- Rich yield as a rule
- Abundant myxochondroid matrix
- Strands and clusters of medium-sized epithelial-like, at times binucleated cells
- Smaller round to oval and polygonal cells with a granular cytoplasm, slight to moderate anisokaryosis, bland chromatin, and small nucleoli
- Large epithelioid cells with an abundant (multi)vacuolated cytoplasm (physaliferous cells)
- Infrequent spindle cells
- Myxoid and fibrillar matrix encircles single cells and small clusters of cells
- Rare pleomorphic cells with prominent nucleoli and multinucleated tumor giant cells

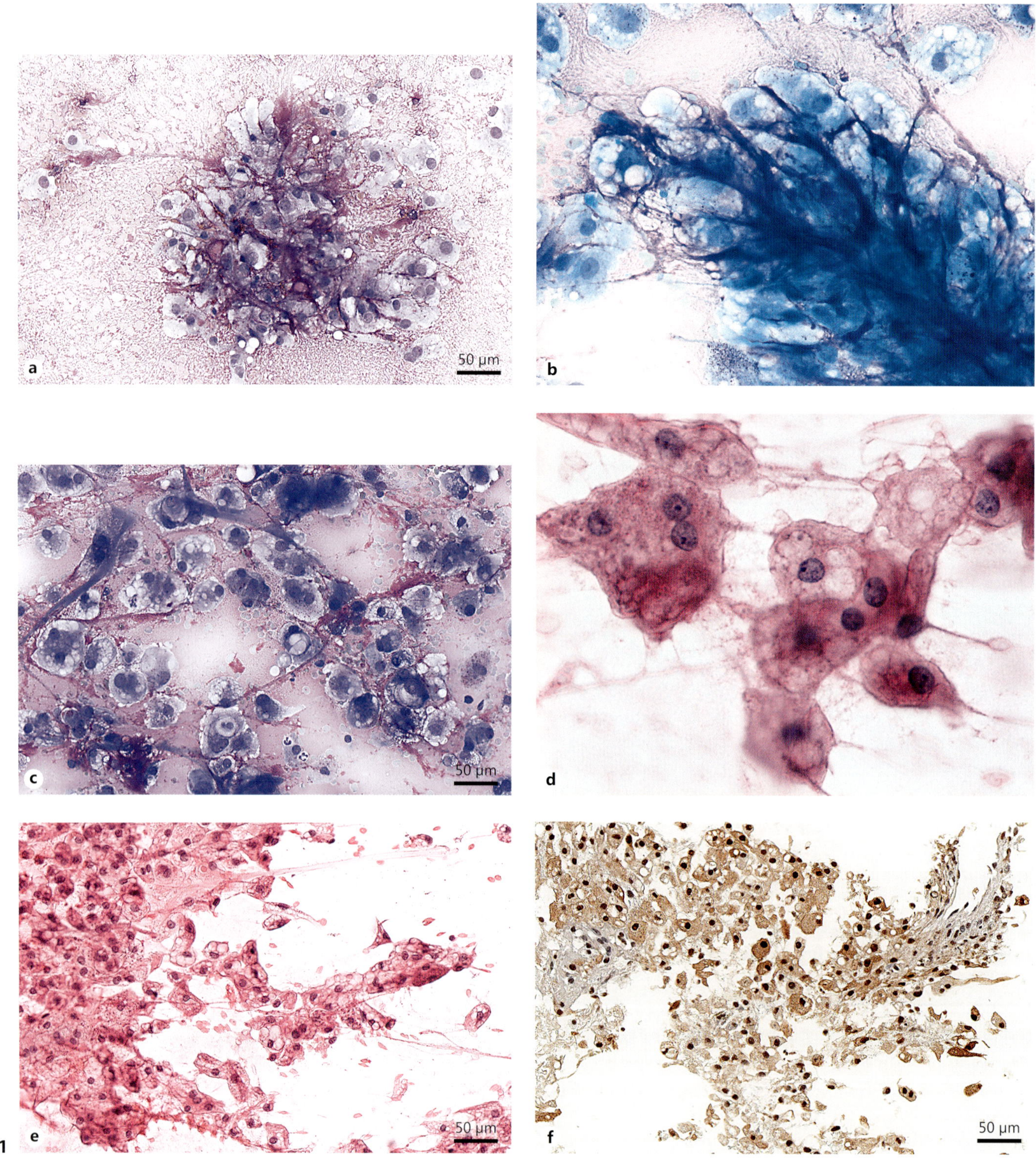

(For legend see next page.)

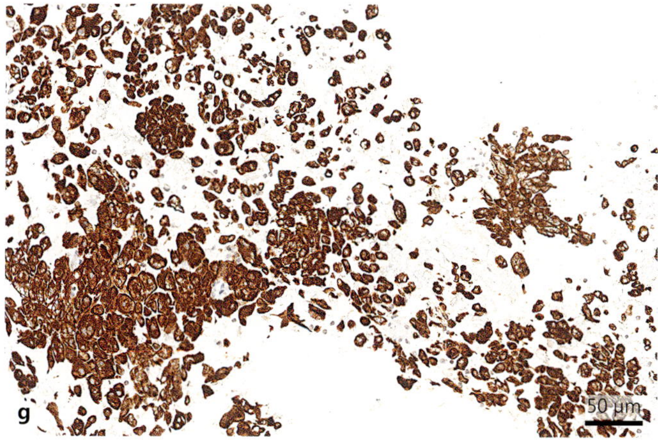

Fig. 1. Chordoma. **a**, **b** Loose clusters of tumor cells embedded in a fibrillary blue-violet myxoid matrix that encircles many single tumor cells. MGG stain. **c**, **d** Large cells corresponding to physaliferous cells, with an abundant, multivacuolated cytoplasm, and uniform, round nuclei with small nucleoli. MGG and HE stains. **e** The background matrix is usually less obvious in wet-fixed smears than in air-dried smears. HE stain. **f**, **g** Tumor cells are positive for S100 protein and keratin. Cell block; S100 and keratin.

Ancillary Tests

Immunophenotype

Chordomas express S100 protein together with epithelial membrane antigen (EMA) and/or low molecular weight keratin. Recently, staining with nuclear positivity has been shown to be highly sensitive and specific for chordomas [1].

Genetics

Cytogenetically, these tumors often display a near diploid or hypodiploid karyotype with numerous structural and numerical changes. Monosomy of chromosome 1 and gain of 7 are common [2]. Loss of 1 or both copies of the tumor suppressor genes *CDKN2A* and *CDKN2B* are also common findings [3]. These changes can be detected with cytogenetics, fluorescence in situ hybridization, single nucleotide polymorphism array, polymerase chain reaction, and next-generation sequencing on available material.

Differential Diagnosis

- Chondrosarcoma
- Clear cell- or mucin-producing adenocarcinoma
- Myxopapillary ependymoma

Although chordoma is a rare primary bone sarcoma, some series and case reports of chordomas examined by FNA have been published to date [4–23]. The distinctive cytologic features, including the abundant, myxoid, often fi-

brillar background substance, which appears like a network, encircles groups of cells and/or single tumor cells (Fig. 1a, b), and the presence of the physaliferous cells with their abundant, "bubbly" cytoplasm allows the correct diagnosis to be made in most cytologically examined cases (Fig. 1c, d). The myxoid matrix is intensely red-blue or violet in May-Grünwald-Giemsa (MGG) and DiffQuick, pale pink in hematoxylin and eosin (HE), and pale green-gray in Papanicolaou stain. However, in wet-fixed smears the background matrix is usually less obvious (Fig. 1e) than in air-dried smears, and this feature together with the presence of vacuolated epithelioid-like cells, sometimes with eccentric nuclei, might lead to an incorrect diagnosis of metastatic adenocarcinoma [24]. Typical physaliferous cells are not seen in chondrosarcoma, nor the fibrillar matrix encircling individual tumor cells. In addition, positive stains for S100 protein together with EMA and/or low molecular weight keratin typically seen in chordomas (Fig. 1f, g) is of great help in distinguishing chordoma from chondrosarcoma and metastatic adenocarcinoma [25–27]. Brachyury increases the sensitivity of chordoma diagnosis to 100% when added to the conventional panel of S100, EMA, and keratins [1]. Sacrococcygeal myxopapillary ependymoma is another, albeit very rare, differential diagnosis [10, 28, 29]. In the few cases of fine-needle aspiration cytology reported of this rare tumor, central mucinous cores surrounded by cuboidal or columnar cells in a rosette-like pattern was a typical finding and physaliphorous cells were not present.

References

1 Jo VY, Hornick JL, Qian X: Utility of brachyury in distinction of chordoma from cytomorphologic mimics in fine-needle aspiration and core needle biopsy. Diagn Cytopathol 2014;42:647–652.

2 Grabellus F, Konik MJ, Worm K, Sheu SY, van de Nes JA, Bauer S, Paulus W, Egensperger R, Schmid KW: MET overexpressing chordomas frequently exhibit polysomy of chromosome 7 but no MET activation through sarcoma-specific gene fusions. Tumour Biol 2010;31:157–163.

3 Hallor KH, Staaf J, Jonsson G, Heidenblad M, Vult von Steyern F, Bauer HC, Ijszenga M, Hogendoorn PC, Mandahl N, Szuhai K, Mertens F: Frequent deletion of the CDKN2A locus in chordoma: analysis of chromosomal imbalances using array comparative genomic hybridisation. Br J Cancer 2008;98:434–442.

4 Castro M, Aslan D, Manivel JC, Pambuccian SE: Parapharyngeal chordoma: a diagnostic challenge and potential mimic of pleomorphic adenoma on fine-needle aspiration cytology. Diagn Cytopathol 2013;41:85–91.

5 Kanthan R, Senger JL: Fine-needle aspiration cytology with histological correlation of chordoma metastatic to the lung: a diagnostic dilemma. Diagn Cytopathol 2011;39:927–932.

6 Permi HS, Kishan Prasad H, Veena S, Teerthanath S: Presacral chordoma diagnosed by transrectal fine-needle aspiration cytology. J Cytol 2011;28:89–90.

7 Hernandez-Leon N, Coll-Mesa L, Rodriguez-Rodriguez R, Garcia-Hernandez S, Brito-Garcia A, Gonzalez-Gaitano M, Martin-Corriente C: Fine needle aspiration cytology of primary or recurrent chordomas. Cytopathology 2011;22:340–342.

8 Moonda AH, Ganesan S: Images in cytology: fine-needle aspiration of a lumbar chordoma. Diagn Cytopathol 2010;38:900–901.

9 Saiz A, de Agustin P, Barrios AP, Alberti N: Fine-needle aspiration of a chordoma and its recurrence 19 years after. Diagn Cytopathol 2006;34:663–664.

10 Layfield LJ: Cytologic differential diagnosis of myxoid and mucinous neoplasms of the sacrum and parasacral soft tissues. Diagn Cytopathol 2003;28:264–271.

11 Kay PA, Nascimento AG, Unni KK, Salomao DR: Chordoma: cytomorphologic findings in 14 cases diagnosed by fine needle aspiration. Acta Cytol 2003;47:202–208.

12 Gupta RK, Cheung YK, Al Ansari AG, Naran S, Lallu S, Fauck R: Diagnostic value of image-guided needle aspiration cytology in the assessment of vertebral and intervertebral lesions. Diagn Cytopathol 2002;27:191–196.

13 Crapanzano JP, Ali SZ, Ginsberg MS, Zakowski MF: Chordoma: a cytologic study with histologic and radiologic correlation. Cancer 2001;93:40–51.

14 Gupta RK, AlAnsari AG: Value of image-guided needle aspiration cytology in the assessment of thoracolumbar and sacrococcygeal masses. Acta Cytol 1996;40:215–221.

15 Hazarika D, Kumar RV, Muniyappa GD, Mukherjee G, Rao CR, Narasimhamurthy NK, Shenoy AM, Nanjundappa: Diagnosis of clival chordoma by fine needle aspiration of an oropharyngeal mass: a case report. Acta Cytol 1995;39:507–510.

16 Das DK, Francis IM, AbuZeidan FM: Fine-needle aspiration (FNA) cytology diagnosis of a sacrococcygeal chordoma and its recurrence. Diagn Cytopathol 1994;10:194–195.

17 Caballero C, Fontaniere B: Sacrococcygeal chordoma: fine needle aspiration cytological findings and differential diagnosis. Cytopathology 1993;4:311–313.

18 Hughes DE, Lamb J, Salter DM, al-Nafussi A: Fine-needle aspiration cytology in a case of chordoma. Cytopathology 1992;3:129–133.

19 Walaas L, Kindblom LG: Fine-needle aspiration biopsy in the preoperative diagnosis of chordoma: a study of 17 cases with application of electron microscopic, histochemical, and immunocytochemical examination. Hum Pathol 1991;22:22–28.

20 Plaza JA, Ballestin C, Perez-Barrios A, Martinez MA, de Agustin P: Cytologic, cytochemical, immunocytochemical and ultrastructural diagnosis of a sacrococcygeal chordoma in a fine needle aspiration biopsy specimen. Acta Cytol 1989;33:89–92.

21 Nijhawan VS, Rajwanshi A, Das A, Jayaram N, Gupta SK: Fine-needle aspiration cytology of sacrococcygeal chordoma. Diagn Cytopathol 1989;5:404–407.

22 Thompson SK, Callery RT: Cytologic diagnosis of a chordoma without physaliforous cells. Diagn Cytopathol 1988;4:144–147.

23 Mondal A, Mukherjee PK: Cytological and cytochemical diagnosis of chordoma by fine needle aspiration biopsy – a case report. Indian J Pathol Microbiol 1988;31:64–66.

24 Chivukula M, Rao R, Macchi J, Ghazala F, Rao RN, Komorowski R, Shidham VB: FNAB cytology of chordoma masquerading as adenocarcinoma: case report. Diagn Cytopathol 2002;26:306–309.

25 Moriki T, Takahashi T, Wada M, Ueda S, Ichien M, Miyazaki E: Chondroid chordoma: fine-needle aspiration cytology with histopathological, immunohistochemical, and ultrastructural study of two cases. Diagn Cytopathol 1999;21:335–339.

26 Gherardi G, Marveggio C, Cola C, Redaelli G: Decisive role of immunocytochemistry in aspiration cytology of chordoma of the clivus: a case report with review of the literature. J Laryngol Otol 1994;108:426–430.

27 Plate KH, Bittinger A: Value of immunocytochemistry in aspiration cytology of sacrococcygeal chordoma: a report of two cases. Acta Cytol 1992;36:87–90.

28 Kulesza P, Tihan T, Ali SZ: Myxopapillary ependymoma: cytomorphologic characteristics and differential diagnosis. Diagn Cytopathol 2002;26:247–250.

29 Kumar ND, Misra K: Fine needle aspiration cytodiagnosis of subcutaneous sacrococcygeal myxopapillary ependymoma: a case report. Acta Cytol 1990;34:851–854.

FNA Cytology of Soft Tissue and Bone Tumors

Domanski HA, Walther CS: FNA Cytology of Soft Tissue and Bone Tumors. Monogr Clin Cytol.
Basel, Karger, 2017, vol 22, pp 175–180 (DOI: 10.1159/000477316)

Lymphohematopoietic and Histiocytic Tumors

Plasma Cell Neoplasm: Solitary Plasmacytoma and Plasma Cell Myeloma

Plasma cell neoplasms of the bone constitute a spectrum of clonal proliferations of plasma cells, including plasma cell myeloma with osteolytic defects of the skeleton and monoclonal protein in the serum, and solitary plasmacytoma of bone, both composed of identical neoplastic plasma cells. The cytologic and immunocytochemical features of cells from solitary plasmacytoma of bone are indistinguishable from those of multiple myeloma of bone. Solitary plasmacytoma and plasma cell myeloma represent the most common primary bone neoplasms. Plasma cell myeloma arises predominantly in elderly patients with a peak of incidence in the sixth and seventh decades of life and is very rare in individuals younger than 40 years of age. Solitary plasmacytoma occurs in somewhat younger patients with a median age of 55 years and a male to female ratio of approximately 2:1. Those lesions are most common in bones with active hematopoiesis such as the vertebrae, ribs, skull, femur, pelvic bones, scapula, and clavicle.

Solitary plasmacytoma of bone is often a well-circumscribed, expansile lytic lesion within the bone marrow and with a geographic pattern. The overlying cortical bone is often thin and a cortical perforation may be seen on CT or MRI. The tumor often looks benign on plain radiography.

Due to cortical bone destruction, plasma cell neoplasms are most often easy to needle and the yield is rich (Fig. 1a). It may be difficult to distinguish reactive plasmacytosis from solitary plasmacytoma/multiple myeloma in bloody, hypo-cellular smears containing only normal-appearing or slightly atypical plasma cells (Fig. 1b, c). A cytologic diagnosis may be even more difficult when the sample is admixed with a prominent component of normal bone marrow cells. Flow cytometric analysis and/or immunocytochemical studies are necessary for a definitive diagnosis.

Cytologic Features [1–3]
- Often hemorrhagic smears
- Predominantly dispersed cells but small clusters of loosely cohesive cells may be seen
- Variable cell differentiation from normal-looking plasma cells to highly pleomorphic (bi- or multinucleated) cells
- Occasionally, cells have a plasmablastic morphology (immunoblast-like cells with prominent central nucleoli)

Ancillary Tests
Immunophenotype
The neoplastic plasma cells express monotypic immunoglobulin light chains and heavy chains and, in most cases, express CD138, CD79A, plasma cell transcription factor MUM1 (nuclear staining) and, in approximately 40% of cases, epithelial membrane antigen (EMA).

Genetics
In the majority of cases these tumors display polysomies with gains of several chromosomes, including 3, 5, 7, 9, 11, 15, and 19 [4]. The remaining cases without the polysomies

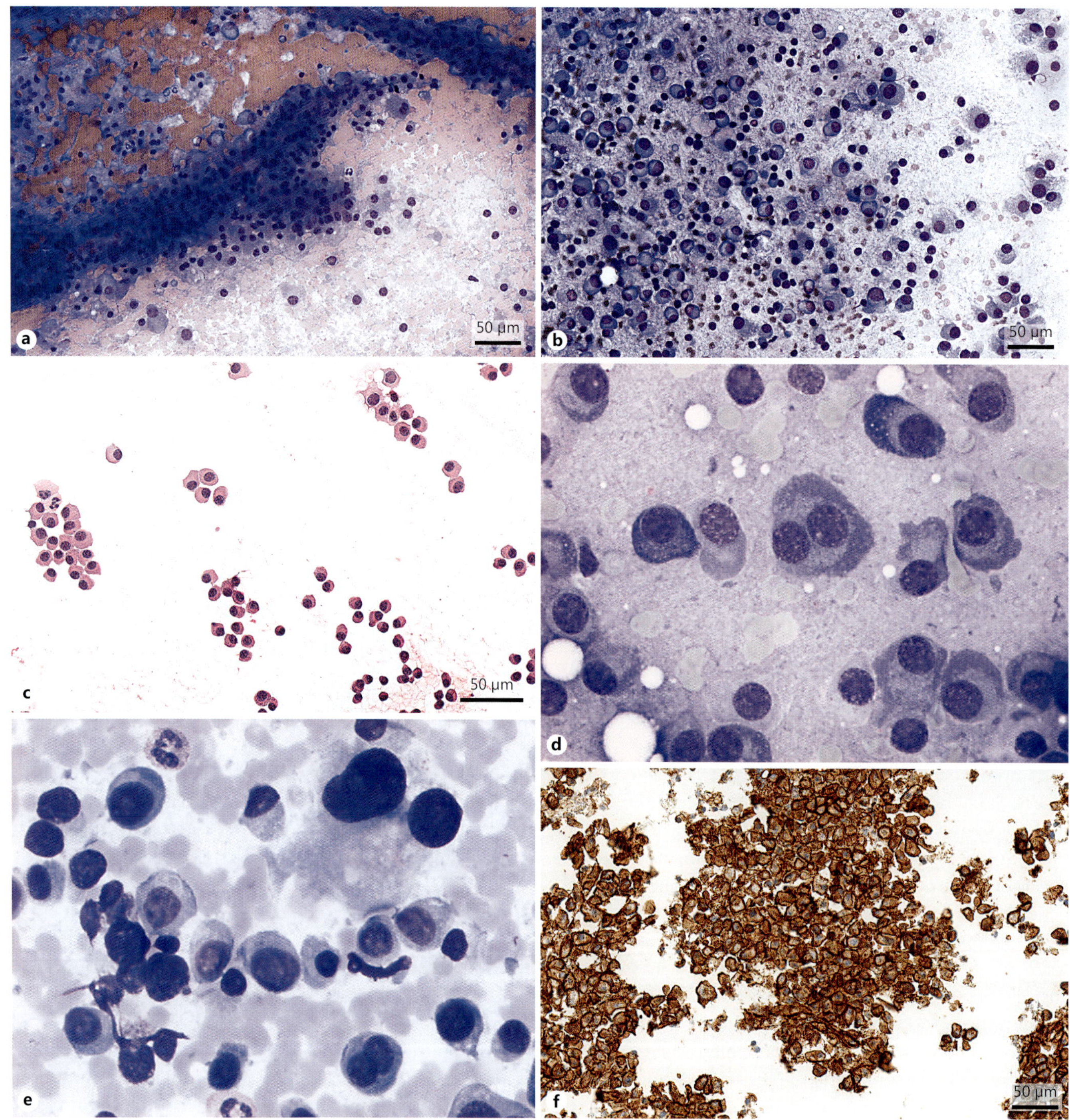

Fig. 1. Plasma cell neoplasm. **a** Hypercellular smears with dispersed cells and small clusters of atypical plasma cells. MGG stain. **b**, **c** Smears containing predominantly dispersed, slightly atypical, neoplastic plasma cells. MGG and HE stains. **d** Atypical plasma cells showing a distinctive paranuclear cytoplasmic "Hof." MGG stain. **e** Smears of low differentiated (anaplastic) plasmacytoma show highly atypical tumor cells. MGG stain. **f** Tumor cells are positive for CD138. Cell block; CD138.

often show translocations involving the heavy chain (IGH) locus at 14q32 and a number of different translocation partners [5]. This can be detected by cytogenetics, fluorescence in situ hybridization, single nucleotide polymorphism (SNP) array, polymerase chain reaction (PCR), and next-generation sequencing (NGS) on available material. Flow-cytometry is useful in detecting monoclonal cells and is a useful diagnostic tool in plasma cell neoplasms.

Differential Diagnosis
- Large B-cell lymphoma of immunoblastic type
- Reactive benign plasmacytosis
- Metastatic carcinoma

The diagnosis criteria of solitary plasmacytoma include a solitary bone involvement and no evidence of plasmacytosis in the bone marrow. Complete radiographic investigation of the skeleton is thus necessary. Osteoblasts resemble plasma cells; reactive osteoblasts may be mistaken for atypical plasma cells. However, the cytoplasmic "Hof" is paranuclear in plasma cells (Fig. 1d). Smears of low differentiated (anaplastic) plasmacytoma show highly atypical tumor cells [6, 7] with variable amounts of cytoplasm and often bi- or multi-nucleated tumor cells lacking a cytoplasmic "Hof" (Fig. 1e).

The neoplastic plasma cells express monotypic immunoglobulin and in most cases it is possible to diagnose a light chain restriction in cell block or cytospin preparations. Compared to aspirates of non-Hodgkin lymphomas of B cell type and carcinomas, the neoplastic plasma cells express CD138 (Fig. 1f) and CD79A, but not CD20 or keratins.

Primary Lymphoma of the Bone

Primary bone lymphomas are rare lesions that are defined as a lymphoma within bone without signs of involvement of lymph nodes or other nonskeletal sites within 6 months after the onset of symptoms. Primary lymphoma of the bone comprises approximately 3–7% of all malignant bone tumors. Lymphomas solely involving the bone account for about 5% of all extranodal lymphomas. The majority of lymphomas occur in the long bones followed by the pelvic bones and the spine. Any age group may be affected but most patients are older than 45 years of age. The vast majority of lymphomas are aggressive B-cell lymphomas (diffuse large B-cell lymphoma). Certain subtypes, such as precursor (lymphoblastic) lymphoma and anaplastic large cell lymphoma, may arise in children and young adults. The radiologic findings are noncharacteristic. There are often multi-

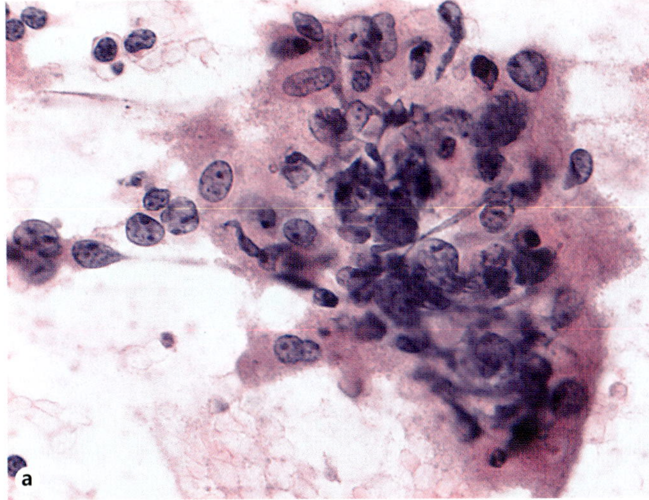
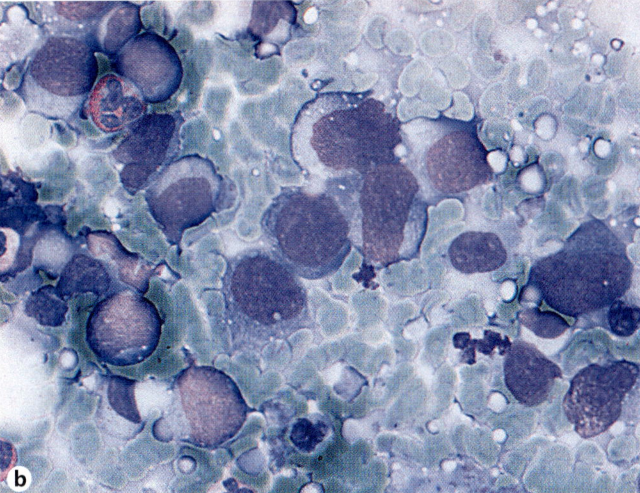

Fig. 2. Non-Hodgkin lymphoma. **a**, **b** Smears of skeletal large-cell diffuse B-cell lymphoma; cytologic features and criteria for diagnosis are the same as for nonosseous lymphoma. HE and MGG stains.

ple osteolytic lesions with moth-eaten or permeative bone destructions. Cortical destruction indicates a soft tissue component. Periostitis may also occur. Both histopathologic and cytologic criteria for diagnosis are the same as for nonosseous lymphoma [3].

Cytologic Features (Fig. 2a, b)
- Cytologic features and criteria for diagnosis are the same as for nonosseous lymphoma.

Ancillary Tests
Flow cytometric immunophenotyping is necessary for the correct diagnosis and subtyping of lymphoma.

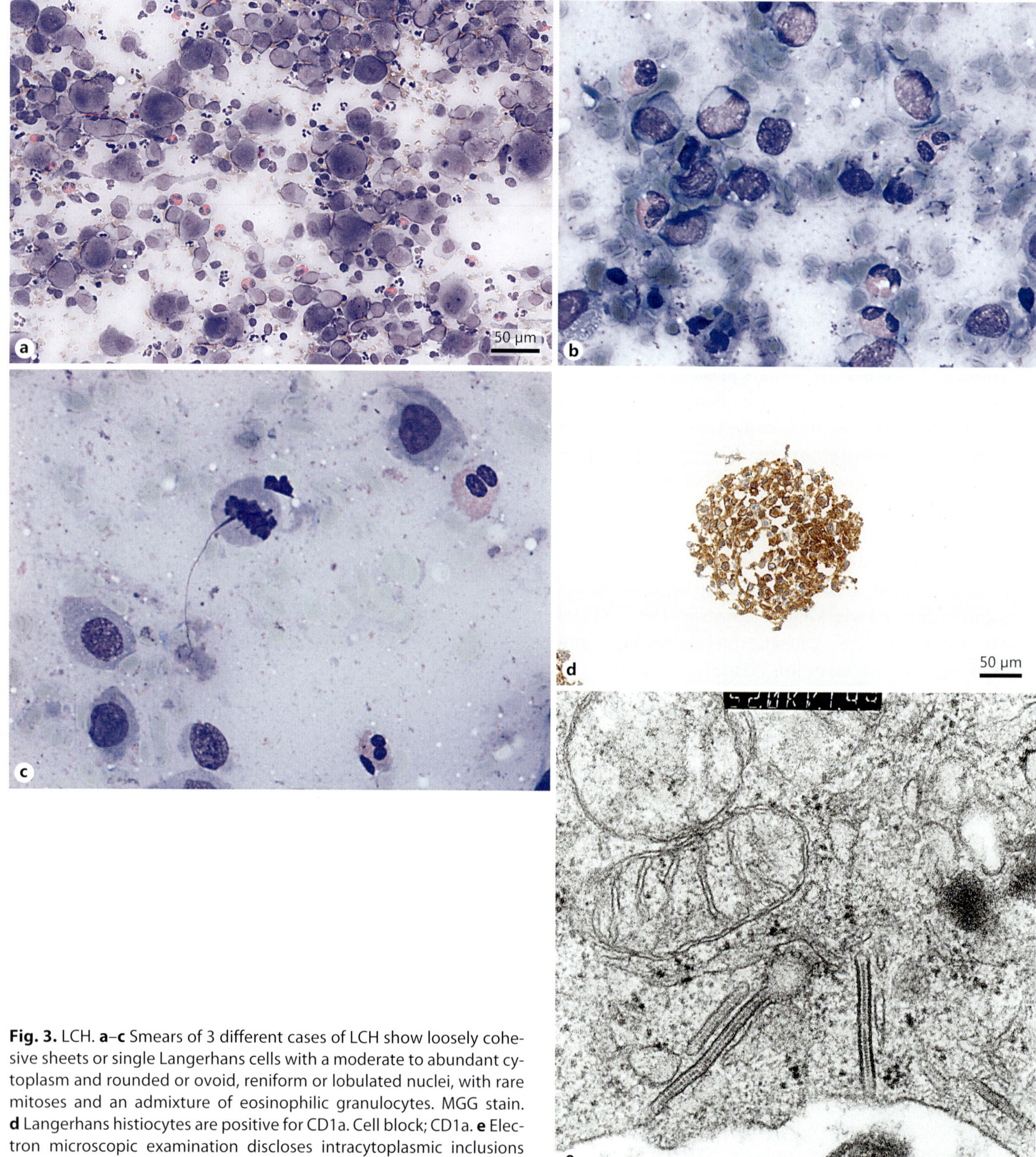

Fig. 3. LCH. **a–c** Smears of 3 different cases of LCH show loosely cohesive sheets or single Langerhans cells with a moderate to abundant cytoplasm and rounded or ovoid, reniform or lobulated nuclei, with rare mitoses and an admixture of eosinophilic granulocytes. MGG stain. **d** Langerhans histiocytes are positive for CD1a. Cell block; CD1a. **e** Electron microscopic examination discloses intracytoplasmic inclusions known as Birbeck granules.

Immunophenotype
Bone lymphomas should be worked up by immunocytochemistry in the same way as their nodal and other nonosseous counterparts. Terminal deoxynucleotidyl transferase (TDT) should be included in the antibody panel when a precursor lymphoma is suspected and CD30, EMA, and Alk-1 should be included to reliably diagnose anaplastic large cell lymphoma.

Genetics
Genetic analyses are guided by what subtype of lymphoma is suspected and no general diagnostic aberrations or analyses are applicable. The same principles used for diagnosing nonosseous lymphomas are valid.

Differential Diagnosis
- Ewing sarcoma
- Immunoblastic or plasmablastic variants of plasmacytoma
- Granulocytic sarcoma
- Metastatic small cell undifferentiated carcinoma

When a non-Hodgkin lymphoma is a diagnostic alternative, ancillary techniques are indispensable to reaching a correct diagnosis. The same diagnostic methods are used as in cases of a nonosseous lymphoma.

Langerhans Cell Histiocytosis (Eosinophilic Granuloma)

Langerhans cell histiocytosis (LCH) is a localized or systemic clonal proliferation of pathologic Langerhans cells. LCH, previously named histiocytosis X, is currently classified according to the extent of involvement and includes the group of localized nonsystemic lesions with single extraskeletal or skeletal organ involvement and multifocal or systemic forms. Multifocal forms represent entities in childhood previously known as Hand-Shüller-Christian disease and Letterer-Siwe disease. The localized form of LCH occurs in the first 3 decades of life with a peak of incidence between the ages of 5 and 15 years. In the systemic form, patients are usually younger than 5 years of age. The most frequent sites of LCH are the bones and skin. The bone lesions might be solitary (most common) or multiple. Although any bone can be involved, the skull, femur, and humerus in children, and the skull, pelvic bones, and ribs are often affected in adults.

The lesions are generally well defined and lytic, as exemplified in the skull and pelvic bones with a central radiodense focus occasionally presenting within the skull lesions, called "button" sequestrum. In the spine, the destruction often leads to a flattened vertebral body, a "vertebra plana." Lesions in the long bones are initially well defined and radiolucent, but with further growth they encroach on the cortical bone, which may lead to periosteal new bone formation. Lesions in the ribs may cause a pathologic fracture.

Cytologic Features (Fig. 3a–c)
- Langerhans cells in loosely cohesive clusters, sheets, or single cells
- Binucleated and multinucleated histiocytes are often present
- Ovoid, reniform, or lobulated nuclei often showing nuclear grooves ("coffee-bean" nuclei)
- Bland chromatin and small nucleoli
- Abundant pale cytoplasm
- Occasional osteoclast-like giant cells
- Variable numbers of eosinophils, neutrophils, and lymphocytes

Ancillary Tests
Immunophenotype
The Langerhans cells stain for S100 protein (nuclear and cytoplasmic) and CD1a and Langerin/CD207 (membranous).

Ultrastructure
Diagnostic features of LCH include the presence of intracytoplasmic inclusions known as Birbeck granules.

Genetics
The tumor cells show no known recurrent cytogenetic abnormalities, but mutation of the oncogene *BRAF* has been noted in over 50% of examined cases [8]. This can be examined by SNP array, PCR, and NGS on available material.

Differential Diagnosis
- Nonspecific osteomyelitis

Cytologic features of skeletal LCH have been infrequently reported [9–18]. The correct diagnosis can be established on routinely stained FNA smears correlated with clinical and radiographic data in the majority of cases. However, according to the Histiocyte Society, a definitive diagnosis should be based on the morphology and immunohistochemical expression of CD1A (Fig. 3d) or the presence of Birbeck granules on electron microscopic examination (Fig. 3e).

References

1 Gill MK, Makkar M, Bains SP: Solitary plasmacytoma of skull: a rare cytological diagnosis. J Clin Diagn Res 2013;7:1702–1703.

2 Soderlund V, Tani E, Skoog L, Bauer HC, Kreicbergs A: Diagnosis of skeletal lymphoma and myeloma by radiology and fine needle aspiration cytology. Cytopathology 2001;12:157–167.

3 Orucevic A, Reddy VB, Selvaggi SM, Green L, Spitz DJ, Gattuso P: Fine-needle aspiration of extranodal and extramedullary hematopoietic malignancies. Diagn Cytopathol 2000;23:318–321.

4 Lai JL, Zandecki M, Mary JY, Bernardi F, Izydorczyk V, Flactif M, Morel P, Jouet JP, Bauters F, Facon T: Improved cytogenetics in multiple myeloma: a study of 151 patients including 117 patients at diagnosis. Blood 1995;85:2490–2497.

5 Tian E, Sawyer JR, Heuck CJ, Zhang Q, van Rhee F, Barlogie B, Epstein J: In multiple myeloma, 14q32 translocations are nonrandom chromosomal fusions driving high expression levels of the respective partner genes. Genes Chromosomes Cancer 2014;53:549–557.

6 Subitha K, Renu T, Lillykutty P, Letha V: Anaplastic myeloma presenting as mandibular swelling: diagnosis by cytology. J Cytology 2014;31:114–116.

7 Stewart JM, Krishnamurthy S: Fine-needle aspiration cytology of a case of HIV-associated anaplastic myeloma. Diagn Cytopathol 2002;27:218–222.

8 Badalian-Very G, Vergilio JA, Degar BA, MacConaill LE, Brandner B, Calicchio ML, Kuo FC, Ligon AH, Stevenson KE, Kehoe SM, Garraway LA, Hahn WC, Meyerson M, Fleming MD, Rollins BJ: Recurrent BRAF mutations in Langerhans cell histiocytosis. Blood 2010;116:1919–1923.

9 Handa U, Kundu R, Punia RS, Mohan H: Langerhans cell histiocytosis in children diagnosed by fine-needle aspiration. J Cytol 2015;32:244–247.

10 Agarwal P, Kaushal M: An unusual presentation of Langerhans cell histiocytosis. J Cytol 2014;31:227–229.

11 Kumar N, Sayed S, Vinayak S: Diagnosis of Langerhans cell histiocytosis on fine needle aspiration cytology: a case report and review of the cytology literature. Patholog Res Int 2011;2011:439518.

12 Kilpatrick SE, Ward WG, Chauvenet AR, Pettenati MJ: The role of fine-needle aspiration biopsy in the initial diagnosis of pediatric bone and soft tissue tumors: an institutional experience. Mod Pathol 1998;11:923–928.

13 Kilpatrick SE: Fine needle aspiration biopsy of Langerhans cell histiocytosis of bone: are ancillary studies necessary for a "definitive diagnosis?" Acta Cytol 1998;42:820–823.

14 Pohar-Marinsek Z, Us-Krasovec M: Cytomorphology of Langerhans cell histiocytosis. Acta Cytol 1996;40:1257–1264.

15 Biswal BM, Lal P, Uppal R, Mallik S: Unifocal Langerhans' cell histiocytosis (eosinophilic granuloma) resembling Ewing's sarcoma. Australas Radiol 1994;38:313–314.

16 Akhtar M, Ali MA, Bakry M, Sackey K, Sabbah R: Fine-needle aspiration biopsy of Langerhans histiocytosis (histiocytosis-X). Diagn Cytopathol 1993;9:527–533.

17 Howell LP, Russell LA, Howard PH, Teplitz RL: The cytology of pediatric masses: a differential diagnostic approach. Diagn Cytopathol 1992;8:107–115.

18 Elsheikh T, Silverman JF, Wakely PE Jr, Holbrook CT, Joshi VV: Fine-needle aspiration cytology of Langerhans' cell histiocytosis (eosinophilic granuloma) of bone in children. Diagn Cytopathol 1991;7:261–266.

Domanski HA, Walther CS: FNA Cytology of Soft Tissue and Bone Tumors. Monogr Clin Cytol.
Basel, Karger, 2017, vol 22, pp 181–182 (DOI: 10.1159/000477317)

Bone Metastases

Metastatic carcinomas are the most frequent malignant neoplasm of the skeleton. Following the lungs and liver, the skeleton is the third most common site with metastatic involvement. Any bone can be affected, but metastatic deposits usually arise in bones with active bone marrow, such as the vertebrae, pelvic bones, sternum, ribs, and proximal femur. Approximately 80% of metastases to the skeleton are from carcinomas of the breast, prostate, kidney, lung, and gastrointestinal tract. Malignant melanoma is not an uncommon metastatic tumor in adults.

In the pediatric age group, the most common neoplasms that metastasize to the bone are rhabdomyosarcoma, neuroblastoma, and clear cell sarcoma of the kidney. When a destructive bone lesion is the first sign of malignancy, fine-needle aspiration cytology is very useful to rapidly identify or suggest the primary site. Many metastatic tumors attempt to recapitulate the original neoplasm [1–3]. Access to ancillary techniques, especially immunocytochemical examinations, is necessary to establish the origin of metastasis in the majority of cases.

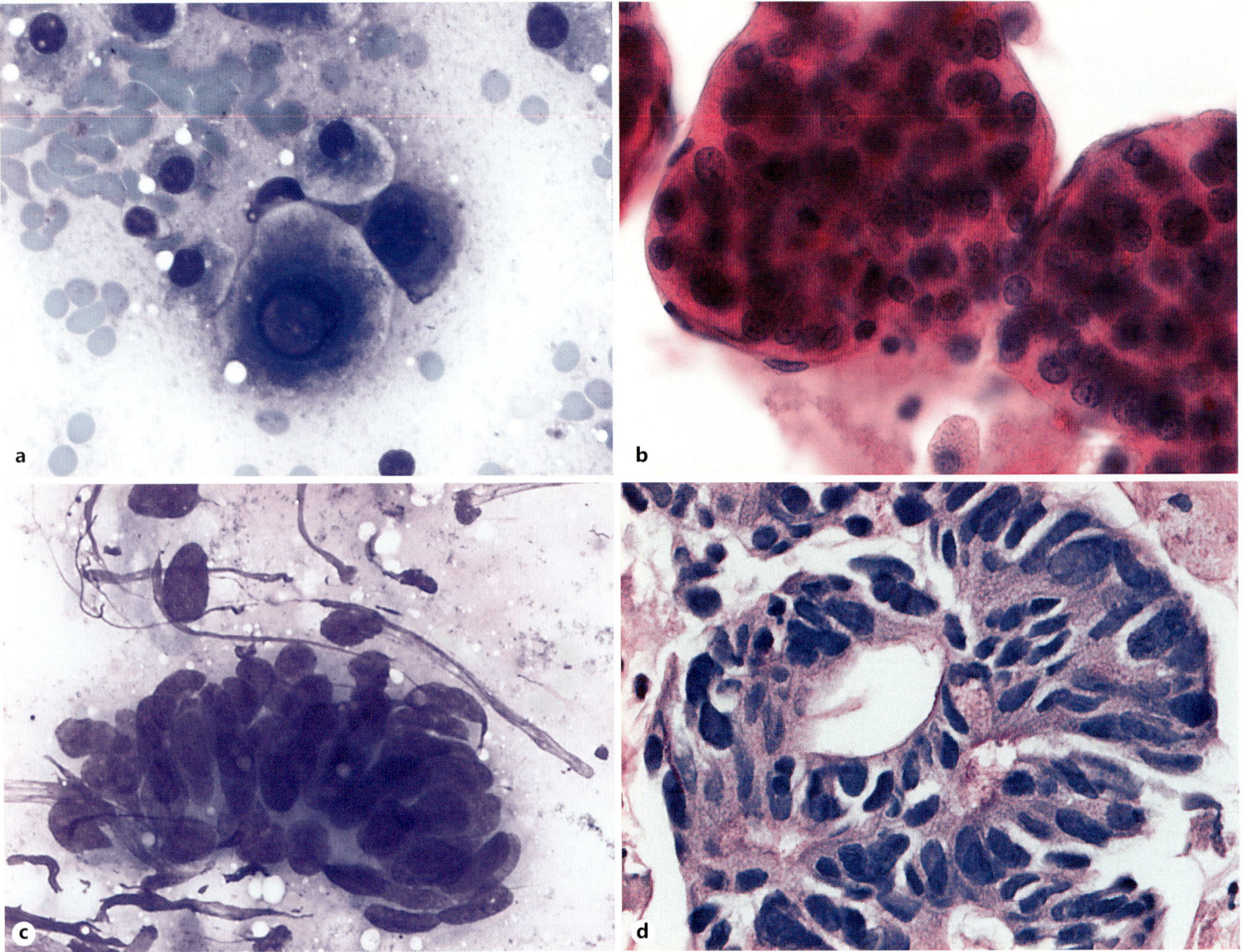

Fig. 1. Bone metastases. **a** Skeletal metastasis of hepatocellular carcinoma: tumor cells in smears resembling hepatocytes. DiffQuik stain. **b** Endothelial lining of smooth edges of cohesive microfragments of tumor cells resembling fine-needle aspiration smears of well-differentiated hepatocellular carcinoma. HE stain. Skeletal metastasis of colonic adenocarcinoma. **c** Tight cluster of malignant cells in a mucinous background suggestive of metastatic adenocarcinoma of intestinal origin. MGG stain. **d** Cell block section; alveolar structures recapitulate moderately differentiated colonic adenocarcinoma. Cell block; HE stain.

References

1 Wedin R, Bauer HC, Skoog L, Soderlund V, Tani E: Cytological diagnosis of skeletal lesions: fine-needle aspiration biopsy in 110 tumours. J Bone Joint Surg Br 2000;82:673–678.

2 Treaba D, Assad L, Govil H, Sariya D, Reddy VB, Kluskens L, Green L, Selvaggi SM, Gattuso P: Diagnostic role of fine-needle aspiration of bone lesions in patients with a previous history of malignancy. Diagn Cytopathol 2002;26:380–383.

3 Suterwala S, Volk EE, Danforth RD: Aspiration biopsy of osseous metastasis of occult hepatocellular carcinoma: case report, literature review, and differential diagnosis. Diagn Cytopathol 2001;25: 63–67.

Domanski HA, Walther CS: FNA Cytology of Soft Tissue and Bone Tumors. Monogr Clin Cytol.
Basel, Karger, 2017, vol 22, pp 183–185 (DOI: 10.1159/000477318)

Bone Lesions Rarely Examined by Fine-Needle Aspiration

Introduction

The major aim of this work was to thoroughly describe and illustrate the most common entities. Cytologic diagnostic criteria have not yet been established in some primary bone tumors/lesions that are not common targets for fine-needle aspiration (FNA) examination, or in some very rare entities.

Adamantinoma

Adamantinoma is a very rare biphasic (mesenchymal and epithelial) low-grade malignant tumor arising in the tibia, occasionally in the fibula. The tumor is composed of epithelial cells surrounded by a fibrous stroma. Adamantinoma constitutes 0.1–0.5% of all malignant bone neoplasms. Two subtypes of adamantinoma have been reported – classical (mainly in children and young adults) and osteofibrous dysplasia-like (mainly in adults). The classic type may show cortical destruction and involve soft tissue, while the osteofibrous dysplasia-like adamantinoma is an intracortical tumor.

Cytologic Features
- Predominantly bland-appearing spindle cells
- Cohesive clusters of basaloid or squamoid epithelial cells

Ancillary Tests
Immunophenotype
Adamantinomas are positive for keratins, especially keratins 14, 19, 5, and 17.

Genetics
These tumors can display numerical chromosomal aberrations with extra copies of chromosomes 7, 8, 12, 19, and/or 21. Structural chromosomal changes, including translocations and marker chromosomes, have also been noted [1]. These abnormalities can be detected with cytogenetics, fluorescence in situ hybridization, single nucleotide polymorphism array, and next-generation sequencing on available material.

Differential Diagnosis
- Metastatic carcinoma

Only single case reports of FNA cytology of adamantinoma have been published to date [2–8]. The clue to the diagnosis is the presence of a double-cell population of spindle-shaped mesenchymal cells and epithelial cells (Fig. 1).

Vascular Neoplasm of Bone

While solitary or multiple hemangiomas most often involving vertebral bodies of the spine are common and usually asymptomatic neoplasms in bone, epithelioid hemangioendothelioma and angiosarcoma arising primarily in bone are uncommon. Most vascular bone tumors are sporadic, although syndromes such as Klippel-Trenaunay and Sturge-Weber may predispose patients to vasoformative tumors. Few reports describing FNA features of primary vascular neoplasms of bone exist [9–16]. The morphology of smears

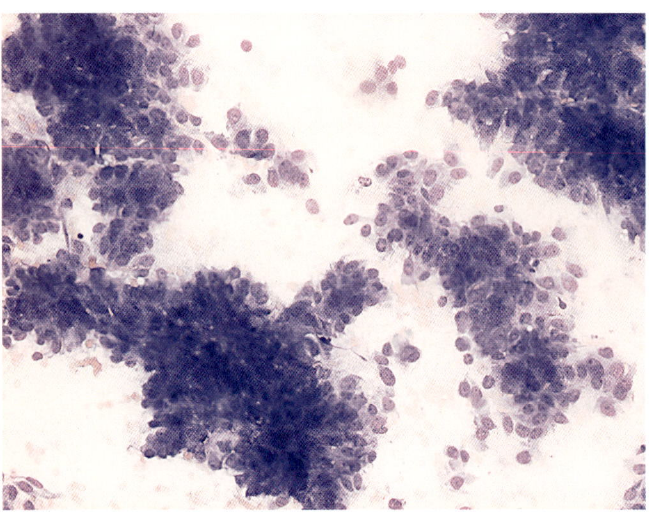

Fig. 1. Adamantinoma. Cohesive clusters of epithelioid cells with a moderate cytoplasm and round, somewhat irregular nuclei with small nucleoli. MGG stain.

from vascular neoplasms is comparable with morphologies in other settings (Fig. 2a, b).

Fibrous Dysplasia

Fibrous dysplasia is a solitary or multifocal intramedullary benign lesion. The solitary (monostotic) type is more common, accounting for approximately 70–90% of lesions. Most cases are diagnosed before the age of 40 years, and the highest incidence is in the second decade of life. Commonly affected bones are the craniofacial bones, ribs, femur, and tibia, although any bone may be involved. Common symptoms are bone deformity and soft tissue swelling, and sometimes pathologic fracture. While histologic sections of fibrous dysplasia display characteristic diagnostic features of cellular fibrous matrix containing a variable amount of irregularly arranged bony trabeculae similar to Chinese characters and with an admixture of osteoclasts, cytologic features are less characteristic, involving a mixture of uniform spindle cells or cohesive clusters of spindle cells with some osteoclasts and occasionally osteoblastic cells. Cytologic findings in single case reports of fibrous dysplasia have been reported [17–19]. FNA smears that contained osteoclast-like giant cells and tissue fragments probably represented woven bone [18, 19]. Presumably, the only indication for FNA cytology is when the presenting symptom is a pathologic fracture.

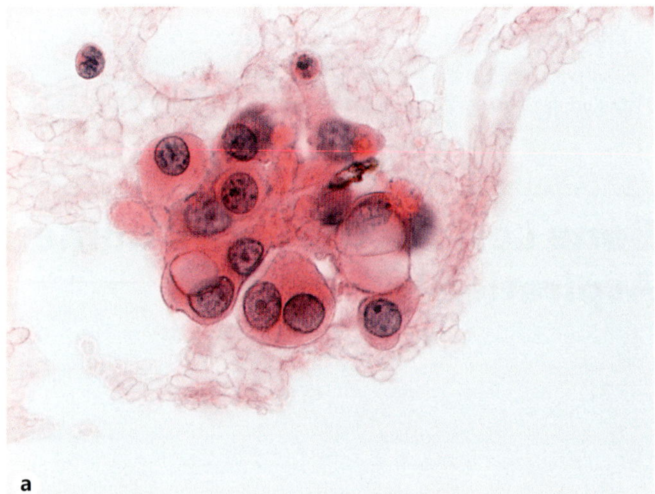

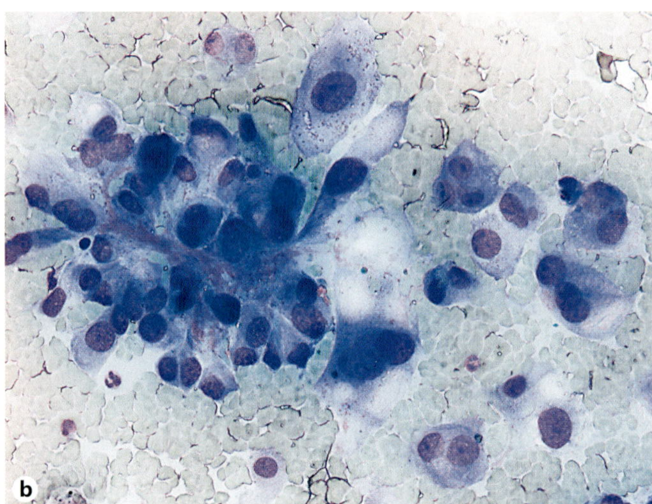

Fig. 2. Epithelioid hemangioendothelioma. **a, b** Small, loose clusters and dispersed single cells with variable-sized, round to oval nuclei and a moderate to abundant cytoplasm with occasional cytoplasmic densities. HE and MGG stains.

Fibrous Cortical Defect (Nonossifying Fibroma)

A fibrous cortical defect is usually an incidental finding involving the metaphyseal region of long bones or the pelvis; occasionally, fracture may be the first sign of presentation. When the tumors extend from the cortex to the medullary cavity, the term "nonossifying fibroma" is used. Predilection sites are the femur and the tibia. The tumors occur in the second decade of life and are virtually never seen after the age of 30 years. The lesions have a characteristic radiographic appearance and morphologic examination is most often unnecessary.

References

1 Camp MD, Tompkins RK, Spanier SS, Bridge JA, Bush CH: Best cases from the AFIP: adamantinoma of the tibia and fibula with cytogenetic analysis. Radiographics 2008;28:1215–1220.

2 Gangopadhyay M, Pramanik R, Chakrabarty S, Bera P: Cytological diagnosis of adamantinoma of long bone in a 78-year-old man. J Cytol 2011;28:28–29.

3 Bishop JA, Ali SZ: Primary tibial adamantinoma diagnosed by fine needle aspiration. Diagn Cytopathol 2010;38:198–201.

4 Flowers R, Baliga M, Guo M, Liu SS: Tibial adamantinoma with local recurrence and pulmonary metastasis: report of a case with histocytologic findings. Acta Cytol 2006;50:567–573.

5 Perez-Ordonez B, Bedard YC: Metastatic adamantinoma diagnosed by fine-needle aspiration biopsy of the lung. Diagn Cytopathol 1994;10:347–351.

6 Laucirica R, Mody D, MacLeay L, Kearns RJ, Ramzy I: Adamantinoma: a case report with aspiration cytology and differential diagnostic and immunohistochemical considerations. Acta Cytol 1992;36:951–956.

7 Galera-Davidson H, Fernandez-Rodriguez A, Torres-Olivera FJ, Gomez-Pascual A, Moreno-Fernandez A: Cytologic diagnosis of a case of recurrent adamantinoma. Acta Cytol 1989;33:635–638.

8 Hales MS, Ferrell LD: Fine-needle aspiration biopsy of tibial adamantinoma: a case report. Diagn Cytopathol 1988;4:67–70.

9 Siddaraju N, Soundararaghavan J, Bundele MM, Roy SK: Fine needle aspiration cytology of epithelioid angiosarcoma: a case report. Acta Cytol 2008;52:109–113.

10 Wong KF, So CC, Wong N, Siu LL, Kwong YL, Chan JK: Sinonasal angiosarcoma with marrow involvement at presentation mimicking malignant lymphoma: cytogenetic analysis using multiple techniques. Cancer Genet Cytogenet 2001;129:64–68.

11 Schindler S, Cajulis RS, Gokaslan ST, Frias-Hidvegi D, Yu GH: Fine needle aspiration of primary angiosarcoma of bone. Acta Cytol 1997;41:1225–1228.

12 Khiyami A, Green LK, Gyorkey F, Landon G: Primary angiosarcoma of the cuboidal bone: a case report. Diagn Cytopathol 1991;7:520–523.

13 Murali R, Zarka MA, Ocal IT, Tazelaar HD: Cytologic features of epithelioid hemangioendothelioma. Am J Clin Pathol 2011;136:739–746.

14 Kilpatrick SE, Koplyay PD, Ward WG, Richards F 2nd: Epithelioid hemangioendothelioma of bone and soft tissue: a fine-needle aspiration biopsy study with histologic and immunohistochemical confirmation. Diagn Cytopathol 1998;19:38–43.

15 Zhu C, Zhu HG, Zhang ZY, Wang LZ, Zheng JW, Ye WM, He Y, Wang YA: Intraosseous venous malformations of the facial bone: a retrospective study in 11 patients. Phlebology 2013;28:257–263.

16 Mondal A, Misra DK: CT-guided needle aspiration cytology (FNAC) of 112 vertebral lesions. Indian J Pathol Microbiol 1994;37:255–261.

17 Gupta N, Gupta R, Bakshi J, Rajwanshi A: Fine needle aspiration cytology in a case of fibrous dysplasia of jaw. Diagn Cytopathol 2009;37:920–922.

18 Huening MA, Reddy S, Dodd LG: Fine-needle aspiration of fibrous dysplasia of bone: a worthwhile endeavor or not? Diagn Cytopathol 2008;36:325–330.

19 Logrono R, Kurtycz DF, Wojtowycz M, Inhorn SL: Fine needle aspiration cytology of fibrous dysplasia: a case report. Acta Cytol 1998;42:1172–1176.

Subject Index